'I neve ... about dying but this ... e-enhanc... Matthew Parris, *The Times*

'Here she shares her experiences and observations from the front line of nursing ... What makes the book bearable is Worth's compassion and a burning mission to remind us that end-of-life care doesn't have to be complex' *Lady*

'Jennifer Worth addresses head-on the taboos that surround death and dying ... Her stories are often poignant and sometimes disturbing, but all show an understanding of the patient's needs' *Nursing Standard*

'Perhaps her most thought-provoking book ... Worth raises challenging questions that are sure to encourage the reader to develop a stronger, more profound view of death' *Church of England Newspaper*

'An honest, moving and sobering account which told me much I did not know – or possibly didn't care to think about too deeply ... I feel fortunate to have read this inspiring book' *The Woman Writer*

Praise for *Call the Midwife*

'Worth is indeed a natural storyteller – in the best sense of the term, with apparent artlessness, in fact concealing high art – and her detailed account of being a midwife in London's East End is gripping, moving and convincing from beginning to end ... a powerful evocation of a long-gone world' David Kynaston, *Literary Review*

'This uplifting story is about love, that of mothers for their children, and the love of God that compelled the nuns to dedicate their lives to the well-being of the poor' *Tablet*

'Funny, disturbing and incredibly moving, *Call the Midwife* opens a window onto the fascinating and colourful world of the East End in the 1950s' *Mature Times*

'Worth's portrait is subtle, skilfully describing a sense of community that no longer exists' *FT Magazine*

'Funny, disturbing and incredibly moving' *Yorkshire Evening Post*

Jennifer Worth trained as a nurse at the Royal Berkshire Hospital, Reading, and was later ward sister at the Elizabeth Garrett Anderson Hospital in London, then the Marie Curie Hospital, also in London. Music had always been her passion, and in 1973 she left nursing in order to study music intensively, teaching piano and singing for about twenty-five years. Jennifer died in May 2011 after a short illness, leaving her husband Philip, two daughters and three grandchildren. Her books have all been bestsellers.

By Jennifer Worth

Eczema and Food Allergy
Call the Midwife
Shadows of the Workhouse
Farewell to the East End
In the Midst of Life

IN THE MIDST OF LIFE

JENNIFER WORTH, SRN, SCM

Clinical Editor
David Hackett, MD, FRCP, FESC
Consultant Cardiologist

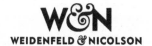

WEIDENFELD & NICOLSON

A W&N PAPERBACK

First published in Great Britain in 2010
by Weidenfeld & Nicolson,
This paperback edition published in 2017
by Weidenfeld & Nicolson,
an imprint of The Orion Publishing Group Ltd,
Carmelite House, 50 Victoria Embankment
London EC4Y 0DZ
An Hachette UK Company

1 3 5 7 9 10 8 6 4 2

ISBN 978 1 4746 0666 0

Typeset by Input Data Services Ltd, Somerset

Printed in Great Britain by Clays Ltd, St Ives plc

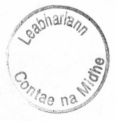

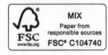

MIX
Paper from
responsible sources
FSC® C104740

www.orionbooks.co.uk

Dedicated to
Lydia, Daniel and Eleanor
and all of their generation

They are the future

CONTENTS

In my beginning is my end;
In my end is my beginning.

— T.S. Eliot

IN THE MIDST OF LIFE WE ARE
IN DEATH

This book assumes that death is sacred.
It is about the mystery, the beauty, the loneliness and the
aspirations of death.
It is about the fear of death, and our inability to handle it.
It is about how we die. Perhaps few people have seen the
Angel of Death approach and depart.
It is about the meaning, shape and purpose of life that will
some day end.
It is about my own search to understand.

Since girlhood I have pondered these mysteries, reflecting
on the deaths I have seen in hospitals and the hopes and
fears of people who have come my way.

This book is about the need for peace in the hour of
our death.
It suggests that death can sometimes be a friend, and is not
always an enemy.
It raises the vexed issue of resuscitation, and the law.
It is about the need to rekindle reverence in the face
of death.
It is about the humility of acceptance.

It is about the spiritual nature of death – God if you like,
or Allah, or Krishna, or Jehovah, or Brahma, or one of a
thousand names given to something we cannot understand.
Or just Evolution, Random Chance, or Biochemistry.

It really does not matter what you think or believe.
Death comes for us all.
How, when and where we die has always been a game
of chance.
Our determination to control it has not loaded the dice
in our favour.
Did anyone ever imagine that it would?

— *Jennifer Worth*

INTRODUCTION

Fifty years of thought, and four years of writing, have gone into the production of this book. The best wine and cheese, we are told, are slow to mature. Let us hope it is the same for books!

It has been written with a strong sense of vocation. 'Modern medicine' was just developing when I started nursing in the 1950s – they were exciting days. I was only eighteen, but could see quite clearly that with every new advance in pharmacology and surgery, the acceptance of death was being transformed into denial.

Only those who have seen death are able to talk about it meaningfully. I was privileged to be of that generation of nurses who were required to sit with the dying, and the insights gained from those experiences inform the whole book.

I left nursing in 1973, and although the earlier stories in the book are now medical history, the moral and ethical issues remain the same. But through the professional journals, friends and relatives, and observation, I have kept in touch with medicine and nursing, as the later stories illustrate. In order to bring this book clinically into the twenty-first century, I have asked three professionals who are currently working to write updates on modern medical practice: David Hackett, consultant cardiologist; Madeline Bass, palliative care nurse and teacher; Louise Massen, ambulance service paramedic and clinician. These papers are to be found in the appendices at the end of the book. Readers who are interested in a serious update on professional papers and government reports and directives can find an extensive reading list, but it must be remembered that these are changing all the time, and almost every month new material is added.

Jennifer Worth,
September 2010

A NATURAL DEATH

My grandfather died in 1956 at the age of eighty-six. I loved him deeply and was very close to him. I saw very little of my father during the war, and in the years after. Every girl needs a man in her life, and my dear grandfather gladly filled that role. I treasure a Bible that he gave me for my twenty-first birthday, shortly before he died, with a loving message carefully penned by a shaking hand, unaccustomed to writing. He was barely literate, having left school at the age of eleven to work in a builder's yard, and was the oldest of thirteen children, born in 1870, when every child in a working class family had to labour from an early age. At fifteen he lied about his age and joined the army, 'So that one of my brothers could have my boots,' he told me. He had about him a quiet simplicity and wisdom that greatly influenced my childhood, and therefore my whole life.

I remember his tenderness throughout my early years; going for long walks in the countryside, my grandfather pointing out and naming birds, trees and flowers. I remember going to his allotment to dig potatoes, him pushing me in the wheelbarrow and me shouting 'Faster, faster!' I remember helping him to polish shoes, clean the windows, clear out his garden shed, clean the grate and chop the wood and get the coal in. And I remember him growing old.

It was a gradual process. First it was the wheelbarrow. However much I shouted, he couldn't go any faster.

'I am getting old,' he would say. 'You get out and run. Your legs are younger than mine.'

As I grew older and stronger, he grew older and weaker, and, after a few years, I was the one pushing the wheelbarrow. Soon, digging for potatoes became too much for him, so I dug up the golden white globes. I had always been told that Grandad was hard of hearing, but I had never noticed it when I was little. I prattled on and he always seemed to understand me. I noticed that his nose dripped.

'Why is your nose dripping?' I asked, pertly.

'Don't be saucy, little madam,' he replied, taking out his hand-kerchief and wiping the offending organ. From an early age I remember pulling his skin and watching with interest as it settled slowly back into place. I pulled my own skin, and it bounced back.

'That's as it should be,' Grandad said. 'When you are as old as me your skin will be like mine.'

'I'm never going to grow old!' I shouted confidently as I raced down the garden path to his shed, which was always a place of wonder.

My grandmother had died in 1943, of a heart attack, I was told. My grandfather and my mother were with her when she died. My mother told me that he held her in his arms during the last half hour of life, tenderly stroking her face and kissing her. She had died as she had lived, in the protection of her husband's love, and, after her death, he lived alone. They had had eight children, and four of his daughters, including my mother, regularly attended to his needs. Cleaning became a problem. I recall my mother saying,

'Dad's getting very dirty. I found two pairs of dirty underpants hidden away in the back of his drawer.'

And, as I grew older, I was aware that his smell had changed. I had always thought of him as a lovely smell of earth and leaves and smoky old jackets. But it changed. Later on I realised the change in the smell was urine. He was never really incontinent, but most elderly men have prostate problems; it was gradual, and never so noticeable as to be offensive.

Two of his daughters had a small sweetshop at the end of the road. At first, after Grandma's death, they had let Grandad serve in the shop. He enjoyed meeting the customers, and 'it gives him something to do,' my aunts said. A few years later he could not be trusted to give the correct change, and, worse still, he did not seem to notice when his nose was dripping, so in the end he had to be steered gently away. He missed the shop, but said acceptingly, 'I'm getting old, now. You young people must take over.'

My grandfather was a Boer War veteran (1898–1902) and he was, therefore, offered a place as a Chelsea Pensioner, but he refused. He preferred to stay with his family – and how grateful I am that he did. My development towards adult life would have been very different, had he accepted.

The doctor came to see him from time to time. My grandfather didn't really need medical treatment, but he got 'chesty' in the winters and so the doctor ordered cough linctus, which probably had no effect. He said, 'There is nothing wrong. Your father's quite healthy. He is getting old, well past his three score years and ten. He will just potter on until he fades away.'

In those days, doctors accepted that people die of old age.

'He shouldn't be smoking that pipe,' said my aunt.

'Let him,' replied the doctor, 'if he enjoys it.'

For years, my grandfather had smoked a briar pipe filled with a villainous black tobacco called Twist, which he cut up himself with a penknife. I remember poking the shards of tobacco into the bowl of the pipe and lighting a coloured spill from the fire, holding it over the bowl as he sucked hard to get the thing going. The smoke was prolific and the odour pungent (to this day I adore the smell of a man with a pipe). The doctor was right. My grandfather enjoyed it, and it certainly never did him any harm, until the day when my aunt found a large burn hole in his bed! After that he was supposed to smoke only when one of his daughters was present. I doubt if he obeyed.

'He won't eat properly,' my aunt said. 'I cook a nice dinner and he only picks at it.'

So the doctor advised a pint of stout a day. My grandfather seemed to live on this, plus a bowl of bread and milk, which he made for himself each night. I wasn't aware of any other treatments prescribed for his failing strength.

Tragedy struck the family when my grandfather's eldest son died at the age of forty. I remember the old man weeping at the funeral.

'Why could it not have been me? My life is over. My only wish is to join my dear wife in her grave. But he, my son, he had everything to live for.'

He was visibly smaller. It was not merely that I was growing up and getting taller. He had been a guardsman, well over six feet tall, and he shrank by several inches until we were the same height. His proud, military bearing seemed to fold in on itself, and his confident step became an old man's shuffle.

He felt the cold more, and needed several layers of woollies to keep him warm. He had a coal fire every day, except in the hottest weather, and always kept a good stock of fuel in the grate, but chopping wood and carrying coals became harder as the years passed, so he made lots of journeys to the coal house, carrying a little at a time, and someone else chopped the wood.

We still went to his allotment on sunny days, he and I, me pushing the wheelbarrow, he prodding the pavement with his stick. But the weeds grew higher and higher and could not be controlled. Eventually, we dug his last crop of potatoes, and he had not the strength, nor indeed the interest, to plant any more.

My grandfather seemed to be withdrawing into himself. He became deafer, which cut him off from conversation, but he seemed perfectly content to sit in the luxury of silence, puffing his pipe, and thinking his thoughts. Sometimes he chuckled quietly to himself. Occasionally one saw a tear in the corner of his eye, but if anyone asked why, he did not respond. He had never been a talkative man, and, as he drew towards the end of his life, speech became even more of an effort, something he did not want to be bothered with. When he had to speak, his words were slow and measured, and somewhat distant, as though his mind was a long way away, and had to be coaxed back into the world around him. Sometimes he spoke of death, saying, 'I will soon be going to my dear wife.' On another occasion he spoke of seeing his dead son again. He also spoke of the Angel of Death approaching. This is an old-fashioned concept, but was very real to former generations.

It was obvious that he was fading away, although he was never particularly ill in the medical understanding of the term. The regular pumping of his heart, which circulates the blood, conveying oxygen to all parts of the body, was becoming irregular, but he never had any pills to control the heartbeat. Without adequate oxygen supply, the internal organs gradually lose their efficiency, and eventually cease to function. The tide of his life was gently ebbing away.

The last week or two of his life came suddenly. One day, he was pottering about as usual, and the next he couldn't be bothered to get up. 'Let me bide,' he told my aunt who tried to chivvy him out of bed. He more or less stopped eating, and took only sips of fluid.

I was nursing then, and lived about forty miles away, but I came back as often as I could to see him. It happened that I was with him on the day of his death. I had seen quite a lot of people die, all nurses have, and I knew what to expect. As soon as I entered the room I could see the change, which is obvious to the experienced eye. In the last few hours of life something mysterious happens, which can best be described as a veil being drawn. The dying person looks the same, but is not the same. Breathing changes, skin colour changes, the eyes change, muscle tone all but vanishes, speech becomes virtually impossible. The nearer one approaches death, the less one has the strength to resist it.

I told my mother to call the rest of the family. By a miracle of public transport, they all arrived, and he died in the evening of that day.

The doctor was not called until afterwards, and then only to sign the death certificate. He asked if we wanted a woman to come in to lay out the body, but I said no, I wanted to do it myself. And so I prepared his body and put a shroud on him, in readiness for his last journey to the grave, as I had been taught in my first year of training.

I do not know what the doctor entered on the death certificate. He knew, and we knew, that the cause of death was old age. But he could not put that. Legally, death has to be the outcome of an illness.

For everything there is a season,
A time for every matter under the sun.
A time to be born, and a time to die.

— *Ecclesiastes Chapter 3, verses 1 and 2*

AN UNNATURAL DEATH

It is rare to predict one's own death, or to meet anyone who has done so. But occasionally it happens, and I knew such a lady.

Mrs Ratski was Latvian, born in the 1880s, and virtually her whole life had been lived under the shadow of military conflict. She was a simple peasant woman, and she was immensely strong, both physically and morally.

In 1941, the German armies marched into Latvia and brutally crushed the resistance. Her husband and four sons were forcibly drafted into the German army, and they all died except Slavek, her youngest child. Slavek survived because he was taken prisoner of war by the British. It was the luckiest day of his life. In England he was a free man, and he worked on a farm, which is where he met Karen. Slavek was a good-looking boy with wide blue eyes, blond curling hair, and an infectious *joie de vivre* that made everyone he met feel good. Karen was a Land Army girl, and the work was hard, the day long, and she was often exhausted at the end of it; but not too exhausted for assignations with Slavek.

After the war, in 1947, they married. He worked as a garage mechanic and she as a hairdresser, and between them they saved up enough money to put a deposit on a terrace cottage and take out a mortgage. They were proud and happy property owners, and they had two little daughters who were six and seven at the time this story begins.

One day Slavek received a letter from his sister Olga, in Latvia, saying that their mother had suddenly announced that she was going to die, and that she must see her only surviving son first. Accordingly, she had applied for a visa to leave the country.

Nothing more was heard for fourteen weeks and Slavek

supposed that the whole thing had been forgotten. He had not reckoned with the resolution of a determined old lady! Alone, and with only a spare pair of boots and an extra shawl, Mrs Ratski had set out to walk across northern Europe, to reach the French coast, and find a boat that would take her over the channel to England.

This sounds a fanciful story, but at that time it was not. Millions of people trekked thousands of miles across the length and breadth of war-torn Europe, to reach a destination they thought might be home, or at least a haven from persecution and danger.

The first that Slavek knew about it was a policeman at the door, saying that his colleagues in Reading had received a phone message from the police in Dover, informing them that an old lady, who spoke no English, had been referred to them by the port authorities. Her only identification was a piece of paper that bore Slavek's name and address. The old lady was his mother.

The following day, the police brought her to his house. The meeting between mother and son was deeply emotional. She clung to him and wept, and blessed him in the name of the Virgin Mary and Jesus Christ and all the Saints in Heaven. 'You are my only son left, my youngest, my fairest, my swan, my hope. To see you again has been my dearest wish. Now I will die happy.' And she blessed him again.

'But you can't be dying. You are not ill!' he protested.

'No, but I am old, and I can see the figure of death, the Reaper. I hear the swish of his scythe that cuts down the old grass so that new may grow. It is the way of life. I am content now, and I ask God for nothing more than to die peacefully under my son's roof.'

Four days later Mrs Ratski developed acute intestinal obstruction. Suddenly, and unaccountably, a loop of bowel twisted on itself, a condition that, if untreated, is fatal. Slavek was the first up that morning, and found his mother in great pain on the sofa in the living room where she had been sleeping. She was leaning forwards, clutching her stomach, moaning and rocking herself. She looked up when he entered, and her face was grey with pain, her lips pressed back over her gums and her eyes dull. He went over to her and took her in his arms.

'Oh, my son, my jewel! It has been a long night, but the morning brings my Slavek, praise be to God.'

Slavek felt himself panicking, and ran to the bottom of the stairs. 'Karen,' he called. 'Come quickly. Something terrible's happened.'

'I must give my blessing to your wife and your children before I go,' said the stricken old lady.

'We must get the doctor,' said Karen.

The doctor arrived and examined Mrs Ratski as best he could, but she was rigid and he could barely move her. He noted her pain and sweat and rapid pulse. Her temperature was very high. 'I will give her an injection of morphine, and then I will order an ambulance to take her to hospital,' he said.

I was a first-year student nurse at the Royal Berkshire Hospital, Reading, when Mrs Ratski was admitted. The year was 1953 and I was eighteen years old. We had been told to prepare for a woman with an abdominal obstruction of unknown origin, possibly a perforation, and peritonitis. The ward sister told the staff nurse to take me with her and to instruct me in preparation for an emergency abdominal exploration.

We made ready a bed, a surgical trolley for the examination, an injection tray for drugs and infusions, a trolley for gastric intubation and suction, and a drip stand for glucose and saline infusion. Our patient arrived and the staff nurse took her temperature, which was high, and blood pressure, which was subnormal. Her pulse was thin and racing, and her skin was white and sweating. Her mouth and tongue were dry, her eyes glazed, and she was deeply asleep, breathing slowly – only about six to eight breaths per minute. Our patient was obviously in a state of shock. I was told to undress her.

Slavek was hovering in the background, so the staff nurse took a medical history from him. He did not know his mother's age, but thought she was between seventy-five and eighty years old. He informed us that she had been a peasant, uneducated, and had worked on the land since she was about seven. She had married, and borne (he thought) nine children. 'Had there been any miscarriages?' He did not know. 'Had she ever been ill?' He thought not – at least, he had never been told of any illnesses. 'Had she ever had an operation?' He didn't think so. 'Was her husband with her?' No, he had died many years ago.

I was still taking off all her black clothes, revealing an emaciated body. Staff nurse was a thoughtful girl, and remarked, 'She looks half-starved, as though she has hardly had a good meal in her life. How did she come to be with you?'

Then Slavek told us the story of her astonishing lone journey across Europe to England. Staff nurse wrote it all up in the notes. 'Amazing,' she said, 'hardly credible. But she is here, so she must have done it. Why did she come?'

'She told my sister, Olga, that she was going to die, and that she must see me first.' Slavek could scarcely get the words out, his voice catching as he choked back the tears.

'Her dying wish, eh?'

'I suppose so. She told me that she was happy to go now that she had seen me.'

Staff nurse was kind and optimistic. 'Don't worry. Your mother is in the right place. We can treat this sort of thing. She will soon be well again.'

'Thank you so much. You are wonderful.'

The house surgeon arrived. He was very young, about twenty-four, and this was his first house job. Like me, he was nervous and a bit hesitant. He checked Mrs Ratski's heart and lungs, looked into her eyes, ears and throat, and checked all her involuntary reflexes. He took blood for crossmatching, set up a glucose/saline drip, and put the gastric suction machine in readiness, but he did not insert the gastric tube. He examined the abdomen, which was hard and distended, and applied his stethoscope to listen for abdominal sounds. 'Hmmm,' he said, looking very wise, 'I will call the registrar.' With that, he left.

I was told to give the old lady a blanket bath, and to put a surgical gown on her. She was so thin, I thought she might break if I moved her. She could scarcely have weighed more than seven stone. Her distended abdomen, hard and shiny, contrasted strangely with the rest of her. I wondered what kind of life she had had back in Latvia.

The registrar came, accompanied by the houseman. The registrar was only about thirty, perhaps less, but five years' experience in medicine can make a great deal of difference. There was no careful hesitation in *him*. He was quick, confident, and arrogant. He tapped the abdomen and listened.

'What do you make of it?' he demanded of his junior.

'Well, em, I, er, could hear abdominal sounds.'

'And what did you make of them?'

'Well, I found, er . . .'

'Can't hear a damned thing that means anything. We'll have to open it up to see what's going on. Go and book theatre. Laparotomy, with exploration. Possible gastrectomy, resection, won't know till we get in there. I'll go and talk to Carter. See if he wants to do it, or if I should.' They left.

Mr Carter, the consultant, arrived with an anaesthetist. He examined Mrs Ratski and read the notes. The anaesthetist was concerned about the patient's emaciation and her state of shock. He ordered a gastric tube to be passed and suction to be commenced immediately. He commented that she would not need a pre-med, because she had had morphine. He said, 'We must have a consent form, and she can't sign it. Is there anyone here who can?'

'Her son is with her,' replied the staff nurse.

'Get him to sign, will you, Staff?'

The two consultants left, and Staff took a consent form to Slavek. 'Your mother must go to theatre for an abdominal exploration. Would you sign the consent form for her, please.'

'Of course,' said Slavek, and signed.

There had been no discussion with Slavek about his mother's condition; no mention of what an exploratory laparotomy means, still less of what a gastrectomy or resection could entail, nor of the post-operative complications that can so easily arise in old people after major surgery. There had been no hint that perhaps the surgery could lead to a death more agonising, and certainly more prolonged, than the abdominal crisis that had occurred in the early hours of the morning. Neither the doctor nor the nurse discussed with Slavek his mother's dying wishes, nor her certainty of her impending demise, her astonishing resolution to get to England to see him, and her acceptance of death once she had achieved this. No one asked him, quietly and sympathetically, if he could project what his mother might want. Whilst all the decisions were made about and around her, Mrs Ratski was in a deep, morphine-induced, sleep. But no one suggested waiting until she roused so that she could speak for herself.

That was when, at the age of eighteen, I started to contemplate death.

A LIFE SAVED

Mrs Ratski was taken to theatre within an hour of the ambulance arriving at Slavek's house, and Mr Carter took the case himself, with the registrar and houseman assisting. The abdomen was incised, and a volvulus was found to be causing the obstruction. Volvulus is the term applied to the twisting of a loop of bowel on itself. The pelvic colon is most commonly involved, and the patients are usually elderly. Manual untwisting of the bowel was performed after deflation of the loop with an aspirating needle, then the gut was examined, and no other abnormality was detected. Gastric suction was continued throughout the operation, and a saline and glucose drip continued. To relieve the pressure on the pelvic colon, a left inguinal colostomy was undertaken, which was intended to be temporary. A colostomy is when a loop of colon is brought out through the abdominal wound on to the skin surface, and retained in position with sutures. An opening is then made into the bowel, and the contents will drain into a bag or bottle.

The operation itself was relatively straightforward, but difficulties arose because of the anaesthetic. The patient was old, under-nourished, and in deep shock. Her blood pressure was very low, hardly sufficient to maintain circulation, so cardiac stimulants and oxygen were given. The patient did not have adequate respiratory drive to breathe, so a tracheotomy was performed. The anaesthetist made an artificial opening through the windpipe, and passed an endotracheal tube directly down the trachea for oxygen and gases to be delivered under positive pressure. The gas used was ether, and Mrs Ratski went into an ether convulsion, which is a serious complication. Antidote drugs had to be given intravenously, the gas was stopped, and a mixture of oxygen and carbon dioxide administered instead. The patient was in theatre for three hours, and for most of that time the anaesthetist was battling for her life. Several times the theatre staff thought she had died, but each time the anaesthetist resuscitated her successfully.

Mrs Ratski returned from theatre to the ward. Post-operative intensive care units did not exist in the 1950s, so the ward sister and her nurses took that responsibility. We had been alerted that the patient's condition was grave, and a small side ward had been prepared. The ward sister received the patient and checked her condition, and a nurse was told to stay with her. There were no monitoring machines in those days. A patient's post-operative condition was maintained entirely by nursing observation and assessment.

Slavek had been obliged to go to work. He had been told to ring the hospital at midday, and that he could visit in the evening. When he telephoned, he was told that the operation had been successful, but that his mother was still under the anaesthetic. He came to the hospital directly from work, but she still had not regained consciousness. The breathing tube in her throat frightened him, so he asked the sister about it, and she told him that it was only temporary and would be removed when his mother had enough strength to breathe normally. He asked about the blood transfusion entering her arm. What was wrong with her blood? The sister quietly explained that it was normal procedure after major surgery to give blood. An oxygen cylinder hissing away beside her bed alarmed him, but at the same time it reassured him – everything possible was being done for her. Everything would be all right. She was sleeping and looked comfortable, so he slipped away.

On the second evening, he was alarmed to find his mother's hands tied to the side of the bed. The sister explained that it was necessary, because his mother had tried to pull the tube out of her throat. His mother turned her head and looked at Slavek, her eyes full of anguish, but she could not speak because of the tube in her windpipe. He stroked her hand and kissed her forehead, whispering, 'You'll be all right, mother. They know what they're doing.'

On the third evening the oxygen cylinders had been removed, but the tube was still in her throat, and her hands were still tied. Slavek asked about the tube, and the sister said that there would be a ward round tomorrow, so a decision would be made then. He felt reassured, and told his mother that the surgeon would see her the next day, and that everything would be all right.

But everything was not all right, and we, the nursing staff, knew it.

In the first instance, our patient's recovery from anaesthetic had been abnormally prolonged. She had not shown any signs of consciousness for more than twenty-four hours, and when she did recover, she seemed excessively agitated. She had attempted to throw herself out of bed, and had to be restrained by two nurses. She tried to shout, but could not make a sound, because of the tube in her trachea, so she tried to pull it out. We nurses had to prevent her from doing this, and we explained that it must stay in place for a few days. Only then did we realise that she neither spoke nor understood English, and it took us some days before we appreciated how difficult this was going to be. She watched us carefully, and when a nurse's back was turned she tried to pull the tube out again, and had to be restrained. The naso-gastric tube, which was attached to a machine for continuous suction, was another focus of worry. Then Mrs Ratski discovered the blood drip entering her arm, and had a go at that, too. The night sister had ordered her hands to be tied to the sides of the bed, because during the night when fewer nurses were on duty she would have undoubtedly succeeded.

Mrs Ratski lay immobile, hands restrained, in terrified silence. Soundless sobs racked her body, and tears streamed from her eyes. She could not swallow, because of the pain in her throat. Her mouth became completely dry and crusted, and had to be moistened and cleaned every hour, but even so her tongue was ulcerated and cracked. She did not pass any urine, so a nurse had to catheterise her, but she held her body completely rigid, to prevent anyone from parting her legs. Did she think she was being raped? I wondered. Maybe she had been, in a prison camp? A muscle relaxant was injected, which she could not prevent, and the catheter inserted.

The house surgeon, registrar and anaesthetist visited frequently to check her condition. On the fourth day Mr Carter did his ward round. These were always elaborate affairs – the consultant, accompanied by the ward sister, followed by his team of doctors, and another team of nurses who were there to do or get things. It was highly ritualistic, like a visit from royalty. The consultant would go round the beds of his patients, asking questions of the sister, checking notes, ordering another test or another path lab analysis, changing a drug, or the dosage of a drug.

Mr Carter approached Mrs Ratski's bed. She lay still, her lips compressed, only her eyes moving, as they flickered from one white coat to another. Mr Carter read through the notes. 'I hear you have had trouble with her, Sister.'

'Yes, sir. She keeps trying to interfere with the dressings.'

'That is why you have tied her hands, I suppose?'

'Yes, sir. It was the only way.'

'Hmm. Well, we can discontinue gastric suction and start fluids by mouth. The blood drip can be removed after this bottle. That will help you, won't it, Sister? I can't give any instructions about the endotracheal tube. That's a matter for the anaesthetist. Everything else satisfactory, Sister? Urine, faecal discharge?'

'Yes, sir. Do you want to see the wound, sir?'

'Yes. Get a nurse to remove the dressings.'

I was at the back of the entourage, so I came forward and removed the dressing. Mr Carter looked at it.

'Hmm. Satisfactory. You can remove one of the drainage tubes, Sister. We'll take the other one out when we remove the sutures – we'll have to take her back to theatre when we close the colostomy. You can do that, Ryder,' he said to the registrar.

'Yes, sir.'

'Well, everything satisfactory, wouldn't you agree?'

'Yes, sir, very satisfactory,' said the registrar.

And they moved on to the next bed. As they went, the tension in Mrs Ratski's body visibly relaxed.

After the round had finished, Staff nurse told me to assist her in the removal of the naso-gastric tube. The blood had very nearly run out from the bottle, so she removed that also. With the removal of the suction machine and the drip stand Mrs Ratski looked more like a human being.

The anaesthetist came and said that he would remove the endo-tracheal tube under local anaesthetic. Staff nurse assisted him, and I was told to accompany her. The young house surgeon also came to watch, because he wanted to know how it was done. At the sight of another surgical trolley and several doctors and nurses, Mrs Ratski became visibly distressed. She could not make any sound, and her hands were still tied, but all her body language was that of panic. The anaesthetist took up a syringe of local anaesthetic, and, as she saw the needle approach her neck, Mrs Ratski's skin lost all colour, and sweat poured from her brow. The anaesthetist retreated. He took her pulse rate.

'It's gone up to one hundred and twenty. I can't proceed like this. She will have to have a general.'

So, for a second time, Mrs Ratski was prepared for theatre and given a pre-med and muscle relaxant. Removal of the tube and suturing of the trachea and outer muscle and skin only took a few minutes, and then the patient was back in her bed.

In the evening, when Slavek called, he was relieved to find his mother's hands free, and all the machines gone. Her throat was bandaged, however, and she still could not speak; this was due to throat ulceration, which is very painful, but ultimately not damaging.

After a few days she *could* speak, but we did not know what she was saying. We were able to sit her up in bed, and she could look around at the other patients. Fear and distrust were always in her eyes, and she reacted with dread whenever a doctor came near. We nurses tried to feed her, but she refused; we could not persuade her even to drink.

'If this goes on, she will have to have another saline drip. She cannot go without fluids,' Sister said. In the evening when Slavek visited she asked him to try to persuade his mother to drink. But even he could not. He told us that she thought we were trying to poison her, and he could not convince her otherwise. If he brought her drinks and food from outside, she would perhaps take it. So he did, and she drank and ate a little for a few days.

On the seventh day her sutures and drainage tube were removed, and her condition appeared to be stable. On his ward round, Mr Carter said that if all went well the colostomy could be closed on the tenth post-operative day. He was confident of a complete recovery.

In the early hours of the ninth day, the night nurse reported extreme restlessness, and signs of pain and distress. The night sister went to the ward and found Mrs Ratski doubled up in pain and moaning piteously. Her pulse was rapid and her temperature high. The abdomen was examined; it had become rigid again. Whilst the night sister was present Mrs Ratski vomited copiously and effortlessly, without retching. Sister was alarmed and called the house surgeon. The time was 5 a.m., and when he arrived only ten minutes later, symptoms of shock were very apparent, and her temperature and pulse had risen again. It all happened very quickly. The patient vomited once more, a green, bile-stained fluid, in a projectile fashion.

The registrar was called and a quick examination was all that he needed.

'This is another obstruction. Acute abdominal dilation with fluid and gas could be due to a paralytic ileus. We'll have to get her to theatre at once. I'll speak to Carter – and Sister, you alert theatre for an emergency abdominal.' He turned and spoke to the houseman. 'Give her a good shot of morphine and get naso-gastric suction going straight away. We will probably need more blood, but have some serum ready until we can get into the blood bank.'

The registrar was at his best in an emergency – quick, confident, decisive, and, above all, commanding. He performed the operation himself. Part of the intestine was found to be paralysed and dilated with gas, and the area of the original volvulus had adhered to coils of the large intestine and showed signs of gangrene. The sigmoid colon and the rectum were removed, and the rectal orifice closed. The colostomy, which was intended to be temporary, was now permanent.

When Slavek visited in the evening he found his mother in the same position as she had been nine days before. The only difference was that she did not have a tracheotomy and endotracheal tube. He was deeply distressed. What had happened? He was simply told that his mother had had to go to theatre for further surgery.

Nothing went right after that. The old lady was in a pitiable state. Two major operations and anaesthetics at her age took their toll. For two weeks she barely clung to life, but we kept her going. The gastric suction was continued for three or four days, and the drip for about a fortnight. Drugs were given by injection, because she would not swallow them. Her abdomen again filled with gas, and a trocar and cannula was thrust into the peritoneal cavity to release the gas. This was done under local anaesthetic and she was too weak to resist. Her mouth, tongue and throat were massively ulcerated long after the naso-gastric tube was removed. The self-retaining catheter had to be changed for cleansing, and she tried to resist, but was too weak to do so effectively. A urinary infection developed, so drugs were given to combat it.

Then she developed a chest infection, so more drugs were ordered – all of which were injected. Her cough reflex was inadequate, so a physiotherapist was called in to stimulate coughing by use of exercises, palpation and postural drainage. Her heart was compromised by her weakened condition, so cardiac stimulants were given. She had been in bed for so long that she developed bedsores, which we treated two-hourly but could not prevent. The abdominal wound, after the second operation, looked as if it was never going to heal and, together with the colostomy, exuded such a foul smell that it was sometimes difficult to go near her.

Doctors came and went. They tapped her abdomen, listened for abdominal sounds, and conferred over their findings and differing opinions. They took samples of blood for path lab reports on haemoglobin levels and white cell counts; took more blood to measure the electrolyte balance; ordered sputum and urinary analysis; probed orifices; and discussed erythrocyte sedimentation rates.

They came and went, and, as the weeks passed, they came less and went more quickly. In my experience, consultants, and particularly surgeons, kept an invisible barrier between themselves and their patients. Before and during the operation their professionalism could not be faulted. But once the post-operative stage was reached they became more remote. The house surgeon, the most junior of the doctors, was the only one who spent any time with our patient.

But, in fairness, there was nothing more that they could have done. They had twice, by emergency operation, rescued Mrs Ratski from certain death. After that, it was up to the nursing staff to help maintain life. And this is what we did, day by day, hour by hour.

One of the most distressing things to witness was her fear of us. Nurses do not usually inspire fear. We asked Slavek if he knew why she was afraid, and he told us that she thought she was in a prison camp where the Nazi doctors carried out forcible experiments on human beings. He tried to reassure her that she was in an English hospital because she had become very ill, and that we were making her better, but it made no difference. She was convinced that we were conducting experiments on her and pointed to her stomach.

'Look what they have done to me. They have cut me up and pulled my insides out (she pointed to her colostomy). They have interfered with my private parts; it is too terrible to say what they have done. You wouldn't believe it if I told you. They cut my throat – you saw it. No, my son, this is a medical experiment, the work of the devil. They have no heart, no pity, no soul. They are machines doing the work of the devil.'

Mrs Ratski was tough, both physically and morally. She had lost almost all her menfolk in wars and insurrections. Political conflict had been her only experience of life, and she had kept going through it all to keep the nucleus of her family alive. During the Second World War she had been in one of the many prison camps, where she must have endured cold, starvation and cruelty. She had been surrounded by death, but somehow survived.

In hospital, she lived through two operations and began to recover; but with increased strength she became more resistant to our efforts to nurse her. She fought us whenever we came near her, even for benign things like bed making. We tried to give her drugs by mouth, but she hit us and spat at us and knocked them to the floor, so the doctors ordered that drugs be given by injection. This required three nurses – two to hold her down, one to inject. She screamed and shouted what was probably abuse at us, then hit us as soon as she could. She tore off her abdominal dressing, and the colostomy bag; she even managed to pull out the self-retaining catheter. We were at our wits end to know what to do, so paraldehyde was ordered. This was a colourless fluid with a distinctive and revolting smell, which emanated from the patient, and could be smelled for a wide area around. We nurses hated having to inject it, because such a large quantity had to be given with a wide bore needle, thrust deep into the muscle. It certainly sedated the patient, but seemed to have peculiar properties, and I wondered if it was hallucinogenic. When the effect of the drug wore off, after about six hours, patients were often wildly excitable and disorientated.

Mrs Ratski had been in hospital for five weeks, and during that time I became increasingly troubled. When the paraldehyde started, I could not contain myself any longer. I blurted out to the staff nurse, 'Why are we giving her this stuff?'

'Because we have to be able to control her.'

'But it's mind-bending! People aren't the same after they have had it.'

'I know, but we have to give it.'

'Why?'

'You are not here to ask questions, Nurse. You had better speak to Sister, if you are worried.'

'I *am* worried, and it's not just the paraldehyde that is worrying me. It's everything.'

It took a lot of courage to speak to Sister. The nursing hierarchy in those days was such that a junior student nurse couldn't speak to a ward sister unless spoken to first, so I asked Staff if she would intercede for me.

A couple of days later, as I was going off duty, Sister called me back.

'I understand you are worried about giving paraldehyde to Mrs Ratski, Nurse?'

'Yes, Sister, and lots of other things, too.'

'What sort of things?'

'Everything, I suppose. Her treatment, the operations, the drugs, like cardiac stimulants, antibiotics – just everything . . .'

The severe aspect of Sister made me so nervous that I could not continue.

'You are not criticising the treatment Mrs Ratski has received in this hospital, I trust?' The words were delivered in such a way that they sounded more like a threat than a question.

'Oh no, Sister,' I said hastily, feeling foolish.

'Good. You may go off duty, Nurse.'

A few days later, in the middle of a morning's work, when all hands were needed to cope with the volume of duties we had to finish before lunchtime, Staff came up to me and said, 'You are to report to Matron's office at once. I will take over your work here.'

In those days, the matron of a hospital was a very powerful and influential figure, and most of them were quite outstanding women with remarkable minds, and great character and moral standing. A good matron knew everything that was going on in her hospital, and had her finger on every pulse. She had a prestige and authority that is quite unknown in nursing today. Many a consultant surgeon had been known to quake in his shoes if he received a message requiring him to report to Matron's office – a junior student nurse might collapse on the spot. Miss W Aldwinkle, OBE was in the top rank.

But I was not afraid. In fact, I was relieved. I had been called to account for myself once before, in an altercation with a consultant who had pushed me, and I had gained the impression she was a wise and understanding woman. I felt I could talk to her in a way that I could not talk to the ward sister.

I approached her door and knocked. 'Please enter,' a voice called.

It was a large and beautiful room, in a fine Victorian building that overlooked a spacious courtyard.

'Sit down, Nurse Lee. I understand that you are worried about the treatment given to Mrs Ratski?'

'Yes, Matron.'

'What exactly worries you?'

'It is hard to put into words. What concerns me is the amount of mental and physical suffering we have put her through. But I think it's more than that, really.'

'We always meet suffering in hospitals.'

'Yes, but this has been inflicted by us.'

'She would have died if she had not come to hospital.'

'But what is so wrong with that, Matron? My grandma died a few years ago, and no one thought it was wrong. She had a heart attack and just died. My grandad and my mother were with her. She didn't have to go through the weeks of suffering Mrs Ratski has endured.'

Matron looked steadily at me in a way that encouraged me to continue.

'Mrs Ratski knew that she was going to die, and she travelled all the way across Europe in order to see her son.'

'Yes, I know the story.'

'So why couldn't she be left to die in peace, like my grandma did?'

I was only eighteen, and my mind was in turmoil. Vague and disconnected thoughts I barely understood myself came tumbling out.

'What's wrong with dying, anyway? We're *all* going to die. If we are born, we must die. The road always goes in one direction. There are no alternative routes.'

Still Matron said nothing. I was getting so worked up I had to stand and walk around.

'You don't know what that poor old lady has been through, Matron. I do. I have been there day after day, and her suffering has been awful. Simply awful.'

'I know the extent of her suffering.'

'And it is all so futile. What has been the purpose?'

'Mrs Ratski is alive.'

'But what sort of life is this? We have turned a vigorous, healthy old lady into a pathetic invalid. She will never recover properly. And it may be that her mind has been damaged. She knew what she was doing before she came to us. Now she doesn't.'

'Sit down, Nurse.'

Matron rang a bell and a maid entered.

'Would you fetch a pot of tea and two cups, please, and some biscuits?'

'Yes, Matron.'

Matron looked at me and sighed.

'I can see you are upset, Nurse, and you raise questions I cannot answer. Nobody can. When I was your age, I was a young nurse in the war working in France. Death was all around us. Millions of young men died in that war. Millions. Yet I remember one who came to us with his face blown apart by an explosion. Where his nose, mouth and chin should have been there was just a great, bloody hole. Still, he was alive, and his eyes moved, and his mind obviously worked, though he could not speak because he had no mouth or tongue. The surgeons patched him up; they grafted skin over the shrapnel wound, and he recovered. But he had been a handsome young man, and was now left with two eyes and a ghastly-looking hollow with a hole in it, and a tube in the hole, so that liquid foods could be passed into his stomach.'

It was now my turn to gaze at *her* without speaking.

'I was about eighteen, and like you I thought: "Why have they done this? Surely life with such a face, if you could call it a face, is worse than death."'

I did not know what to say. There was a knock at the door and the maid entered with a tray.

'Thank you, Bertha. Put it here, please.'

Matron poured tea.

'These are deep and terrible subjects, Nurse, to which there can be no answers. I know you are upset, and I understand.'

'That is a terrible story, Matron. I would not want to live with a face like that. What happened to him?'

'He lives in an ex-servicemen's home. He cannot live in the community, because everyone stares and points at him.'

'So he is still alive! Is he happy?'

'I do not know. He seems content – he is a gardener, and gardeners are always happy people. And he has a dog. When I was your age I thought as you do. You have just said: "I would not want to live with a face like that." But I very much doubt if that man would say that he would rather be dead.'

'But he was *young*, and he had a whole future in front of him, even with such an affliction. Mrs Ratski is old, she has come to the end of her life. She said she was going to die; she achieved what she wanted to do, and then said she was content to die. The obstruction in her intestines would have meant her suffering would have lasted only a few hours, and she would very likely have died in her son's arms, like my granny died in my grandad's arms.'

'But the medical and nursing professions cannot allow anyone to die, if it can be prevented.'

'But who are we doing it for? For the benefit of the patient, or the benefit of the medical profession? We say that the welfare of the patient comes first, but I am not so sure. The practice of medical skills and techniques seems to come first.'

'I am certain that Mrs Ratski has been treated for the best of motives – to preserve life.'

'But for the rest of her days she will be a decrepit old invalid who will be a burden to everyone!'

'Human life is precious.'

'And human death is sacred. Or at least it should be – and would be, if we allowed it to be. In the short experience I have had, sitting with the dying, I can say that the last few hours are always peaceful, almost spiritual. Wouldn't you call that a sacred time?'

'Yes, I agree, Nurse, and I have had thirty-five years of nursing experience. I don't really know what is meant by the term "death agony" because I have never seen it.' She paused and thought, then added, 'Perhaps, in a few people, I have seen what can be described as a struggle with death, and it can be distressing to behold. But for the vast majority of people death is gentle, tender.'

'Well, it's not like that for Mrs Ratski. The agony has been going on for five or six weeks, and it will continue. She has been deprived of a gentle death.'

Matron said nothing, but I blundered on.

'She thinks she is in a concentration camp, you know, and that we are using her as a guinea pig. She can't understand what we are doing, or why. She is terrified all the time, terrified of *us*.'

'Yes, I know. That is something no one could have anticipated.'

'But she has lived in fear, Matron, for weeks. It is tragic, terrible. I can't bear to see it.'

I was getting tearful, and had to stand up and walk about again. 'And there's another thing. All these injections she's having. Dozens of them, daily. And now we've started paraldehyde. It's mind-bending, Matron. It replaces one madness with another, different sort of madness.'

I walked the length of the room and back, then sat down.

'And there is another thing that worries me, Matron. All this business about "she must have". It is written in her notes. "If drugs are refused, to be injected." And we, the nurses, have to inject them. It seems wrong.'

'A nurse must obey medical orders.'

'She does refuse drugs, all the time, so we hold her down and inject them. Isn't that assault? And who commits the assault? The doctor who orders it, or the nurse who does it?'

'I cannot answer these questions. Perhaps a lawyer could, but I doubt it. If life-saving drugs are to be given, they *must* be given, and any court of law would uphold the medical necessity to save life.'

'Well, I don't agree with the law!'

'Nurse, you are young and passionate. You are trying to under-stand a subject too deep for understanding. Death used to be as you have described it – your grandmother had a heart attack and just died in her husband's arms. That is how it used to be for the vast majority, but not any more. Medical science has found hundreds of death-defying tactics, and, as this century unfolds, thousands more will be available to us. We do not know where it will end. Perhaps we will come to a point when human beings are unable to die.'

'That is a frightening thought, Matron.'

'Yes, it is.' Matron stood up, all four feet eleven inches of her, indicating that the interview was over.

'I advise you, Nurse, not to talk too freely with other people on this subject. You will not be understood. In fact you may be positively *mis*understood. All sorts of sinister interpretations could be drawn from your remarks. It is a dangerous subject.'

UNABLE TO DIE

Hospitals in the early 1950s were small, enclosed worlds, especially for nurses. We lived communally in the nurses' home, and all our meals were taken together. Consequently, we exchanged news of hospital life all the time, so whilst I did not directly look after Mrs Ratski after the first five or six weeks, I was able to keep up with her progress, and made a point of doing so.

Mrs Ratski recovered sufficiently to go to the convalescent home attached to the hospital. It was a lovely house, with gardens sloping down to the Thames, which she seemed to enjoy.

The nursing staff tried to teach her how to manage her colostomy, but she did not understand, and seemed incapable of learning. She just muttered to herself, and poked it (the gut has no nerve endings, so can be touched without causing pain). She seemed intrigued, but quite incapable of understanding how to cope with it. After three weeks in the convalescent home, it was decided that she could return home under the care of a district nurse.

A hospital car brought Mrs Ratski home. Her daughter-in-law, Karen, watched with dismay as the driver helped the old lady out of the car, up the garden path and into the sitting room. She went straight to the sofa, muttering to herself, and pulling her shawls round her shoulders.

The district nurse arrived, kindly and helpful.

'Where is she going to sleep?' she enquired.

'I don't know. She slept on the sofa before.'

'She can't do that now – this sofa is not suitable. I can arrange to have a bed sent from the social services. It's wonderful what this new National Health Service can provide, isn't it? I'll go now, and come back this afternoon.'

A hospital-style bed arrived and the men put it up; the sofa was put in the garden shed. Karen watched the whole proceedings, and bit her lip. Her nice sitting room was ruined.

The district nurse returned in the afternoon.

'I've got sheets and pillowcases, and cotton blankets that can easily be washed, and all free from the NHS. Isn't it wonderful?'

Karen was not so enthusiastic. Washing blankets was not something she had anticipated.

Mrs Ratski sat on the edge of the bed looking uneasy, and still muttering.

'I don't know what you are saying, dearie, but let's get these clothes off you, and into bed, shall we?' The nurse turned to Karen. 'I've got to show you how to clean a colostomy.'

'What's a colostomy?'

'Oh, dear. Didn't anyone tell you she's got a colostomy? Well, briefly, the rectum has had to be sealed, and the colon is opened on to the skin surface and the body's waste product goes into a bag. I've brought a supply of colostomy bags with me to leave with you.'

Karen didn't fully understand until she saw her mother-in-law's abdomen. Two huge and angry-looking scars ran the length of the wrinkly old skin, and on the left hand side a pink, protruding thing burst on to the surface. It was covered with a plastic bag containing brown liquid and had sticky stuff around the edges. Mrs Ratski looked at her abdomen, and poked the bag, and tried to pull it off.

'No dear, don't touch.' The nurse pulled her hand away. 'She's been doing this all the time in the hospital, they tell me. They can't get her to understand that the bag has to be left in place. Have you seen one of these before?'

'No, and I can't bear it! I just can't bear it. I think I am going to be sick.'

'You'll get used to it, dear. The first sight is always the worst. The bag has to be changed when it gets full. It's not so difficult when you get used to it. And anyway, I'll be coming in morning and evening to help you.'

The nurse pulled the bag off and wrapped it and its contents in gamgee paper tissue. The huge pink thing, raised from the surrounding skin, looked like a sea anemone attached to a rock, thought Karen, as she watched rigid with horror and disgust.

'It is important to clean the area carefully, otherwise the skin can get very sore,' said the nurse helpfully. 'Watch me.'

Deftly she cleaned around the colostomy with sterile water and applied zinc cream. 'I'll leave this with you,' she said.

'I can't do that!' said Karen in horror.

'I think you will have to, dear. Usually a patient learns to do it herself. But from what I have read in the patient's notes, I doubt if your mother-in-law will ever be able to.'

'I can't, I know I can't,' said Karen plaintively.

'Well, perhaps I can come in at lunchtime to help you out for the first few weeks.'

'Few weeks!' Karen was alarmed. 'How long will this go on for?'

'I can't say, dear. No one can. But she will have the colostomy for the rest of her life. Now, we must talk about other things. What is she going to do when she needs a wee? She can't get upstairs. What did she do before?'

'She went in the garden.'

'Oh, so you've got an outside lavatory. That's useful.'

'No, we haven't. She went behind the blackcurrant bushes.'

The nurse was shocked. Karen explained how she'd wondered where the old lady did her business and had been totally horrified when she first spotted her crouching outside. She'd tried talking to Slavek about it, but he'd been unwilling to broach the subject with his mother.

'Well, she can't do that sort of thing now. She will have to have a chamber pot. Have you got one?' Karen shook her head. 'Then I will get one from NHS Supplies.'

The nurse packed up her bag. She was kindly, and saw Karen's agonised expression.

'Don't worry, my dear. The first few days are always the worst, and I'll be popping in every day. You'll soon get used to it.'

Karen went upstairs to her bedroom, and threw herself on the bed, and cried as she had never cried before.

The days stretched into weeks, and Karen never did get used to it. She could not bring herself to touch the colostomy, so Slavek did. He did not find the task difficult or nauseating. He had cared for farm animals in his youth, had attended birthings, squeezed teats, cut abscesses, applied poultices, and a colostomy was much the same. Added to which, he wanted to spare Karen the burden. The district nurse was true to her word, and came in twice a day, often three times.

Karen kept the children away from their grandmother as much as possible. After school they went up to their bedroom to play, and she joined them. To reach the garden they had to pass through the living room and kitchen, so she discouraged this, taking them to the park instead. Slavek did not like it, and thought her determination to keep the children away from his mother was wrong, so he asked her why she did it.

'I don't want my girls to see that sort of thing. They are too young.'

'They're not. Children need to see everything in life. Old age, sickness, birth, death, everything.'

'It upsets them.'

'That's only because you tell them not to be upset. *You* put the idea into their minds first. If you said nothing, they would take it in their stride. Children always do.'

Karen changed tactics.

'Well, anyway, they can't talk to her.'

'But if you let them they would learn some Latvian.'

But she wouldn't. He watched with sadness as Karen shepherded the girls carefully around the opposite side of the living room, as far away from their grandmother as possible, and upstairs to their bedroom.

One day she said: 'I'm going to ask the nurse to get a screen from supplies.'

'What for?'

'To put around the bed, so I don't have to see her using that chamber pot. And I don't think the girls should have to see it, either.'

He sighed. 'You'll do more harm than good trying to protect them like this.'

But in the evening he came home to find screens around the bed, and his mother completely hidden from the life going on around her. The girls, being children and endlessly curious, would peep behind the screens and stare at their grandmother, as though she were an animal in a cage. Then they would giggle and run away.

He could see that Karen was growing increasingly resentful, and discussed it with the nurse. He felt guilty, and was bewildered by his feelings of guilt. Even though he and the nurse attended to the colostomy Karen had a lot of extra work, with washing, changing the bed, emptying the chamber pot, cooking. He was a practical man, and saw life in practical terms. What he did not see was that Karen's main resentment was that she did not have the house to herself. He had been brought up in a large, gregarious family. They had had only one large room for everything – living, sleeping, cooking, eating. Babies were born in that room. Illness was nursed there, and he remembered, from long ago, his grandfather – his mother's father – dying in the room. And now, here was his own mother dying in *his* room, but completely cut off from his family. He felt guilty about it. Guilt seemed to come at him from all sides: Karen, his mother, the girls. He had let them all down. But how? What had he done wrong? The nurse listened but could only sympathise.

And what of Mrs Ratski in all this? She was the most pitiable figure. Within the space of three months she, who had been a vigorous, determined old woman, had been reduced to an invalid. And her mind and character had subtly changed also, Slavek noticed. The strong, wise matriarch whom everyone in the family looked to for guidance had gone, and a whining, querulous old woman he did not recognise had slipped into her place.

Mrs Ratski was turning in on herself more and more each day. Her thoughts seemed to be centred entirely upon her colostomy. She spent hours muttering to herself, picking and poking at the bag. The old lady who had been the strength of her family throughout decades of war, suffering and foreign domination; who had survived a prison camp; with all her strength, all her resolution to get to England; all that she had endured in hospital; everything was reduced to a pinpoint of focused attention – her colostomy.

There was no doubt that her mind was slipping away from her. She could not understand where she was or why she was there. Probably the acute illness, the anaesthetic, and the drugs had affected her mind, however, the cultural isolation must have had something to do with it, too. The language everyone around her was speaking confused and bewildered her. But it may be – in fact it probably was – that her brain cells, together with all the other cells in her body, were growing older day by day, week by week, and dying, as all living things must die.

One can hope that she was losing her mind, because it would have been a merciful release from loneliness. She had lost all that was familiar, her home, her daughter Olga and grandchildren, her friends, her country and the rhythm of her life, her language and her Church. Everyone around her was doing things to her that she could not understand. No one, apart from Slavek, showed her any love, and she loved no one. The hope must be that senile dementia was laying its kindly hand on her mind, inducing confusion and forgetfulness. Awareness and remembrance of loss would have been more cruel.

The year was drawing to its close, and the nurse was behind the screens tending Mrs Ratski when a quarrel erupted between the young couple.

Karen unexpectedly said: 'I've decided to take the girls to my mother's for Christmas.'

'Why?' asked Slavek guardedly, although he already knew the answer.

'I can't face Christmas here, with your mother in the room.

How can I put up a Christmas tree and hang paper chains? We can't have presents under the tree and a nice Christmas dinner in there; I can't invite people in. No, we're going to Mum's this year. I've told the girls and they are looking forward to it. You can come, if you like.'

'But your parents don't really like me. They won't want me for Christmas.'

'Well, you can please yourself. Mum says you'll be welcome if you want to join us.'

'But I can't leave my mother here on her own!'

'It's not my responsibility. I'm doing what I think is best for the girls. I want them to have a good Christmas.'

He became angry.

'How can it be a "good Christmas" if you take them away from their father? That's not goodness, that's selfishness.'

'Don't you call me selfish! I want—'

He butted in before she could finish the sentence.

'I remember when I was a boy, my grandfather died in our home. It was Christmas time, and all the family were there. We were children, and we just accepted it. We all played, and had a "good" Christmas.'

'Don't you keep reminding me of how you were brought up! Peasants, that's what you were, peasants. No wonder my mother doesn't like you! Well, I'm not a peasant, thank you very much. I was properly brought up, and I'm going to see to it that my girls are, too.'

'I don't know what your "proper upbringing" means, if it means denying the girls their grandmother. And she *is* their grandmother. And they are not just *your* girls. They are *my* girls too.'

'She's not *like* a grandmother. She doesn't do things with them. She can't take them out or play with them like grannies do. She just sits there, muttering and mumbling, and poking that "thing". I can't stand it any longer, all the washing and trying to get it dry, in this weather. And the smell! I can't stand it any more. However much I wash, it's still there. The nurse says if she didn't keep poking at that "thing" it wouldn't leak and the bed wouldn't get dirty, but she won't stop. She keeps poking and picking, and I can't stand it, I tell you, I can't stand it!'

Karen had worked herself up into a hysterical frenzy and was sobbing. Slavek put his arm around her and she became calmer.

'Why doesn't she die, Slav? Why can't she just die? That's what she wanted. That's what she came here for.'

'I know. I've thought about it a lot. She nearly died that morning in August. But we called the doctors, and now she's alive, and can't seem to die.'

'If only I hadn't gone to the phone box.'

'You only did what you thought was right. I did worse. I signed the consent for operation form.'

'Why did you?'

'Well, there wasn't really any time to think. There was a sort of pressure to sign. No one said anything, but it was expected of me, so I did.'

He brooded gloomily for a while, and neither of them spoke. Karen could see his unhappiness and felt sorry for her outburst. She squeezed his hand, and saw his manliness crumble into tears that he tried to hide.

'If I had known what was going to happen,' he continued, 'I would never have let them do it to her. But I didn't know. How could I?'

'If you had refused to give consent for the operation, would it have made any difference, do you think?'

He thought for a bit, and wiped his eyes and blew his nose.

'No, I'm not sure that it would. I think they would have operated anyway.'

'Then you can't blame yourself.'

'But I do. I feel guilty all the time. Guilty because I've made life hell for her, and guilty because I've made life hell for you.'

'Is it wicked of me to wish that she had died last August, Slavek?'

'I don't think so. Death is natural. It comes to us all.'

'Can she go back to Latvia?'

'I can't see how. How could we get her there?'

'She'll have to go into a home of some sort.'

'That's what I'm beginning to think. I didn't want it, but I can't see any alternative.'

Slavek and Karen discussed it with the district nurse who made enquiries. Two local council-run old peoples' homes were full and agreed to put Mrs Ratski on a waiting list, but warned that it might be a year or two before a place became available. They could enquire about private nursing homes in the area, but were told that Mrs Ratski would upset the other residents.

Christmas came. As soon as the school holidays started, Karen took the girls to her mother's. Slavek was left alone with his mother. He attended to her physical needs, and the district nurse called as before. Then Karen decided to stay with her mother – Slavek was devastated. He was lonely and missed his little girls most dreadfully. On Christmas Eve he got drunk and slept for two days, with a couple of bottles of vodka by his bed.

He was awakened by repeated banging on the front door. He staggered downstairs, unkempt, unshaven, and wrapped in a blanket. It was the district nurse.

'What's been happening? I tried to get in this morning. I saw your bike was here, but you didn't answer, and I knocked and knocked.'

'What time is it?' His voice was slurred.

'It's four o'clock. I haven't seen your mother for days. Has she been away with you?'

'No. She has been here all the time.'

'Well, I must see her now.'

They went into the sitting room.

'It's bitterly cold in here. Hasn't the poor old lady even got a fire? And it smells dreadful. Who has been looking after her? Where is your wife?'

'My wife has gone to her mother's and she's not coming back.'

'Not coming back? Oh dear, that won't do. I will have to report that to my supervisor. The old lady can't be left alone all day while you are at work. But I'm sure arrangements can be made to care for her – Meals on Wheels, a home help – yes, there is a lot of support we can give you.'

'I don't want your bloody support! I want my wife and daughters. They're not coming back, I tell you.'

'There is no need to shout, young man. I heard you, and don't use bad language to me!'

'She will have to go into an old peoples' home.'

'That's not so easy, as you well know. The Council Home is full, and your mother is on the waiting list. Have you tried private nursing homes?'

'Yes, and they won't take her. Each one we tried said she would be disruptive and would upset the other residents.'

'Well, all I can do is organise as much home support as possible for her. Now, I must clean her colostomy. She's in a dreadful mess, faecal discharge everywhere. When did you last attend to it?'

'I can't remember. A few days, perhaps . . .'

Muttering words of disapproval, the nurse started work.

'And what has she been eating recently, if your wife has not been here?'

'I don't know. Porridge, I suppose. She likes porridge.'

'Well, it's not good enough. We can't allow her to live on porridge. Meals on Wheels will be arranged as an emergency, from tomorrow. And I advise you to light a fire, young man. It's freezing in here.'

Clucking her disapproval, the district nurse left.

Slavek did not light a fire. He went to the pub and got blind drunk.

Days passed, day after desolate day, and Slavek was utterly alone. Hatred and resentment built up inside him and he could hardly bring himself to go near his mother – stupid, useless old thing. Why hadn't she died when she said she would, why was he stuck with her now, a miserable old bag of bones with no mind? Why couldn't she just *die*? Every day, when he got home from work, he was hoping against hope to find her dead – but she wasn't. She was always there, in Karen's nice sitting room, where the children should be playing by the fire, and having crumpets toasted on the red coals, and stories read to them before bedtime. Every evening he spent in the pub, drinking until closing time.

Men in Slavek's position – having lost wife and children, heart-broken, lonely, angry, frustrated, drinking more and more – can quickly spiral into a crisis from which they cannot escape. Self-neglect, repeatedly arriving late for work with a hangover, unreliability, led to warnings from the management, which were only half-heartedly observed, then ignored. Slavek was dismissed. He was too ashamed to tell Karen that he had been given the sack, so he drew his dole money, sent half to her, and spent the rest in the pub. He had never been a good manager; Karen had always handled the family finances. Perhaps he thought that he was doing enough by sending her money each week; perhaps his brain, fuddled by drink, refused to accept the inevitable consequences of the fact that no money was going into his bank account.

In March he received a letter from the bank manager, saying that there was insufficient money in his account to pay his monthly obligation to the building society. Slavek ignored it. April brought a similar letter. He didn't even open it. Each month a letter arrived, but was ignored.

Karen knew nothing of all this. If she had, she would have done something about it. But by the time August came and Slavek was six months in arrears with the mortgage, the sum outstanding was so huge that there was nothing she could have done to rectify the situation.

In September, the building society obtained an order for distraint. The house would be repossessed and sold to recover the loan the society had made. Slavek didn't really understand what had happened until the bailiffs arrived and ordered him and his mother out of the premises. The district nurse arrived at the same time, and, as no provision had been made for the old lady, she took control of the situation and a week's grace was allowed.

The Court Order was the first news Karen had of the financial crisis. She was utterly distraught and rushed over to see Slavek. How had it happened? It couldn't have happened suddenly. There must have been warning letters. Where were they? Slavek rummaged around amongst a pile of unopened letters and produced a couple.

'You fool!' shouted Karen. 'Why didn't you let me know? Why did you ignore them? Now look what's happened. We are going to lose our home. Don't you understand? They are going to take our home away and sell it. We will be homeless.'

At last Slavek understood. But it was too late. There was nothing either of them could do. Karen returned to her mother, and stayed there. Slavek moved into a men's hostel, and drink took over his life.

As soon as the nurse informed the council of the eviction order, they assumed responsibility for Mrs Ratski. She was taken to a short-stay home for the elderly, but was terrified by the new surroundings, and became so disruptive that she had to be moved. This was a pattern that repeated itself several times. With each new move she thought she was going to be poisoned and wouldn't eat or drink. With puny strength she fought the staff and other residents and had to be forcibly restrained.

Mrs Ratski ended up in a psycho-geriatric ward where she could be kept under nursing care and more or less continuous sedation. All her fear, suspicion and aggression faded away and she became quiet and docile. She no longer resisted the nurses, and meekly swallowed the tranquillisers, and everything else that was given to her. Every so often she developed a chest infection or a kidney infection and obediently she swallowed the antibiotics. She lived like this for three years, not able to understand where she was, or how she had got there; maybe not even who she was. She could not speak to anyone, nor comprehend a word that was said to her. She had no visitors. The hospital chaplain arranged for a Latvian priest to come, but she stared at him strangely and did not speak. Her loneliness and isolation were more total and more terrible than if she had been transported to a distant planet inhabited by aliens.

The end came in 1957 when she fell out of bed and broke her pelvis. It was virtually impossible for the pelvic bone to mend because it could not be immobilised. An operation was performed to try to pin the bone, but the wound did not heal, and staphylo-coccal infection developed, which did not respond to antibiotics. Generalised septicaemia set in. From this, Mrs Ratski died, alone, in the brittle whiteness of an English hospital.

This is a family tragedy that could only have been prevented by the old lady's death. Yet there is not a doctor in the civilised world who would fail to treat a simple intestinal obstruction. Nor, I think, are there many lay people who would say, 'Leave her alone – she must die.' No one could have foreseen that it would lead to the break-up of a family, and the downfall of a good man.

RETIREMENT

It's some years since
I felt my servant's discontent;
The vigour of his service seemed to pall.
I noticed this without undue dismay
At first.
The sometime faltering foot
Or wheezing breath
Or jack-knife on the exit from a car —
All brushed beneath the carpet
Of my mind —
An easy-going master.
But the incidents grew more
Till, patience fled, I turned on him,
Upbraided him with negligence, or worse.
He said: 'Your lifetime, now
I've been your faithful slave,
Attending to your every need,
Drew in clean air for you
And made your blood,
Remodelled you from food,
Ejected what was not required,
Enabled you to see and hear
This varied world;
Gave you mobility,
Produced your thoughts and passions.
But now, at last, I'm weary,
Wish to rest,
Return to earth and air

Which nourished me,
As all things must,
While you go free.
What say you, master?
Will you grant me my release?'
'That is not mine to do,'
I countered;
'I serve too;
I serve one who
Would rage at my presumption
If I gave you leave to go.
He is the great Disposer.
For Him, it's you who must depart,
Give notice, go,
Not wait for your release.'
And so it was;
My servant went
And left me here and everywhere,
No longer part but whole.

— *Philip Worth*

THREESCORE YEARS AND TEN

My grandfather's death has an idealistic quality about it. His span of life had run out, he was cared for by his family, and he died peacefully in his own home. We would all wish to die like that. But, half a century later, we have to face the stark fact that for most of us it is unlikely.

Not so long ago old age was seen as the natural winding down of life, but somewhere along the way that attitude has changed. Now our waning years are viewed as a series of illnesses requiring medical intervention. A GP can prescribe drugs to arrest the symptoms of ageing, but a time will come when this is not enough and, at that stage, the elderly person is taken into hospital for treatment. This is almost compulsory these days; consequently, the majority of us will die in hospital or an institution of some sort.

It is a strange fact that a doctor cannot sign a death certificate having entered the cause of death as 'old age'. This is illegal, and a doctor who did not conform would be censured. Death has to be caused by a named disease. In countries where births and deaths are registered, this is required by all governments, and endorsed by the World Health Organization. It is unlawful to die of old age. This is illogical, but as Mr Bumble the Beadle famously remarked in *Oliver Twist*, 'The law, Sir, is a ass.'

We who are growing old know that we are. We feel it each day in our bones, in our joints, in our balance, and our slowing down; we see it in our hair and wrinkles; we find that little things we used to do without thinking have become difficult, and the struggle gets harder as the years go by. Strength, eyesight, hearing, memory, all begin to fail us. This is ageing, and we accept it because there is no alternative. Although we try to shut it from our minds we know that death is approaching; we 'know not the day nor the hour', but we know it will come.

We all react differently. In earlier generations it was time to 'take to one's bed', for those who could afford it, and I have known many people who did exactly that. No doubt a bed, an armchair by the window and no exercise shortened life, but no one expected to live beyond the age of seventy. I don't know of anyone who would want to do that now. Life has lengthened, thanks largely to drugs, but also to diet, general health, attitude and expectations. We know that the Horseman of Death is fast approaching, and it seems to have stimulated a collective desire to cram as much as possible into the few remaining years. Thousands of old people, with the help of medication and artificial hips and knees, are gadding about all over the world, doing things they have never done before, and enjoying life hugely. In 2005, to celebrate my seventieth year, I aimed to cycle one thousand miles for charity, and achieved fourteen hundred. This sort of crazy venture is not unusual. The organisers of activity holidays, such as a trek in the Himalayas, or perhaps the Road to Katmandu, often find that the majority of their clients are between sixty and ninety years old. Such activity would have been unthinkable a generation ago.

Active old age is wonderful, but it is entirely dependent on good health, which is a gift of God, or if you prefer, the luck of the draw, and not a right of man. We all know that any day, at any hour, something catastrophic could happen – a stroke, a heart attack, a broken hip – that would put an end to the life we have built. And then we would be dependent on others. A chill of fear enters the heart. The medication that has given us an extra decade of active life can still keep a tired and ageing heart pumping; can maintain sufficient pressure to keep the blood circulating and prevent it coagulating; can make liver and kidneys continue to function. Medication can help us for a long time, even when the body is manifestly worn out. Legs cannot function, a tremor affects the limbs, eyesight and hearing go, voluntary and involuntary control deserts us, the brain ... well, let us not speak too much of the brain, for that is the most frightening thought of all. 'I would rather be dead,' people say.

Not so. The instinct to live is far, far stronger than the rational mind, and when the time comes, instinct will win. People will consent to operations that will keep them alive for a bit longer, or take pills that they know will prolong their infirmities, though they know in their hearts that it is the fear of death that drives.

In the natural course of events, the period when death is taking over a body is fairly brief. My grandfather (who had no medication) had about a fortnight of this period in his life. Today it can drag on for months or years.

I spent twenty years in medicine, and I loved every minute of it. For me, it was a vocation and a privilege, working with the sick and the dying. To cure the sick was a joy, and exhilarating. To ease the process of dying was a sacred duty. I respect and admire the medical profession more than can be expressed. And I lament the sublime irony that the profession that has cured so much disease, and enhanced the quality of life for millions of people has, through its own success, been the instrument of distress at the end of life.

Healing the sick used to be described as 'the art and science of medicine'. Recently I have heard it called 'the science and technology of medicine'.

In the last fifty years medicine has changed profoundly. The scientific advances in pharmacology, made by multinational drug companies, are mind-blowing. The technology of medical treatment has advanced exponentially, and this will continue. Surgery and anaesthetics are such that staggering things can be achieved. And all is directed towards preserving life. This is what most people want, expect and sometimes demand, as though we have an intrinsic right to good health. In a post-religious age we place vast and unmerited confidence in the powers of medicine. When someone goes into hospital, it is expected that the doctors will be able to cure whatever is wrong. If they cannot, there is often a sense of outrage amongst aggrieved relatives. Even if someone is ready to go, relatives often feel that death cannot simply be allowed to take its course. They do not realise how quickly active old age can slip into extreme old age and imminent death.

If you look out for it, you will find in many local newspapers an indignant relative telling a story to an editor, who can see a good front page headline: 'Hospital allows Dad to Die!' This will be accompanied by a picture of a tearful woman holding up a photo of Dad. Then follows the story that the old man was around ninety, had had a heart attack or a stroke, or perhaps had broken a major bone, which had led to immobility, and in consequence he had developed a lung or kidney infection and died. The relatives claim, 'It shouldn't have happened. It was sheer neglect. He was in good health, enjoying life. He shouldn't have been allowed to die like that. I blame the hospital.'

Doctors and nurses are the first to see the futility of strenuous intervention, but the fear of legal action can drive them into what is known as 'defensive medicine'. This is bad medicine. The beleaguered doctors and nurses feel unable to make a decision based solely on professional judgement. They must always temper it with the thought that a decision or action might lead to an accusation of professional incompetence or neglect, or worse. Hospital practice today is driven by this necessity, and even if death is inevitable, doctors and nurses must be able to *prove* that they made every effort to prevent it. This is widely expected, nay demanded, by the general public and the law.

If people were with their elderly relatives all the time, day and night, as nurses are, they would be able to see for themselves the suffering and manifold indignities caused by the strenuous efforts to maintain life. Then perhaps they would be more inclined to say, 'Enough is enough – and no more.' Such a statement from a layman to a medical team is, I know, incredibly difficult. But the professions will usually accept it, and frequently with relief and gratitude.

Not infrequently an elaborate game of double-bluff is going on. Medical teams find it hard to suggest 'no more, this is futile' because they fear the reaction of relatives; at the same moment, relatives are perhaps thinking the same thing, but feel constrained from saying so in case someone thinks them callous or avaricious. No one will speak openly and truthfully. And whilst this is going on, a helpless old person at the end of life is unable to die.

Death, of course, will win in the end. But not the old-fashioned Angel of Death, nor even the dark Reaper, with the swish of his scythe. No, it will be the modern, hospitalised death, accompanied by the hum of a hydraulic airbed, and the bleeping of electronic monitors fixed to our fragile hearts and arteries, of flashing lights and drugs and drips and suction machines. All the paraphernalia of modern technology will guide us to our graves. We, who are growing old, cannot expect our children, and still less our grandchildren, to be with us at the hour of our death. We cannot, realistically, expect even a nurse to be with us. Machines do not need a nurse, unless the red light flashes on the central monitor, indicating that a drop in blood pressure or cardiac arrest has occurred, and then it is more likely to be a resuscitation team than a nurse that comes to watch and to wait.

I swear by the music of the expanding universe
and by the eloquence of the good in all of us
that I will excite the sick and the well
by the severity of my kindness
to a wholeness of purpose. I shall apply my knowledge,
curiosity, ignorance and ability of listen.

I shall co-operate with wondering practitioners
in the arts and the sciences,
with all who care for people's bodies and souls,
so that the whole person in relationship
shall be kept in view, their aspirations and their unease.

The secrets of the universal mind
I shall try to unravel to yield beauty and truth.
The fearful and sublime secrets told to me in confidence
I shall keep safe in my own heart.

I will not knowingly do harm to those in my care,
I will smile at them
and encourage them to attend to their dreams
and so hear the voices of their inner strangers.

If I keep to this oath I shall hope for the respect of my teachers,
and of those in my care and of the community,
and to be healed even as I am able to heal.

— *David Hart*

This poem was commissioned by the *Observer* newspaper to be a rewriting of the Hippocratic Oath, and was published there in July 1997. It was reprinted in *Setting the Poem to Words* (Five Seasons Press, 1998).

DR ELISABETH KÜBLER-ROSS
(1926–2004)

Elisabeth Kübler was born in Switzerland, one of triplets, weighing only two pounds. No one expected the tiny baby to live, but from the start Elisabeth was a survivor. She fought for life, and survived to be the author of the seminal work *On Death and Dying*.

She was thirteen years old when the Nazi armies marched into Poland, ruthlessly crushing the unprepared Polish Army as they attempted to defend their homeland, then rounding up hundreds of thousands of Jews, forcing them into trains and then taking them to . . . well, at the time, no one knew where. Elisabeth was a young girl, listening to a scratchy old box-radio with her family, and she bristled with anger as she heard the news. She made a silent promise to God that, when she was old enough, she would go to Poland and help the people to defeat their cowardly oppressors. Her father and brother later witnessed Nazi machine gunners shooting a human river of Jewish refugees as they attempted to cross the Rhine from Germany to the safety of Switzerland. Few made it to the Swiss side. Most of them floated down the river – dead. These atrocities were too great and too numerous to be hidden from a young girl already inflamed by the outrages, and she renewed her promise to God.

Yet she didn't really believe in Him. Not the God of the Lutheran pastor who taught and terrorised the Sunday School children, anyway. The pastor was a cold, brutish, ignorant man, unloving and unchristian, whose own children turned up at school with bruises all over their bodies, and were always hungry. The other children gave them food, but when the pastor found out he beat his children savagely for eating it. After that they didn't dare accept. Elisabeth didn't believe in the pastor's God. Maybe there was another one somewhere who loved little children. That Lutheran pastor turned Elisabeth against organised religion for the rest of her life. But she never ceased searching for the God of Love in whom she could, and eventually did, believe.

From an early age she was determined to be a doctor, but her father would not allow further education for girls, so she left school at fourteen to become a maid. After a year of skivvying for a rich woman she ran away and arrived at a hospital, offering to do anything. In those chaotic war years she was taken on and told to work as an assistant on the VD wards, in which all the patients were dying. Syphilitic patients were feared, shunned and locked away, but Elisabeth found them to be pathetic creatures who were warm and pleasant, and simply craved friendship and under-standing. She opened her heart to them, and it was this mutual affection that prepared her for worse that was to come.

On 6th June, 1944, the combined allied forces landed in Nor-mandy and the war changed. Thousands of refugees from all over Europe streamed into Switzerland. For days, then weeks, they marched, limped, crawled or were carried. The very old, the very young – all were half starved, ragged and verminous. Virtually overnight, the hospital was inundated with these traumatised victims of war.

For weeks, Elisabeth worked entirely with children who were mostly orphans, frightened and lost. De-lousing and disinfecting them was the first job, then finding clothes, then the search for food. She and another girl stole most of the food from the hospital stores, which seemed like a good idea at the time, but nearly had serious consequences. She was saved from the wrath of the outraged authorities by a Jewish doctor, who quickly arranged for the Zürich Jewish community to refund the cost of the food. He proved to be a powerful influence on her young life. He was a Polish Jew, and he told Elisabeth the horrifying stories of the concentration camps that had been built in Poland, and of the need for dedicated young people to go to his sad country to help with rebuilding. His words were another clarion call to Elisabeth.

On 7th May, 1945, all the bells of all the churches rang out in every country across Europe. People rejoiced, sang, danced, partied in the streets, got drunk. The war was over. It had lasted for six years, but the rebuilding would take much longer. Elisabeth joined the International Voluntary Service For Peace, and for four years worked with medical teams in some of the worst areas of devastation. When a team was assigned to go to Poland to set up a first aid station, she joined them, and went to Majdanek, a death camp, where 300,000 people had been gassed alive. She saw with her own eyes trainloads of children's shoes and clothes, and trunks full of human hair that had been destined for Germany to make pillows. She smelled the sweet odour of the gas sheds, the smell of death, and the all-pervading stench of rotting corpses. She saw the barbed wire, the guard towers, the spotlights, and the rows of barracks in which men, women and children had spent their last days while they awaited their call to strip and form a line to enter the gas chamber, to fulfil the quota of exterminations for that day. She wandered around, numb with shock, and saw to her amazement, sketched on every wall of every barrack, hundreds of butterflies. What, in the name of Heaven, could impel people waiting in such conditions for their inevitable death, to depict the form of a butterfly? She did not know, none of us will ever know, but it was a concept that would fill her imagination, and haunt her for the rest of her life. It was this image, and the symbolic message sent out by these doomed people, that would eventually lead her to a belief in the God of Love.

It was only after four years of this voluntary work that Elisabeth returned to Switzerland, more determined than ever to become a doctor. She had to start night school in order to learn the basics of science from scratch. There was no help from her father or her tutors, who told her to go and be a housewife, a maid, a seamstress – academia was not for girls. But she had been trained in the harsh school of life and she knew the value of persistence. In 1957, at the age of thirty-one, she passed her final examinations and became a country doctor in the mountain villages north of Zürich. It was a happy time.

It is interesting to speculate on how life turns out for each of us, and how chance plays its part. Elisabeth always said it was the hand of God guiding her. If she had not met and fallen in love with a handsome American doctor, she would have remained a contented family doctor in rural Switzerland, probably married to a respectable burger, happy to settle down after the hectic adventures of her youth. Instead, she married Emanuel Ross, went to America, and entered the maelstrom of American hospital medicine. This was where her intellectual life, coloured by her early experiences of suffering, began. She had found her vocation.

Elisabeth had never really wanted to go to America, still less did she want the post of psychiatric resident at Manhattan State Hospital, but it was the only job she could get. She worked with the mentally ill for nearly two years, and learned a great deal about the psychology of the human mind, its dark recesses and closed doors.

One day her chief asked her to examine a man who was supposed to be suffering from psychosomatic paralysis and depression. The man also had an incurable degenerative disorder. Elisabeth examined him, and spoke with him at length. She had seen this state of mind before in the ravaged towns and villages of Europe, and she knew what it meant.

'The patient is preparing himself to die,' she reported.

The neurologist not only disagreed, he appeared embarrassed, and ridiculed her diagnosis, saying that the patient just needed the right medication to cure his morbid state of mind. Days later the patient died.

This encounter started Elisabeth thinking, watching, and noting her observations. She saw that most doctors routinely avoided mentioning anything to do with death, and the closer a patient was to dying, the more the doctors distanced themselves. She asked questions of her medical colleagues, but they avoided giving her direct answers, and she gained the impression that very few of them had been present at the bedside at the actual moment of death. 'That's not my department; I leave that sort of thing to the nurses,' was the implied response. She questioned medical students and found that they were taught nothing about death and how best to handle a patient with a terminal illness.

At first she was intrigued, and not a little amused by the head-in-the-sand attitude of her colleagues, and wondered how it would be defined in the school of analytical psychology. But then she began to wonder what effect it had on the patients themselves; and she gravitated towards those who were the most sick and the closest to death. Her experience in war-torn Europe made it easy for her to talk to these people, and she would sit with them for hours. What she discovered, mainly, was the grief of loneliness and isolation. Very often a patient had first learned of the gravity of his condition by the altered behaviour of those around him – avoidance, evaded questions, lack of eye contact. The silence of physicians added to their fears. Relatives and friends, it seemed, were also engaged in a massive game of 'let's pretend', thereby closing the door on empathy and understanding. There is not a single dying human being who does not yearn for love, touch, understanding, and whose heart does not break from the withdrawal of those who should be drawing near.

What she was observing was so at odds with her upbringing in her village in Switzerland, where a dying person was treated with love and compassion, that she thought it must be something peculiar to New York. But in 1962 the family – by now they had two children – moved to Denver, Colorado, and she and her husband got jobs at the University Hospital. Quietly, she continued her observations and discovered, to her astonishment, that the medical and social attitude to the dying was exactly the same in Colorado as in New York. Throughout America, apparently, death was a subject no one wanted to deal with.

'This is a national sickness, more serious than anything I have seen on the schizophrenic wards,' she opined.

Her new job was working on liaison between psychiatry and general medicine, covering all disciplines. The team was headed by a professor whose main interest was in measuring the relationship between the mental, emotional and spiritual with the pathology of physical illness. Elisabeth and the professor were on the same wavelength, and she was able to discuss with him the effects that rejection and non-communication had on terminally ill patients.

He was the first doctor with whom she had been able to express her concerns, and he understood, and encouraged her to continue her quest.

The professor was a brilliant and charismatic lecturer, and he drew large crowds to his weekly seminars, at which he discussed with students of all faculties how psychology and psychiatry could be applied to general medicine. One day, in 1964, he called Elisabeth to his office and said that he would soon be travelling to Europe for a period of time, and that he would like Elisabeth to take over his lectures.

'I don't follow a syllabus. You can choose your own subject. You have two weeks to prepare,' he said.

Her first reaction was blind panic. She would never be able to take the place of this brilliant man, and hope to hold the attention of his audience. But it was an honour, and she knew she had to do it. Her subject would be death.

Her thesis was simple: doctors would be more comfortable dealing with death if they understood it better, and if they simply talked about what it was like to die.

She went to the university library to research the subject but found nothing that would help her. There were a few obscure and difficult psychoanalytical treatises, and a few anthropological studies about the death rituals of American Indians, Eskimos, Hindus and Buddhists, but nothing more. She had to write her own lecture, with no precedent and no references.

But a greater problem faced her. The professor's lectures were two hours long – an hour for the lecture, then a break, and then an hour presenting empirical evidence and taking questions. How on earth could she present empirical evidence to support a thesis on death? It was impossible. Yet without it, her lecture would be a failure.

Elisabeth was still devoting her spare time to dying patients in the hospital, talking with them to try to ease their fears and loneliness. A young girl called Linda impressed her deeply. She was sixteen, and at an advanced stage of leukaemia. The direct and focused way in which she discussed her condition was impressive.

She was comfortable and unembarrassed about it, and suddenly it dawned on Elisabeth that, if Linda could talk to the medical students, she would be the ideal person to tell them what it was like to be dying at the age of sixteen. Linda readily agreed to participate.

On the day of the lecture, Elisabeth was a nervous wreck. She stood on the podium and read from her notes. The students' behaviour was inexcusable: they chewed gum, chatted, leaned back with their feet up, and sniggered; but, as the lecture drew to its close, their behaviour became more respectful. During the break Elisabeth brought in her brave sixteen-year-old and wheeled her into the centre of the auditorium. The girl was pathetically frail and thin, and she could not stand, but she was nicely dressed and her hair looked pretty. Her clear brown eyes and determined jaw showed that she was perfectly in command of herself.

The students sat nervously in their seats. No one spoke, no one put his feet up, no one even chewed gum. They were obviously feeling uncomfortable. Elisabeth introduced the girl, explained her condition, and said that she had generously and bravely volunteered to answer their questions on what it was like to be terminally ill, and to know that you have only a short time to live. There was a slight rustle as people shifted awkwardly in their seats, and then there descended a quiet so profound it was disturbing. Elisabeth asked for volunteers but no hand was raised, so she selected a number of students, called them on to the stage so that they would be close to Linda, and instructed them to ask questions. All that they could think of was muttered questions about her blood count, the size of her liver, and other clinical details.

Until then, Linda had been calm and was even smiling, but at that point she lost all patience with the students, and in a passionate fit of anger the floodgates of her frustration and loneliness opened.

'That's all you people ever think of – tests, tests, tests. No one ever thinks of *me*, as a person. You people hide behind your tests and charts so that you don't have to talk to me. Me, who is dying, who is younger than any of you, but will never go to college, never go out on a date, never get married and have children. No one ever talks to *me*, to try to know my thoughts and feelings. Until Dr Ross came the only person who wanted to talk to me was the black cleaning lady in our block. She is very poor, and all her people are poor. She was never taught to read or write, but she understands me and sees what I am going through, and she tells me not to be afraid – death is an old friend for her people, and is not so very frightening. Until Dr Ross came she was the only person who talked to me.

'You people never talk to *me*. You stand by the bed and talk *about* me, as though I wasn't there, and call me "she". You won't even look me in the eye. Are you afraid of me? Am I infectious? Do you people think you will catch death off me if you come too close? Even my family can't mention the subject. If I try to speak of my dying to my mother, she changes the subject. Does she think I'm morbid or unnatural to think about death, when it's with me every minute of every day? Do you know, she even put an article in the paper, advertising my leukaemia, and asking people to send me "Happy Sweet Sixteen" birthday cards. Hundreds of silly cards came to the hospital, all from strangers.'

She held up her frail arms to her spellbound audience, her cheeks flushed with anger and her eyes bright. 'I don't *want* silly meaningless cards. All I want is someone who understands what I am going through, who shows me they want to be with me, and who can tell me what is going to happen when the time comes for me to die.'

Linda was exhausted, so Elisabeth wheeled her back to her bed, and when she returned to the auditorium something had happened to the students. They were sitting absolutely still, in stunned, almost reverential silence. Some had been moved to tears. Elisabeth knew that no further words were needed. The girl had said it all.

The impact Linda had on the students quickly resonated throughout the University Hospital, and when she died, her short life had not been in vain, because the lessons she taught on that memorable day became a new teaching in the medical world.

★

Elisabeth was asked to conduct more seminars in the same way, by interviewing dying patients in public lectures. Over the next five years, hundreds of people volunteered. The auditorium was always packed, and a larger venue had to be found. It was a completely new departure in medical teaching. Some said it was exploitative of vulnerable people, others that it was tasteless and unnecessary. Indeed, most of her colleagues were hostile to what she was doing, and her audience was mostly made up of medical and theology students, nurses, paramedics of all disciplines, sociologists, priests, rabbis and counsellors.

Elisabeth became a powerful lecturer. There was something about her that was magnetic. Perhaps it was the sincerity of her passion and conviction, mingled with a waspish wit and pithy humour; perhaps it was her ruthless honesty. Who can say, exactly? But whatever it was, with her incisive attack, and cut-glass delivery, she made a tremendous impact.

Her fame began to spread, and in 1969 Macmillan Publishing asked her to write a book. Her mind was so full of the mental, emotional and spiritual needs of dying people, that she completed the book in two months. When it was finished, she realised that it was exactly the kind of work she had hoped to find in the university library when she was researching her first lecture.

On Death and Dying is still considered to be the master text on the psychology of the subject. It is required reading at medical and nursing schools and is recommended reading for most graduate schools of psychiatry, analytical psychology, theology and sociology.

On Death and Dying is such an extraordinary book that it would be futile for me to try to describe it; such an attempt would only distort and diminish it. It is written with passion – and a depth of understanding that could never be summarised. The best advice I can give anyone is to read it for yourself, and to read between the lines as well as the words on the page. It is written in beautiful English, easy to understand, by a psychiatrist who has studied in depth the mental turmoil that goes on in the human mind as the knowledge of impending death draws closer. It is full of insights into our thought process – shock, disbelief, anger, fear, depression and loneliness. Hope is explored, and the meaning and purpose of life. Most important of all, is the final reconciliation and acceptance. The integrity of the work is indisputable, because much of it has been taken from the public lectures or interviews she gave with dying patients – all of which were recorded by the hospital authorities. Some of the accounts are so moving it is scarcely possible to read without tears. And virtually all of them hold up a mirror in which we can see ourselves, and our loved ones, in the final chapter of life.

By 1980, medical science predicted that within a couple of decades doctors would be able to conquer all disease. Then, in 1981, a brief paragraph in the American Morbidity Report referred to the death of forty-two young men in New York from an unknown disease that appeared to be related to faults in the immune system. By 1983, thousands of such deaths had been reported. The AIDS epidemic had hit a horrified and terrified America. By 1985, babies were being born with AIDS.

Elisabeth was sixty, retired from hospital work, but running clinics, retreats and workshops for the dying in her own property in Virginia. She had around twenty acres of land, with large buildings and numerous helpers. In 1986 she received a letter scribbled on a torn scrap of paper:

> Dear Dr Ross,
> I am dying of AIDS. I have a baby son who has AIDS, and I can no longer take care of him. No one will take him or touch him. How much would you charge to take care of him?

Elisabeth took the child for no charge and cared for him herself. A stream of letters from desperate parents arrived in her mailbox that year, all saying much the same thing – no one would take the children. One mother said that she had approached more than seventy agencies and been turned down by them all. She died without ever knowing her daughter was safe.

Elisabeth, ever emotional, ever passionate, boiled with rage at the paranoia in society, which impelled people to turn their backs on these children. She opened up her home and made it into a hospice for AIDS babies. The respectable and wealthy community of Virginia was in uproar over her work. They called her the Antichrist, the AIDS lady who was trying to bring this dreadful disease into their homes. A town meeting was called and thousands of people tried to get into the tiny Methodist church; they tried to force closure of the hospice, they yelled and booed and hissed, and refused to listen to reasoned speakers. The police closed the meeting at midnight, and Elisabeth was given a police guard to prevent a lynching.

The hospice remained, but she was persecuted by the locals. The Ku Klux Klan burned crosses on her lawn, and terrorised her helpers; bullets were shot through her windows and her car was repeatedly sabotaged. She was a woman of spirit, and virtually fearless, but she was getting older, running out of fire, energy and health, and a year later the hospice for AIDS babies was closed. However, not defeated, she marshalled her considerable resources to try to find other people who would adopt or foster the babies. The word spread and soon hundreds of AIDS babies were adopted by loving families who welcomed these unfortunate children. The work continues.

In 1995 Elisabeth suffered the first of a series of small strokes. Undeterred she pressed on with life, overcoming the physical difficulties with characteristic resourcefulness. She always said, 'I am ready to die,' and when, in 2004, a massive stroke occurred I feel sure she was happy to be released from the earthly life to which she had given so much.

DAME CICELY SAUNDERS
(1918–2005)

If I were asked to nominate one woman as the genius of the last century, I would say Dame Cicely Saunders. At the age of twenty she started nursing at St Thomas's Hospital in London, where she was horrified by the neglect of patients who were dying. Many times she heard doctors say, 'There is nothing more we can do,' and watched them walk away. She saw cancer patients with constant, intractable pain screaming for pain killers and being denied them for the specious reason that 'the effect of the drug will wear off as the body gets used to it and increased doses will be required, and we will be creating drug addicts'. Ten years later, in the early 1950s, I also witnessed this sort of attitude. Doctors were trained in diagnosis and active treatment. If cure was not possible, the medical approach was, 'There is nothing more to be done.'

Four years into her career, Cicely Saunders injured her back and had to leave nursing, so she trained as an almoner – what we would now call a medical social worker. During this time she saw another side to dying – family involvement, or lack of it, and the effect this had on the dying person. She saw that loneliness, or the feeling of rejection, causes a spiritual pain, which can be as bad, or worse, than the physical pain.

Cicely Saunders was a deeply religious girl and faith in a loving God was the core of her life. Religious conviction is comparatively rare, and a 'calling' even more so. Dimly at first, but inexorably, she felt that she was being called by God to work with the dying, and to lead others in the same path. Prayer and meditation led her to examine the work of the Catholic Order of the Irish Sisters of Charity at St Joseph's Hospice for the Dying in Hackney, London. She worked with them as a volunteer, whilst continuing her paid work as an almoner.

At St Joseph's she saw that, as a patient drew near to the terminal stage of an illness, far from there being 'nothing more we can do,' there was a great deal more to be done: bring comfort in relaxed surroundings, look after the physical, emotional and spiritual well-being of the patient, give medical care if possible, but if not, meticulous nursing in the last stages of life. However, she saw that the nuns were just as hampered as hospital nurses in giving pain relief for cancer patients, because the medical staff had control of drugs.

During the next six years her vision developed and she realised that the medical profession must change, not just in its attitude to pain relief, but also in the wider context of recognising the needs of a dying patient as an essential part of the physician's work. What an awesome task for a young girl in her twenties – to change the medical profession! She was 'only' a nurse and a social worker. What could she do? A calling from God is always hard and demand-ing, but it can never be resisted, whatever the cost to the individual.

None of us lives or works in isolation, and Cicely was constantly talking to like-minded people; what emerged was the advice that she should train to be a doctor. She did not have the scientific background required, but intensive study got her up to standard, and, at the age of thirty-two, she was accepted by St Thomas's Medical School in London. Six years later, in 1952, she qualified. She was nearly forty, and had travelled a long road from student nurse to qualified doctor. But a longer, more difficult road lay ahead.

Cicely Saunders was the first doctor to devote her entire pro-fessional career to the care of the dying. Many have since followed, inspired by her example and teaching. Her inspiration is with us still, and widening all the time in the hospice movement that she created, and that became international in scope.

As a newly qualified doctor she was determined that her first task must be research into the control of pain. The medical director and the nuns of St Joseph's Hospice gave her the facilities to test her theory that pain in cancer could be fully controlled by the regular, four-hourly use of analgesics. The idea was revolutionary at the time and, by the 1960s, she had proved, beyond a shadow of doubt, that drugs given in this way did not create zombie-like drug addicts, that the dose did not have to be increased to maintain effectiveness, in fact it could sometimes be decreased, and that patients became calm, comfortable and, in every way, happier because the pain had gone.

Sixty years ago, only about four per cent of cancer patients survived; today, around forty-eight per cent can be cured. Pain is nearly always part of the disease, and we take it for granted that pain can be controlled. But it took a nurse-turned-doctor to prove the fact – and point the way for others to follow.

I remember so clearly a woman I nursed at the Royal Berkshire Hospital in 1953. She had a sarcoma, an aggressive type of cancer. The seat of the cancer was probably in her ovaries, but it had spread to her bones and she was in the orthopaedic ward because one of her legs was broken. It was altogether the wrong ward for her, because most orthopaedic patients are relatively young and feel quite well, but this lady was dying. Whilst they hobbled around on their crutches she lay in bed, unable to move. One could see that she was trying to hide the pain, but every so often sweat would break out on her forehead and she would bite the sheets and grip her hands so tight the knuckles became white. Through clenched teeth she would articulate in a strangled voice:

'Can't you give me something, Nurse – another injection? I can't stand much more.'

Ward sister would say something like:

'Not just yet, dear, it's too soon after the last dose. Try to hang on till the night nurses come on duty. Then you can have an injection for the night.'

In speechless agony she would nod, her eyes frantic with fear and suffering, then say: 'I'll try, Sister, I'll try. How long must I wait?'

'Only another couple of hours, dear. I tell you what; I can give you a couple of codeine. That will ease things until you have your injection.'

The ward sister was not being stupid or callous; this was no better and no worse than the norm. It was accepted practice.

When I was a ward sister in 1963, at the Marie Curie Hospital in Hampstead, this would never occur. We gave analgesics, four hourly, day and night, and every dose was different, tailored to individual needs and the patient's level of pain. Dr Saunders' studies had been so successful, and her teaching disseminated so widely, that uncontrolled pain had become a memory.

Dr Saunders did not rest on her laurels, however. Great souls never do; there is always more to be accomplished. She felt that her calling was to create a hospice that would be a working/teaching model for the medical profession. This imaginative approach would not only ensure pain relief and meticulous nursing, but also maintain a patient's self-respect and dignity, enhancing the remaining period of that person's life, however short it might be.

A hospice for the dying was unknown and unacceptable to the decision-makers of the National Health Service in the 1960s and they would not support it, so private money had to be found. Fundraising was a massive task. Millions had to be raised, a building site found and purchased, architects instructed and planning permission obtained. Dr Saunders had many helpers and admirers, people who were also aware of the neglect of the dying, and who were inspired by her visionary outlook and inexhaustible energy. Money was raised, obstacles overcome, and in 1967, nearly thirty years after the young nurse first heard her calling, St Christopher's Hospice was opened in Sydenham, Kent.

Planning, building, fundraising – that was the easy part. Even research into the control of pain was easy, compared with the next part – the need to change medical and social attitudes to death.

The primary objective of the hospice movement was, and still is, to show to the world that death need not be a time of suffering, but a time in which to achieve fulfilment. This does not mean a grand ending to a brilliant life; it encompasses the quiet, unsung lives of millions of ordinary people who have lived simply, within a small circle, doing their best and achieving great things in small ways. My mother-in-law was such a person. She had done nothing spectacular in her life, but she was a good woman and, in human understanding, she was one of the wisest people I have known.

She died in her daughter's arms, quietly and peacefully, as she had lived. This is what I mean by the fulfilment of life.

The hospice movement strives to achieve this, working towards the mental, physical, spiritual and emotional well-being of each patient as he or she approaches the end.

Meticulous, skilled nursing is the most important part of the care of the dying, and the nurse becomes a central figure in the patient's life. Dr Saunders knew this – had she not been a nurse herself? Most nurses are by nature kind and compassionate, but they need special training, and Cicely Saunders' series of six articles on the Care of the Dying in the *Nursing Times* (1959–61) were seminal in the development of the profession and it has been found that those who specialise in palliative care usually find it so rewarding that they do not want to return to mainstream medicine.

Death is a family affair – or should be – just as a new birth involves the whole family. But dying at home often needs professional help, and this was another part of Dr Saunders' vision – to maximise home visiting. St Christopher's Hospice trained nurses to work in the community and, today, practically every hospice in the country has its own specialised nurses working in people's homes so that a dying patient does not have to go into a hospital or even a hospice. In addition, we have, in the UK, over three thousand Macmillan Nurses who have had five years of training and who work exclusively with cancer patients and those who wish to die at home. This work is mostly funded by charity donations. The National Health Service provides about twenty per cent of the total cost.

Dr Saunders' achievement was truly staggering. 'The Care of the Dying' is a fairly common phrase now, and most people do not realise that it is a relatively recent branch of medicine, with its own specialist training, research and disciplines. Today. around two hundred and fifty Hospices for the Care of the Dying exist all over the country, and this does not include specialist palliative care units in most general hospitals. It has become an international movement – over one hundred countries now have their own hospice care, and look to the teaching of Cicely Saunders as to how they should be run.

Dame Cicely Saunders died of cancer in 2005 at the age of eighty-seven, in St Christopher's Hospice.

It is interesting to compare the lives of Cicely Saunders and Elisabeth Kübler-Ross. They were about the same age – Cicely the elder by eight years – and they died within a year of each other. They both had war experience, when death was all around. With no known contact between each other, they both saw the needs and suffering of dying patients in English and American hospitals in the post-war era. They both identified the cause as the widespread denial of death by the medical professions and society at large. The work undertaken by both of them was groundbreaking.

It is one of those fascinating instances where two people with brilliant, insightful minds identify the same problem at the same time and work towards different but complementary solutions. Cicely started the hospice movement in 1967 when St Christopher's Hospice was opened. Elisabeth published *On Death and Dying* in 1969. The contribution they made to medicine and to society was immeasurable.

DR CONRAD HYEM

In 1957 I worked in Poplar, East London, with an order of nursing nuns and was required to visit a Mr Hyem, who lived in one of the tenements known as Canada Buildings. They were densely populated and regarded as slums.

I climbed the stone stairs, went along the balcony to his flat, and was taken aback by a small brass plate on the door stating: 'Dr Conrad Hyem, Doctor of Philosophy and Psychology'. The day book had called him 'Mr Hyem', so I assumed the 'Doctor' was the wit of some Cockney joker, to amuse himself and his mates. I raised my hand towards the knocker, but at that second the beautiful soaring tones of a violin sounded from within. I stood outside the door, holding my breath, staring unbelievingly at the door. A woman called out:

'Go on. It's only the Doc. 'E's lovely, 'e is. 'E gives us all a toon. Jus' knock. 'E'll soon stop.'

I shook my head and put my fingers to my lips, breathing 'ssshhh', and leaned closer to the door. The music was beautiful, full-bodied and rich, filled with that plaintive yearning which of all instruments the violin can achieve to perfection.

'Makes yer wanna cry, 'e do, sometimes,' the woman sniffed appreciatively. 'But jest give 'im a knock, 'e won't mind, 'e'll soon stop, 'e will.'

Again I shook my head. How could I disturb such a musician, his inner thoughts and emotions? He might never recapture that moment. The final cadence approached, and the last note died away, and I rapped on the knocker.

A tall, silver-haired gentleman opened the door. He was well-built and solid, but not fat. He smiled at me, and the gold fillings in his teeth gleamed in the sunlight. He was wearing well-cut trousers, a plain, high-necked jumper and thick horn-rimmed glasses, and when he smiled, his eyes crinkled attractively at the corners. His hands were beautiful; white and smooth, with polished nails – certainly not the hands of a dock labourer. Nor was he the Cockney humorist I had imagined. I knew at once that he really must be a doctor – of some sort.

'You must be the nurse I was told to expect.'

He spoke beautiful English with a soft guttural accent, which I took to be German.

'A small matter concerning my diabetes?'

He opened the door wider and with a slight bow said, 'Be pleased to enter.'

If I had been surprised to find a musician and scholarly gentleman in the seedy purlieus of the Canada Buildings, it was as nothing compared with my astonishment on entering his rooms. It might have been the study of an Oxford don. Every wall was lined with books from floor to ceiling, thousands of them, mostly leather-bound, some of them with gold tooling down the spine. In front of the window stood a kneehole desk, probably antique, with a beautiful surface of red leather, tooled in gold. A red, leather writing chair stood before the desk and the room held no other furniture save a rosewood music stand. All the shelves were made of warm mahogany, and the lovely smell of wood and leather filled the room. Dr Hyem noticed my reaction, and his eyes crinkled at the corners.

'You like my sanctuary, then? This is my retreat. A man can live very comfortably and quietly in such surroundings.'

A ship's hooter blasted out a long, low note, and a shrill siren sent a warning across the water. Men shouted as the lock gates opened, and a huge, ocean-going cargo boat made its way from the Thames to its quay in the East India Docks. I spoke for the first time.

'It's lovely, here in this flat. Perfect, in fact. But I wouldn't call it quiet!'

'Perhaps not, but tranquillity has more meaning if the hum of life is all around. From my bedroom window I look out over the docks and see the trading vessels of all the world come and go. I see the men, thousands of them, labouring daily, and I contemplate the insatiable appetite of trade for manpower. From my desk I look out over the courtyard of Hudson Buildings, and see the smaller, but no less important, world of the women, and I observe and meditate upon the endless tasks of child-rearing and homemaking. All life surrounds me. Here I can work. "We need more understanding of human nature, because the only real danger that exists is man himself." Do you know who said that, Nurse?'

I shook my head.

'Carl Jung, my friend and mentor.'

'I don't think I've heard of Carl Jung. Who is he?'

'Carl Jung called himself a psychologist, but I regard him as a philosopher. I was his humble student and disciple in Zürich, thirty years ago.'

I murmured, 'I don't think I know anything about him.' Nor, in truth, was I very much interested. Thirty years ago seems an awful long time past when you are twenty-two, and, like most young people I was convinced that nothing of much interest or importance had occurred before the year in which I was born!

But I had a morning's work to do and sharply reminded myself of this. The visit to Dr Hyem was only one of a long list, and I had to get on. I questioned him about his diet and fluid intake, about his lifestyle and his symptoms. Checking his medical notes I observed that he had suffered weight loss, polyurea and glycosuria, and had had the good sense to go to his doctor. We, the nurses, had been asked to visit twice daily for a fortnight to test his urine for sugar and ketones, and to balance the insulin level against the sugar, carbohydrate and fat in his daily diet.

I asked if he had kept an early morning urine sample. Yes, he had, and he led me through a tiny kitchen to an even smaller lavatory.

'This is the best part of my flat,' he said, 'a lavatory. To have the luxury and privacy of one's own lavatory is worth all the gold in Arabia. It was here when I came. It must have been installed in an earlier decade, and water also in the kitchen. As soon as I saw the lavatory, I took the flat.'

I tested the urine specimen.

'There is certainly sugar present,' I said. 'We shall have to check your diet carefully.'

We sat side by side at the leather-topped desk in order to discuss the diet sheet. I ran my fingers over the surface of the desk and felt the pleasing corrugation of the gold tooling along each edge. Placed centrally on the desk was a small picture in a silver frame of a pretty young woman and four young children. We discussed calorie intake and the need to weigh all foods and to have a daily insulin injection, whilst the books and accumulated wisdom of centuries observed us from the bookshelves. It was elegant and peaceful in the little flat, and I felt reluctant to leave, but I had other work to do and said goodbye.

I stepped out into the noisy sunshine of Canada Buildings, and a football travelling at high speed hit my legs, nearly knocking me over. Dr Hyem grabbed my arm to steady me. A woman screamed at a wayward child, who screamed back, so she boxed his ears until he howled.

Dr Hyem suppressed his laughter so as not to offend his neighbours, whom he greeted courteously and charmingly, addressing them all by name. Everyone seemed to know him, and a woman shouted out,

'Whassa trouble, Doc? Piles, boils or blisters?'

He responded gravely, 'It appears that I have developed diabetes, madam, which, with the assistance of this good nurse, I am sure can be controlled.'

And he made a slight bow to the woman, who giggled loudly. His formality and textbook English seemed so out of place in his surroundings that I giggled also, and when I turned to shake hands on leaving I saw that his eyes were full of laughter. I was going to enjoy visiting Dr Hyem twice a day for the next fortnight.

Thereafter, each evening I carefully placed Dr Hyem last on my list of visits so that I did not have to dash off to see someone else, but could linger if I wanted to. I was hoping to hear more of his violin.

It was a beautiful summer evening as I cycled around, with no wind, and just a few clouds moving lazily in the sky. The stairwell seemed quite light and cheery as I climbed up to level 4, and I came out on to the balcony in the full blaze of the evening sun. At almost every door a woman was sitting, some nursing a baby, some chivvying toddlers, some pruning their tomatoes, scrubbing potatoes or cutting up beans; most of the others quietly and contentedly knitting. I made my way along the balcony, and was much surprised to see Dr Hyem sitting outside on his only spare chair, deep in conversation with a woman. He was listening intently, looking down at the floor, nodding his head as though he understood completely. Every so often he would glance up and look into her face, then make some comment, after which she would continue talking. I saw that she was twisting her apron in her strong hands. The sunlight fell on them both, as it did on everyone, but whilst the relaxing warmth seemed to liberate others' good humour and sociability, these two seemed to be locked in a private world of trouble. I felt reluctant to intrude.

The same woman who had spoken to me in the morning noticed my hesitation.

'Oh, go on, ducky, jest chip in. 'E won't mind. 'E's lovely, I tells ya. An' she'll 'ave to wait, poor soul, she wiv 'er troubles. You got work to do, so jest chip in.'

I approached and coughed. Dr Hyem looked up.

'Good evening, Nurse. I was expecting you. Mrs Robins, you will have to excuse me. We will continue our conversation later.'

He stood up and opened the door to his flat for me. A blind was pulled down over the window and it seemed quite dark inside after the bright sunlight of the court.

'I have to keep the blind down,' he said. 'I cannot risk the sun damaging my books.'

I tested the sample of urine in the kitchen and it was high in sugar again. I told him that a trace of ketones had been found in the specimen that I had analysed in our clinical room, and that as soon as he could give me his exact weight we would start insulin. He promised to go to the surgery the next day.

His violin and bow were resting in a corner away from the sun, and music was open on the stand. I had to ask.

'I have loved music since I was a tiny child. Would you play for me?'

He looked at me with some surprise, but simply said, 'Yes, of course. It would be a pleasure.'

He lifted a corner of the blind to give more light, then took up the violin and bow and turned the pages of the music.

'This is a pavane by César Franck. I think you will like it.'

Then he started to play. He was a beautiful violinist – I could tell that by the quality of the tone and phrasing – and I felt tears coursing down my cheeks. I had to control myself, but too late; he turned and saw me crying.

'You really love music, then?'

I could scarcely speak, and managed a cracked, 'Yes'.

'It was music that saved my life. Without it, I think I would have gone mad, or committed suicide.'

I didn't like to ask him how music had saved his life – it seemed too personal and intrusive – but I wanted to. So I said instead,

'You have played all your life, then?'

'Yes, since early childhood. We all played, my parents and brothers and sisters. It was expected of us for that was the way of life for a good Jewish family in Vienna at the turn of the century. My sister Freya was the most talented. She was the most beautiful violinist I have ever heard.'

'I suppose she is a professional now?'

'No.' He stopped, and turning his back on me, opened the violin case, slackened his bow and put the instrument away. He turned and closed the music book, before saying: 'No, Freya is dead. She will not play again.'

'I'm sorry to hear it. Was it an illness?'

He hesitated, then picked up the music stand and placed it in the corner.

'I suppose it must have been. The body can stand so much and no more. But I'm not really sure. Come now, shall we go outside? On a beautiful evening like this I am going to sit by my door and watch the world go by.'

'And I must return to the convent.'

We shook hands on parting, then I said, quickly and shyly, 'You will play for me again, won't you?'

'It will be more than a pleasure, it will be a privilege.'

On the following morning as we were going through the day list I asked Sister Julienne, the head of the order of nuns with whom I was working, if she knew anything about Dr Hyem. She said,

'I only know that he is an Austrian Jew who came to this country shortly after the war. The Jews from all over Europe were looking for somewhere to settle.'

I remembered the photograph of a young woman and four little children, and his saying, 'I'm not really sure how they died.'

'Do you think he or his family were in concentration camps?' I asked Sister Julienne, who knew everything, I always felt.

'I do not know, but it is very likely. You must remember that over six million Jews died. I doubt if there are any European Jews alive today who have not lost relatives. We must all pray for healing.'

Later I learned that Dr Hyem had tragically lost his wife and four children to starvation in an ill-fated attempt to return to Vienna to save his sister Freya.

It became a real joy to me, visiting Dr Hyem. Controlling his diabetes was not difficult, and we always found time to talk about other things that interested us both. One day I had the sauce to ask him, 'Why do you live in a place like this. You are a cultivated man. Surely you could find somewhere better?'

His eyes wrinkled at the corners in the way that was so attractive.

'Now that, Nurse, is where you are wrong. I do not think I could find anywhere better in the world to live. I have two rooms, which are waterproof, and I have a roof over my head. I have my very own private lavatory. What more can a man ask? And for all this, I assure you, the rent is very low.'

'But the environment, the people ... They are just not your type.'

'Again, my dear young lady, you are wrong. From my eyrie I look over the docks, a fascination I had not thought possible until I proved it for myself. The light falls upon the water at different times of day and shows me a thousand different beauties, which are never repeated, but always changing. The cargo boats come and go. The men toil and the women work. As for the people, I like them. Canada Buildings can be described as a microcosm of all life, and humanity is my study.'

Once, when I was showing him how to inject his own insulin, and watching his ham-fisted attempts to insert the needle, I said, 'You are obviously not a real doctor, then?'

'If by that you mean a doctor of medicine, no, I am not. I am a doctor of analytical psychology.'

'A psychiatrist?'

'No. A psychiatrist in this country must first be a medical practitioner, which I am not. Thirty years ago I studied in Zürich with Dr Carl Jung, the greatest thinker and interpreter of the human mind of the century, in my opinion.'

'So that was your job?'

His eyes crinkled again and he gave me a funny look.

'Yes, that was my "job", as you so accurately describe.'

'Do you do it now?' (What a sauce the young have!)

'No. And I know your next question will be "why?" So I will tell you. Frankly, in this country, under your new National Health Service, I do not think I could earn a living. I am not qualified to practice in this country. So I earn my living as a translator.'

'What do you translate?'

'Mostly psychoanalytical treatises and papers for journals in French, German, Italian and Dutch.'

'You are very clever to speak and write so many languages.'

'In my father's house we all had to learn the principal European languages. My mother was Swiss and had been brought up to speak three languages fluently, and she taught her children likewise.'

I walked around the room and ran my fingers over some of the leather bindings, which were beautiful to the touch. The titles were in several different languages, including English, but there was a collection that looked like nothing on earth to me.

'What are these?' I asked.

Again he gave me that funny look, his eyes smiling.

'That is my Greek collection. It is necessary for an educated man or woman to be conversant in Latin and Greek. These two are the fundamental languages of civilisation.

I must have looked thoughtful, because he said: 'What are you thinking?'

'I love your books, I love your music; I love your elegant rooms . . . everything.'

The Wigmore Hall was crowded. I felt a tap on the shoulder and turned round. Dr Conrad Hyem was smiling at me.

'What an unexpected pleasure,' he exclaimed.

It was truly delightful to see him. We had not met for three months because he was controlling his diabetes satisfactorily by injecting himself, and he did not need our visits. I regretted the loss of his wonderful company, and would have liked to continue seeing him, but that was just not possible. As a nurse, I could not visit the flat of a single gentleman who had formerly been a patient, without bringing disrepute not only to myself but also, which was far more important, to the order of nuns for whom I worked. But meeting at the Wigmore Hall, quite by chance, was a different matter.

We went to the bar and he offered me a drink.

'Well, only water, at the moment. I never drink alcohol before or during a performance because I like to keep my wits about me to listen to the music. But I'll have a drink later, if the offer is still there.'

'It will be a pleasure, and I'll hold you to that. But for now we will have water. I myself can never understand people who come to hear beautiful music then dull their minds with alcohol.'

After the concert, Dr Hyem said:

'Do not forget you are going to have a drink with me, and would you like a little supper also?'

'That would be perfectly lovely. Thank you!'

Dr Hyem and I had a delightful supper in a small restaurant in Upper Regent Street. He, being diabetic, had to be careful about what he ate, but I had no such constraints, and ate more than he did. He watched me, I thought, with amusement, because his eyes were crinkling at the corners. Then he said,

'You have never been hungry?'

'Me? Don't you believe it. I'm *always* hungry. I eat a huge breakfast most days, cakes or biscuits if I can get them at eleven, a huge lunch with two puddings if possible, tea with more cakes or biscuits, supper at seven – and I'm still hungry. That is why I can eat a second supper now, at eleven o'clock.'

The moment I had spoken I was aware of my callous insensitivity to a man who had lost his entire family from starvation.

'I'm terribly sorry,' I faltered. 'That was a dreadful thing to say. Please forgive me.'

He smiled. 'There is nothing to forgive. It is only natural that the young should follow their instincts and I'm sure I was always hungry when I was your age. Would you like another pudding?'

My cheeks were burning with embarrassment, and I suspected he might be mocking me.

'No. No, really. But I must go, it's getting late and I will be on duty at eight o'clock.'

'Then we will leave together.'

He paid the bill and held my coat for me to slip my arms into.

Over the next six months or so we attended many concerts and recitals together. It was delightful. He introduced me to the rarefied world of chamber music. He obviously had an extensive and detailed knowledge of the subject, and it enhanced my enjoyment if he analysed a quartet before the performance. But he sometimes looked so sad, and once, after a Schubert quintet, he just sat for ages with his head in his hands. The lights had gone up and everyone was moving about. He muttered to me:

'You go to the bar, Jenny. I will join you in a minute.'

But he didn't come, and when I returned he was still sitting in exactly the same position, and I knew that he was thinking of his wife and children. My heart ached for him, but there was nothing that I could do or say, so I sat down and took his hand, and he gripped it fiercely. Such depth of suffering and loss cannot be shared; it must be endured alone.

That night Dr Hyem and I travelled back together on the tube and bus. We did not talk much. He was locked in his thoughts and memories, and I did not know what to say. What *can* you say to someone who has suffered and lost everything? I fell asleep, and was wakened by a voice.

'Time to wake up. We have reached the Blackwall Tunnel.'

His eyes were smiling as I tried to adjust myself to the waking world and he took my arm to steady me. We stood on the pavement as the bus rumbled off. I looked across the road, and the church clock said a quarter to one.

Just at that moment the clouds parted behind the spire and the moon appeared in all her silver glory. My hair blew across my face.

'Isn't that just beautiful,' I said. 'Have you ever seen anything more beautiful?'

I stood gazing at the moon, and he was looking at me. Then I suddenly remembered that I would be on duty at eight o'clock.

'I must go. I've got a long day tomorrow.'

I held out my hand to shake his and say goodnight. He took my hand, and then pulled me towards him.

'Come back with me ... Don't go ... Come to my flat.'

I stiffened with surprise.

'Just for a little while – I need you so.'

I tried to pull back.

'What do you mean?'

'You know quite well what I mean.'

He pulled me closer and tried to kiss me, but I didn't want it, and turned my head away.

78

'Don't turn away! Why did you take my hand in the concert then, if you were going to turn away from me now?'

I should have said, 'From pity, nothing more, just pity'. But I didn't. Feebly I said, 'I don't know.'

'Well, I do, so come with me now. Just come. I can't go on like this. It's been fifteen years since I've known a woman. I shall go mad.'

He pulled me tight to his body and I felt him hard against me.

I tried to pull away.

'I've got to get back to the convent. I will be working in a few hours.'

'You prissy little convent girl,' he snarled. 'You have no understanding of the needs of men.'

'That's not fair!' I shouldn't have said it, but I added, 'I just don't fancy you, that's all.'

He jumped back as though I had shot him, and a strange, strangled cry came from his throat. I freed myself and, sensing my power, I had the cruelty, not to mention the bad taste, to add, 'Anyway, you are too old for me.'

I walked away without turning. It was twelve years before I saw Dr Hyem again.

Judith, aged seventeen, died of a brain tumour. Her mother writes:

'That night, as I prepared for bed, Judith said – "Mom, why don't you put the light on? It's getting so dark."

'"I can manage, dear," I replied. I didn't tell her that the light *was* on. As usual, I pushed my bed alongside hers and lay on the top in my dressing gown. We held hands, and with a soft pressure on mine she said, "You've been a lovely Mum." Shortly after she drifted into a last sleep and a blessed unconsciousness.

'During the night Cheyne Stokes breathing took over and, as day broke, I crept into my husband's room and switched off his alarm clock. He stirred and looked up enquiringly. "You won't be going to work," I said. "Judith will die today."

'Later in the morning, the rhythm of her breathing changed. Quickly, I knelt beside the bed and slipped my hand into hers. Her fingers curled automatically around mine, like those of a sleeping babe, and she suddenly became so very young and vulnerable, like a creature emerging from a chrysalis into a new life. It was a beauty so fleeting I held my breath in wonder – and in the room there was no breathing at all. The dying need only a hand to hold and a quiet in which to make their departure.'

— from *Nurse on Call* by Edith Cotterill (Ebury Press, 2009)

THE MARIE CURIE HOSPITAL

In the early 1960s, I was ward sister at the Marie Curie Hospital in Hampstead, London. It was part of the Royal Free Hospital, and was reserved for specialised radium treatment. It had originally been built as a cottage hospital around 1900, and was small, consisting of only thirty beds. The hospital was divided into two halves, a twelve-bed ward and three small side wards for the men, and the same for the women. A similar amount of space was occupied by the radiotherapy machines, which were huge, and required a lot of room. We dealt only with radiotherapy – all operations were carried out at the Royal Free. We also had our own dispensary. A matron was in overall charge of the hospital, and I was ward sister in charge of therapeutic cases. I had two staff nurses, five or six student nurses, two ward orderlies, and a ward maid.

Cancer is a word that evokes fear in the minds of most people, and fears linger in the twenty-first century, although medical research has enabled cures for many forms of the disease. In the 1960s, the fear was even more justified. Chemotherapy was still at the research stage; radiotherapy was crude, but sometimes effective; drugs were highly toxic, and frequently created more distress and suffering than the cancer. The most reliable treatment was the surgeon's knife, but whilst the central growth could frequently be cut away, the secondary tumours often could not be removed, nor could the encroachment into the blood, lymph and skeletal systems be prevented.

Staff nurse and I were preparing Mrs Cox for her third treatment. Heaven knows, it was hopeless, but if the radium could reduce some of the growth, and dry up a little of the exudate from an ulcerated breast that was virtually sloughing away as the malignancy digested her chest wall, it would be worth it for her.

Until the early part of the last century, when mastectomy became a common operation, thousands of women fell victim to the ghastly 'stinking death', as this type of cancer was sometimes called. Women afflicted with breast cancer would hide it beneath blouses and shawls, saying nothing. Perhaps a daughter would be let into the secret, but 'women's matters' would be kept strictly away from the men. Very often a husband did not know of his wife's condition, until the smell of the sticky black exudate became so overwhelming that eventually he noticed, or, reluctantly, his wife confessed. The word 'confessed' is used deliberately in this instance, because often women were ashamed of their bodies and even more ashamed if something went wrong. I have seen many a woman with a uterine prolapse hanging down halfway to her knees, yet uttering no complaint. A prolapse was common with multiple childbirths, and one woman had kept hers up with an apple for years, she told us, before she eventually had a pelvic floor repair.

Mrs Cox was typical of her generation: patient, uncomplaining, enduring passively all that was heaped upon her. She was in a side ward, with the windows kept open at all times, and a fan continually blowing the air in the room away from the corridor, and hopefully out of the window. But still we could not prevent the dreadful smell from penetrating the corridor. Mrs Cox barely spoke; her dull eyes flickered from the massive erupting growth, as large as a dinner plate, to the other breast, where a few smaller sores had started to discharge and bleed. Like many women of her age, she had withdrawn from her friends and family to await death, but a daughter had insisted on calling a doctor, an older GP who had seen this sort of thing before, and was unsurprised. An oncologist was consulted, who said that surgery was impossible, and advised radium treatment, which might dry up some of the exudate, and hopefully reduce some of the growth.

If we, at the Marie Curie, could make the last weeks of her life more comfortable, the treatment would be worthwhile. We were also able to administer drugs to relieve the pain. The Brompton Cocktail was frequently given, which contained morphine, cocaine, belladonna and gin. Every four hours Mrs Cox drank it gratefully. She was grateful for everything – a glass of water, a clean sheet, a face wash, or a hair brush drawn through her stringy grey hair. She did not express her thanks in words, but her eyes showed it. I often performed these small tasks myself, because I could see how close to death she was, and I knew that the young nurses, who were of another generation, and had seen nothing like Mrs Cox's ulcerating cancer before, were afraid to go near her. We could not cover the excoriated breast with any surgical dressing, because dressings have to be changed when they become soaked in body fluids. This occurred frequently and quickly, and when we pulled the dressing off, lumps of decomposing flesh and cancerous material came away with it, causing pain. It is not surprising the nurses are afraid of her, I thought, and I wondered how the radiographers, two healthy young men, viewed this tragic woman.

'Your treatment is helping, isn't it, Mrs Cox?' I said as I handed her the Brompton Cocktail. I did not say 'making you better', as we were taught to say, perpetuating the lie that modern medicine makes everything better.

She nodded. 'And you will have another on Friday,' I continued, 'that makes four. When you have had six treatments I'm sure you will feel a lot easier.'

Again she nodded wearily.

'Your daughter said she would come and see you tomorrow.'

Her lips moved, but any words were unrecognisable. I did not want to say any more about the daughter, who might or might not come, and I suspected that her sons never would. Mrs Cox would probably be left to die alone.

But in this I, as ward sister, had control. I had no control over the inexorable course of the disease, nor over the treatment, nor had I any influence over the sons and daughters whom she had borne and brought up, and who were now rejecting her, but I was absolutely determined that she would not die alone. In those days it was regarded as an essential nursing duty to be with a person throughout the time of dying, especially at the actual moment of death. It was regarded as a disgrace to the ward sister, or staff nurse in charge, if a patient died alone.

We prepared Mrs Cox for her third treatment with radium. Two porters came and lifted her on to the trolley and I went with her to the radiotherapy unit, holding the sheet above her breast so that the men would not have to look at it.

Half an hour later I accompanied her back to the ward. The radiographer told me that her blood pressure had dropped during treatment. Her skin was even more sallow than it had been before and her pulse was very weak, her blood pressure barely perceptible. Although her eyes flickered when I spoke to her, and she gave a little moan, she did not appear to be conscious. The porters wheeled her back to the ward and lifted her on to the bed.

We never knew whether the radium treatment had made her more comfortable, because that afternoon, peacefully, quietly, Mrs Cox accepted death with the same uncomplaining resignation that she had accepted life.

'Dinners is hup, Sister.'

Gladys, the indispensable ward maid, stood in the doorway, arms folded, legs apart, her face expressionless. She knew more about the hospital and how it functioned than anyone, but she never intruded, never grumbled, and above all, never gossiped. One could rely on her discretion, something that, in a cancer hospital, where most of our patients would die, was essential. Thoughtless remarks, a hint or a nudge here or there, could spark off an atmosphere of uncertainty that could escalate, causing patients and their families distress.

The morning had been hectic with, as usual, a shortage of staff, too many duties, and too little time in which to get them done: dressings to change; a drip to install; blood to take; patients to prepare, take to, and return from therapy; the drugs to take round and DDAs to check; a couple of admissions; a patient discharged, with her drugs and treatments to organise and explain to the daughter who was collecting her; the linen arriving from the laundry; someone needing catheterisation; another a bath which he could not manage himself. Morning coffee had been disrupted by three or four radium patients vomiting; the telephone ringing, with a message from dispensary – a drug was available, could a nurse come and collect it? But why could the dispenser not send it up to the ward? They were too busy, the woman said. Does no one ever imagine that the ward is too busy? As we had needed the drug badly for two days, I sent a nurse to get it. And in the rush of work the oncologist – the Chief, we called him – arrived to see a new patient.

He found me in a side ward, washing the mattress of a patient who had died during the night.

'This is a surprise, Sister. Haven't you got a nurse or an orderly to do that sort of thing?'

'All the nurses are busy, and one orderly is off sick. Anyway, a sister should never be too grand to do the menial tasks. I want this room for Mr Waters because I don't want him to die in the main ward if it can possibly be avoided – it's unsettling for the other patients. None of them see themselves getting to that state.' I cleaned the sides of the mattress. 'There, it's done now, and I'm with you.'

Together we went to the bedside of the new patient. Hospital protocol required that I should stay with the consultant whilst he remained in the ward, but Hannah appeared in the doorway with her 'dinners is hup, Sister', and a look of command on her heavy features.

'Then I had better not delay you, Sister,' the Chief said. 'We will be doing the full ward round tomorrow morning.'

I walked swiftly to the kitchen, to the ward orderly in pink, the half circle of nurses in blue, each holding a tray, the electric food trolley plugged into the wall, waiting my attention. It had always seemed extraordinary to me that the serving of patients' dinners occupied such a large part of a sister's duties (the whole process took the best part of an hour), and that all nursing staff looked to her for the lead. It was a relic of the old days, when drugs and surgery were in their infancy, and when so many people who came into hospital were chronically malnourished, so that the dietary needs of each patient were important.

I tucked the tea towel into my belt to protect my uniform from gravy splashes, and removed the aluminium lids from each container. I served a full dinner for several patients, which the nurses took, returning a few minutes later with empty trays.

'Take this to Mrs J. and see that she can manage. Stay with her, if necessary.'

'Yes, Sister.'

'Mr P. doesn't like carrots, so give him this one.'

'Yes, Sister.'

'Special diabetic diets for Mrs D. and Mrs H. Don't get them mixed up, Nurse.'

'No, Sister.'

'There's enough left over for the walking patients in the day room. Take it through to them please, Nurse, and see if anyone wants seconds.'

'Yes, Sister.'

'And Nurse . . .'

She turned, her voice bright and buoyant. 'Sister . . .?'

'Your cap is incorrectly folded. Attend to it before the afternoon, please.'

Her smile vanished, and her mouth tightened.

'Yes, Sister,' she muttered.

I knew just how she felt, having spent all my early nursing years kicking against the rules and regulations, but discipline had to be maintained . . .

The routine continued like clockwork, I, hopefully, remembering everyone's needs and fancies. But one thing I never forgot whilst serving lunches was the mayhem I had caused one dinner time when I was a student nurse.

I was eighteen, nervous and clumsy, awkwardly trying to do my best, and failing at every attempt – every ward sister's nightmare. I felt like a fish out of water in the rigid female hierarchy.

The sister of the ward on which I worked required a cannula that she did not have, and asked me to go to another ward to see if one might be borrowed. Filled with the importance of my commission I walked quickly (we were *never* allowed to run!) to

Sister Collins' ward. It was lunchtime, and no one was in sight. Assuming that the sister would be serving lunches I rushed eagerly into the kitchen. Sister and Staff were not there, but the food trolley was. The porters had left it crosswise to the kitchen door, which I was not expecting. I rushed in, and my whole body collided with it, causing the trolley to topple over and hit the floor. Dinners – meat and gravy, fish in white sauce, potatoes, cabbage, carrots, rice pudding, prunes, egg custard, stewed apple, jelly – *everything* shot across the kitchen floor and slithered under the sink. Horrified and rooted to the spot, I gazed at the scene. The trolley wheels turned slowly in the air; I turned and ran – yes, ran! – from the ward. Still no one was about, no one had seen me enter the ward or leave, so no one could possibly associate me with the disaster. Once round the corner, I slowed to a fast walk and went to another ward to request the loan of the cannula required by my ward sister. An hour later, in the nurses' dining room, everyone was talking about the extraordinary upturning of a hospital food trolley full of dinners. I could never serve dinners without thinking of this, and if nurses saw me smiling, or heard me giggling quietly to myself, they must have wondered why . . .

After lunch I went to the male ward to supervise the moving of Mr Waters to the side ward. Not before time, I thought; that dreadful cough had been unsettling for the other men, but now his inability to cough was worse. Phlegm bubbled and rattled in his chest. Struggling with asphyxia, Mr Waters would die as hard as a man can die, unless drugs were given. I pulled the curtains around his bed and used suction to try to remove the excessive fluid bubbling up from his lungs.

'I'm sorry about this beastly sucker, but it will make you feel better,' I said, trying to avoid his panic-stricken eyes. His lungs were struggling under some terrible oppression and breathing was an intolerable strain. Any respiratory death is distressing to watch, but a natural anodyne – a sudden dimming of consciousness due to oxygen starvation of the higher centres of the brain – comes at the peak of suffering, and mental and physical deterioration descends as swiftly as a hawk dropping on its prey.

'Mr Waters, we think you would be better off in the small room. It has two windows, and they can both be open all the time. It will make your breathing easier,' I said softly. He nodded, and picked at the sheet. I was alone with him, but I could sense a figure hovering beside me. Could he see or feel this ghostly presence? None of us will know until we get there.

I had called the porters, and they arrived with a trolley.

'I think it will be better if we move the whole bed, rather than lifting him on to a trolley, and then on to another bed,' I said. It would be more difficult for them, because the corners were awkward, but they did not question my instructions.

Not an hour too soon, we moved him. Two days earlier he had been sitting upright in bed, leaning forward a little, his cheeks flushed, his lips tinged blue as his chest heaved tumultuously at four times the normal respiration rate. His eyes had been clear and his mind alert, as he noted people and things going on in the ward. Now the struggle to live had departed, and weariness had overtaken him.

I called a junior student nurse, and showed her how to fix up the oxygen and the sucker, and how to use them, and explained the details, which were so much better than ten years previously when I had been a student nurse. I told the girl (she was barely more than a child, with fresh features and the downy skin of youth) to stay with the dying man whilst I went to fetch the injections. What huge responsibility we place upon a nurse's shoulders, I reflected, as I went to the dangerous drugs cupboard. So often they come straight from school, the classroom, the hockey field or the gym, and we expect them to remain with the dying, a task that the majority of mature people would run away from in fear and revulsion. Does this give nurses a heightened sensibility of living, to be so closely acquainted with death? Certainly, nurses always seem to be full of life and vitality, with an inexhaustible capacity for laughter. I had found in nurses none of the lethargy and self-absorption that one often noticed in young girls, contrary to what one might expect, given the nature of our work.

Radiotherapy could not help the malign growth in Mr Waters' lungs. It may have halted the progress of the cancer by a hair's breadth, but it made no real impression on the inexorable course of the disease. Mr Waters had smoked himself to death, and there was nothing that medicine could do to reverse the destruction. For two days he flickered in and out of consciousness, his lungs bubbling and gurgling as he slowly drowned. But his suffering was not as great as appearances suggested, because he received devoted nursing care – and the Brompton Cocktail every four hours. His mind was not conscious of his condition, or of his surroundings, and he showed no signs of pain. We did not try to bring him back from wherever he was, by forcing him to drink this or to take that, nor any of the multifarious futilities of energetic medicine. His perceptions were so dimmed by weakness and weariness that his life was ending slowly, in a dream state, rather than in true awareness.

Each morning when I came on duty I expected to find the side ward empty, but for two mornings he was still there. How extraordinary is life, that one can hang on in that condition, neither alive nor dead? But on the third morning the room was empty, and the night nurse reported that the flickerings of life had given way to the smothering curtain of death.

FAMILY INVOLVEMENT

Mr Elias Roberts had an enormous family, which seemed to expand with each passing day. They were Jamaican and had immigrated to England in the early 1950s, seeking a better life, better education, and better prospects for their children. They had stepped off the boats in their Sunday best, raw and hopeful, into an exhausted and war-torn England. A better time was a long way off. Jobs were plentiful because rebuilding Britain was a priority, but finding somewhere to live was near impossible. Mr Roberts had eventually found a single room at the top of a derelict house for himself, his wife and their two youngest daughters, but the older boys and girls had had to make their own way.

Mr Roberts was admitted to the Marie Curie Hospital suffering from prostate cancer, which had been treated by prostatectomy in the Royal Free Hospital. He had come to us for radium treatment but the widespread metastasis in the bones was clear evidence that the treatment had come too late.

When I was a young girl, I was told that men who had difficulty urinating carried a catheter coiled in their hatbands. When they needed to pass water, they catheterised themselves. At first, they would inevitably develop an infection, but the body's immune system is built to fight that, and once these men had got over the initial bouts of infection, the body became immune to the germs lurking in the hatband.

Testing for cancer was not routine. Some men went to a doctor, but the treatment was fairly rudimentary – diuretics, potassium citrate, no alcohol, barley water – none of which was effective. Later, in the 1940s, the female hormones oestrogen and pro-gesterone were prescribed in the hope of reducing the enlargement, but it is doubtful if these treatments did much good. Consequently, a great many men developed such massively distended bladders, filled with retained urine, impossible to pass normally or by catheter, that abdominal entry was necessary and a supra-pubic catheter had to be inserted to drain the fluid. I was in theatre once as the 'runner' – the lowliest member of the team – when a man was wheeled in with a massive lump in his lower abdomen; it was his bladder. He had not been able to pass urine for weeks. It was impossible, even under anaesthetic, to get a catheter past the enlarged prostate, so a supra-pubic insertion was made and more than a gallon of urine was drained off. The man died from surgical shock.

That was an extreme case, and the worst I have seen, but a great many men had to endure weeks in bed with indwelling catheters, twenty-four-hour drainage, daily bladder irrigation, uraemia, antiseptics and antibiotics before a prostatectomy could be attempted. Sometimes I felt that the catheter in the hatband would have been the better option.

This was all embarrassing and unpleasant for a sensitive man because there were very few male nurses in the profession; so young girls almost always performed such tasks. Incidentally, nursing procedures were comparatively basic. The following is taken from Wilson Harlow's *Modern Surgery for Nurses* (1956):

> There are various means of retaining an indwelling catheter in the male urethra. A common method is to attach four pipe cleaners, or two pieces of tape, to the catheter. The ends, which should be 4–6 inches long, are then brought up and fixed to the penis by a piece of Elastoplast or bandage. A similar retainer can be constructed out of a piece of sheet rubber fitted with holes and collar studs to fasten it to the penis and catheter.

I do not know what humiliations Mr Roberts had been subjected to before or after the prostatectomy, but when he came into the Marie Curie, the cancer was widespread, and there was no hope of cure. Nonetheless, the Chief decided on six doses of radiotherapy to try to control the spread, and eight if the results were favourable.

Mr Roberts' wife and two of their eldest sons came with him. She was an unexceptional woman, apart from two trusting brown eyes that forced the word 'integrity' into your heart. She said that they would prefer to look after her husband at home, but they had only one room and had to climb sixty-four stairs to reach it. The Chief said that we would look after him well, and that they could visit any time, day or night. Doctors, I have found, make these rash comments without the slightest thought to the practicalities involved!

Mr Roberts said, 'My days are numbered, so I thank you, kind doctor. My family will continue my life that is running away from me.' He squeezed his wife's hand and said 'The Lord giveth and the Lord taketh away. Blessed be the name of the Lord.' His wife whispered, 'Blessed be God in his wisdom.' The two boys said 'Hallelujah' and then one of them let out a howl. His mother said: 'Abraham, you stop your noise right now. The good sister no want your noise in her nice quiet ward, you hear me?' From such a small woman the effect was surprising and instantaneous.

The Chief smiled and left, saying, 'I leave it in your capable hands, Sister.' The wife left also, as the two youngest girls were due home from school, but the two young men said they were doing the night shift at a nearby warehouse, and could stay. As it was close to visiting hour, I agreed.

In those days, visiting hours were very strict. Too strict, I felt, but hospital discipline had to be maintained. I was glad to relax the rules when I could, but the Chief's comment about unlimited visiting day or night was going a bit too far. Three o'clock came, and the visitors who had gathered outside were admitted. One or two wanted to see me, but mostly I was left in peace to check the drugs and equipment and to complete what little paper work there was to be done. At four o'clock I asked a nurse to ring the bell to inform people that visiting hour was over; almost simultaneously the clip, clip of high-heeled shoes was heard in the corridor, and three women walked straight into the ward. The eldest one was smartly dressed in a suit, and the two younger women wore pretty dresses. They all had hats and white lace gloves. I called to them, and they turned.

'We come to see our daddy,' one of the girls said.

'But visiting time is over,' I replied, ineffectually.

'We come any time, day or night. The doctor, he say.'

'Yes, but—'

The older woman stepped forward and folded her arms.

'No but! Who are you, anyway?'

'I am the ward sister,' I said, hoping I sounded confident.

'You!' she said scornfully. 'You too young to be ward sister. In Kingston, ward sister is a big, strong mamma, fifty years of age, a woman who know how to handle men. Not skinny girl like you, no way.'

I was completely squashed.

Visitors were beginning to leave and we were blocking the doorway. I stepped aside and the three women took it as a sign that they should proceed to Mr Roberts' bed. The two men stood up. One of them kissed the two younger girls, calling them sister Faith and sister Mercy, and the other said to the older woman, 'Well, well, Aunt Adoration, what you doin' here? Long time no see,' and he shifted on his feet with a smooth, boneless motion.

'You no smirk at me, nephew Zachariah. I come to see my brother Elias, is sick man. You no smirk, or I wipe that smirk right off your silly face.' The boy sat down and shrugged effortlessly, his shoulders moving like running water.

They brought a chair for the woman, who sat very close to Mr Roberts.

'Brother Elias, the Lord, He send a visitation—'

'Is you the visitation, Aunt Adoration?' said the boy.

'You be quiet, saucy puppy. Brother Elias, the Angel of Death come visit you, but you be strong in the Lord and be not cast down, hallelujah.'

'Hallelujah,' chorused the girls.

Several visitors, still lingering, looked at them. It was time to intervene.

'It is ten past four, and visiting hour is over. We have work to do, so I must ask you to leave.'

The older woman settled comfortably in her chair, and took off her gloves, before replying.

'The doctor, he say we can visit any time, day or night, his wife tell me. I come all the way from Notting Hill to sit with my brother Elias.'

She removed the pins from her hat and stuck them into the felt, and removed her hat, a gesture loaded with meaning. 'No way,' she muttered. 'Skinny girls, huh. Mercy, pass me my bag.'

From the bag she removed two small cushions, one of which she sat on. The other she placed comfortably at her back before glaring at me.

'No skinny girl tell Adoration Consolation da Silva what to do,' she announced, and waved her hand to shoo me away.

The girls giggled behind their hands, exchanging glances. The boys looked up to the ceiling and whistled silently. I was floored. It was time to see Matron.

'What!' she exploded, 'the Chief said these people might visit any time, day or night?'

'Yes. I was present when he said it.'

'Doctors! We could run this place very much better without doctors,' she muttered, as she accompanied me back to the ward.

It was a fighting start, but unequal from the outset. Matron had the advantage of being the older woman, but she was also a softie, and no match for Mrs da Silva, who won on points. Eventually, it was agreed that when essential work had to be carried out, the ward would be closed and the family could wait in the visitors' room, which was on the ground floor.

The five people disappeared downstairs, and I went to Mr Roberts' side. He was a very sick man, and looked exhausted and grey. He could hardly move, but he murmured, 'Thank you, Sister.' I checked his urine drainage bag, which was heavily bloodstained, and resolved he must have more potassium citrate and more fluids. I examined his supra-pubic wound, which looked clean and comfortable. I asked if he had any pain, and he breathed, 'No more than usual.' What did that mean? Pain is unquantifiable, and no one can assess the degree to which another feels it. He seemed to me to be a man of great courage, and as time went on we all began to recognise his outstanding qualities. Later, the Chief said to me, 'I have seldom seen a man approach death with more nobility.'

We had finished serving supper, the drug round and the essential bed changing and dressings, so I thought I would go to the visitors' room to see if any of the relatives were still there.

There were now not five people, but eight. I said that two could come upstairs to say goodnight to Mr Roberts, and Aunt Adoration stood up. But at that moment Mrs Roberts came in, accompanied by two younger girls aged about thirteen or fourteen, so I said that she should come up with her daughters. The aunt blustered about being first, but Mrs Roberts said quietly, 'Hold your peace, sister Adoration. Do you not remember our dear Lord's words "and the first shall be last, and the last shall be first"? Hold your peace. Come with me, Daffodil, and you also, Ruby, and we go softly, not to disturb the quiet of the evening.'

Mrs Roberts was the only one who seemed to understand that a dying man needs rest and tranquillity, and, above all, peace in which to approach the ending of life.

That was only the first day. During the next three weeks the stream of relatives was constant. One woman, a cousin I think, turned up with three small children, who were sweet and pretty, but a perfect nuisance. I couldn't let them into the ward, so they raced around the ground floor. We let them out into the gardens, which were normally reserved for ambulant patients, and they shrieked and whooped as they chased each other around, to the anger of the gardener who regarded his garden as a sanctuary for the sick. We tried to limit visitors to two at the bedside, but frequently there were four or five. Brothers arrived from Birmingham, a sister from Bradford, and the sons and daughters who lived locally came every day.

Poor Mr Roberts had no peace, but he never complained and,

as far as we could see, never showed any irritation. He was always courteous, and even though he could barely move or speak, he would open his eyes and smile, and perhaps murmur, 'It is kind of you to come. You are welcome,' and then drift away again to where senses and perceptions are beyond our understanding.

We all knew what would happen, and it did. Other patients, and particularly their relatives, started to complain. 'Why is he allowed unlimited visiting time, when we are confined to the specified hours? It's not fair.' And it wasn't, I had to agree.

It was difficult for us, because at the same time we had a similar problem with Mr Winterton, who was an alcoholic. Alcohol is not allowed in hospitals, but you cannot withdraw all supplies from a true alcoholic and expect his body to adjust overnight. He will go berserk. So, a daily dose of whisky was measured out for Mr Winterton at each drug round. This soon attracted the attention of the other men, some of whom called out good-naturedly, 'Come on, Nurse – splash it around, be a sport.'

Others complained, 'If he can have whisky, why can't we?'

'Alcohol is not allowed in hospitals.'

'Yes, but . . .'

It was a circular argument. We even turned a blind eye to his wife bringing him extra supplies in a hip flask. She was a glamorous and interesting woman – an actress, who earned a lot of money on the stage – and she was devoted to him. Mr Winterton had real charisma, and all the nurses, myself included, felt it when he turned on the charm.

One day I had a telephone call from a woman enquiring about Mr Winterton. You have to be guarded about supplying information to anyone who rings up, so I said that the patient was comfortable and that his wife had just visited.

'I *am* his wife,' replied the voice.

Silence from me!

'Yes, *I* am Mrs Winterton. The woman who has just left is not his wife. Did she tell you that she was?'

'Yes.'

'Well, she isn't. I am. What does she look like?'

I described her.

'I know her. She's an actress, and a very good one at that. She is also either a saint or a fool, I don't know which. She has kept that worthless man for years, moving him from one hotel to another along the coast. When the police pick him up drunk and disorderly, she sorts it out and pays the fine, then moves him on to another seaside resort. She has saved me a lot of trouble.'

It's hard to know what to say to a story like that. After deep thought I said, 'Oh.'

'Well, I had better give you my address and telephone number, so that you can inform me when he dies.'

That was the end of the conversation.

We still called the glamorous woman who brought in illicit bottles of whisky Mrs Winterton, but I looked on her with very different eyes. A saint or a fool, which was she? And is there much difference? The Orthodox Church has a concept of the Holy Fool – one who is a fool in the ways of the world, but wise to the ways of God. Are we all 'fools to love'? Not so; I think the opposite – that the lover is all-wise and sees in the beloved the goodness that no one else can see.

We could not halt the metastases in Mr Roberts' emaciated body. The treatment was proving to be worse than the disease, so after three doses of radium the Chief proposed a halt. He spoke to Mrs Roberts, who said: 'I know. God's will be done. The Lord God say, "Can you command the sun to rise, or the sun to set? Can you move the moon from her course? Did you set the stars in motion? Can you number the days of a man?" I know what you saying, and I see it clear. He is my husband and the father of my children, and I will speak with him. He is ready to die, and will be grateful.'

We stopped all active treatment and increased his sedation and she asked us: 'Is it always right to reduce pain? I am not sure. We are born in pain and some of us will die in pain – is this wrong? If there is pain and suffering in this world, there must be a meaning to it. Some of us have to learn this meaning.'

I said, 'We always try to relieve suffering.'

'Yes, I know, and because I am not sure about the right or the wrong, I must leave it to you to decide.'

Then she laughed, a big chuckle that surprised me.

'There is one thing, Sister, that I am quite, quite sure about. Quite sure. He does not need food. Your nurses bring him food, they try to feed him, and he push it away, he turn his head. They try again. It is a nonsense, a child's game. He cannot eat, and does not want to eat.'

She chuckled again, and her face creased with merriment.

'Does a man need porridge or scrambled eggs when he come to the Pearly Gates? No way. He need a clean mind and a pure heart.'

I laughed with her, and said that it was hospital practice to feed patients, even to the point of force-feeding.

Her merriment vanished. 'You not goin' to force-feed my husband,' she said emphatically.

'We will not try to feed your husband any more, I assure you. But what about drinking?' I asked.

'I give him water, it trickle out his mouth. A nurse give him water, he try to swallow, but the water, it choke him. Does he need water, Sister?'

I said we all need water to live.

'But he is dying, not living. It is different.'

I said that if he had no water his death would come more quickly.

'But does that matter?' she asked innocently.

I had to pause. What a question! Does it matter? I had asked myself that question many times but never dared to voice it. Hearing the words spoken aloud by this woman was a shock. Do we try too hard to keep people alive? And what are we doing it for?

I said, 'I cannot allow a patient on my ward to die of thirst. It is against all my teaching, principles and practice.'

'Yes, Sister, I understand you,' she said quietly.

'If he has no water his kidneys will make less urine, and there will be more blood and infection in what little urine is in his bladder. It will be very bad for him.'

'I understand,' she said.

'We planned to put up a drip today.'

She jerked up and looked me straight in the eye. 'No. No drip.'

'Why? Does your religion forbid it?'

'No. We are Methodists, not Fundamentalists. I don't think it is forbidden. It just seems wrong, unnatural.' Her face dissolved in tenderness. 'He is at the point of death, Sister. He is a good man, and has led a good life. Let him rest in peace.'

I said I would discuss the matter again with the doctor. But I also said that, as he could take very little fluid by mouth, it was important to keep his mouth and throat clean and moist, and that one of the nurses would show her how to do this with swab sticks and moistening solution.

After that conversation, his wife never left him. The family, varying at different times between eight and twenty people, more or less camped downstairs, but Mrs Roberts strictly controlled the number of people who saw him. We put him into a single room, and no drip was installed. The family was assiduous in keeping his mouth and throat moistened, and he took a few ounces of water now and then. Some of the younger members of the family helped the nurses to clean and change his bed, and to attend to pressure points. They liked doing so, and almost fought for the privilege.

The family brought food for Mrs Roberts, and we provided cups of tea and coffee from the ward kitchen, for which she always thanked us most graciously.

It was a busy morning, and she carried her empty cup into the kitchen, saying, 'I see you are busy, I do not need to trouble you to collect my empty cup,' and she put it on the draining board.

When she got back her husband was dead.

It happens this way, time and again. So many people will say something like, 'I only went to answer a knock at the door, and when I came back she was gone,' or, 'I just went to the window to draw back the curtains and look down at the garden, and when I turned round, he was dead.'

Why does the person so often die during the minute or two when the watcher is absent? There must be a reason. It happens this way far too frequently to be a coincidence. Dying is not passive. Dying is not something that happens to you without your knowledge or control. Dying is an active process, in which the soul is the leading actor.

There is more, much more, to human life than mere flesh and blood, bones and brains. There is a living spirit that is the spark of life, and when it knows that the flesh, which it has animated for a while, is decaying, the soul wants to slip away quietly, when no one is looking.

FORGET-ME-NOTS

'Show us your wedding ring, Sister.'

I held out my hand for the ladies in the day room to admire.

'It's lovely, dear. You look after it, and your man. Keep them special.'

'What's he like, Sister? Tell us about him.'

They crowded round, the female interest in love and marriage alive in the face of death. I had brought the photo album of our wedding for the ladies to see.

'He looks nice,' said one.

'You can't trust men,' said another.

'Oh, don't be a sourpuss. There's good and bad everywhere, and I'm sure Sister's chosen a good one.'

'Mine broke my arm for me.'

'Mine could never stop. Fifteen pregnancies I had. Even on his deathbed he was after it. He's gone now, good riddance. I'll bet he'll ask the angels for it.'

A burst of laughter among the women. I loved them all, and was glad to see they still retained their sense of humour. We nurses were always told that we should keep alive an interest in life, tell the patients about our days off, our interests, families, boyfriends and the dances we went to. I even encouraged nurses to flirt with the men – anything to divert their minds. Cancer patients often feel surprisingly well, in spite of the malignancy, and keeping up hope was an important part of our work.

I tried to tell them about my young husband.

'He's very clever. He's a schoolmaster.'

'Oh, fancy that. A schoolteacher, eh? That's nice. Did you hear that, dear? Sister's new hubby's a school teacher.'

'Uh?'

'A schoolteacher, dear, Sister's new hubby. Oh, she's not with us, poor soul. It's a shame.'

'What's he look like? Tell us.'

'He's tall and good looking, very distinguished,' I said.

'Ooh, that's nice,' from the cheerful one.

'Handsome is as handsome does,' from the sourpuss.

'Blue eyes or dark?'

'Blue.'

Little Mrs Merton looked up wistfully. She had not spoken, but had been twisting her wedding ring round and round her finger. She was very small, and had a childlike quality that you sometimes meet in the very old. Her eyes were particularly appealing. They revealed patience, kindness and sadness, but also humour. We knew she had a sarcoma that was consuming her bones, but she thought the pain was due to rheumatism, and we let her think this.

'My Bert's eyes were blue,' she said, 'forget-me-not blue. He was a lovely lad, my Bert, no one like him. Before he went, I gave him a little picture. It was a woodland scene of forget-me-nots growing under chestnut trees. He always said my hair was chestnut brown, so it was like a little picture of us both, you see.'

'That's nice.'

'That's pretty.'

'What a nice idea,' the ladies chorused.

Mrs Merton looked pleased and flattered.

'I thought so, and so did he. He took it with him when he went off to the Great War. I've got his likeness here. You can look at it. I'm that proud of it.'

She took a locket from around her neck, and opened a small silver clasp.

'That's my Bert.'

She handed it around lovingly. Boyish features with smiling eyes looked out at us.

'He was such a lovely lad, always laughing, always happy, proud of his uniform – oh, I can mind him now, marching off.'

She smiled as she took the locket back and hung it around her neck. 'I'm never parted from these – my wedding ring, and the likeness of my lovely lad. He was nineteen when we were married in 1915, and two months later he marched off to the war. Oh, I can mind him still, waving and smiling, and marching off.'

'Did he come back?'

'No, he never came back. Smiling and waving, he was. But my lovely lad, he never came back.'

The clock ticked on the wall, and the evening sun cast long shadows through the window. Traffic could be heard in the street, but in the day room no one spoke. Fifty years of love, still burning after only two months of marriage, could be felt by all the women.

Then Mrs Merton spoke again.

'When I got a telegram saying "missing presumed dead" I knew he was gone for ever. I cried for two years, and for ten years I ached all the time. All the time – just here.' She put her hands up to her chest. 'Here it was, the ache. It was terrible. Terrible it was, far worse than the rheumatics.' She chuckled and looked around her. 'Rheumatics is nothing compared to the pain of losing your only love. A great wound, it was, open and bleeding just here.' She pressed her hands on her chest again. 'I can't explain the ache, the feeling, but it was there all the time, never went away, ten years, the ache, ten years . . .' Her voice trailed away.

There were sighs of compassion among the ladies.

'Wicked it was – half our lads gone.'

'War's a crime, I say.'

'My aunt lost four sons.'

Mrs Merton spoke again, her bird-like features eager. 'And then, after about ten years, something happened. I can't explain it, but it did. One morning I woke up and – d'you know what?'

She looked around brightly. We shook our heads.

'No. What?'

'The pain was gone. Quite gone. The wound had healed over, and my Bert was there inside me.'

She hugged her chest protectively.

'Here, inside me, my Bert with his forget-me-not eyes.' She chuckled. 'And I've never been alone since. He's always inside me, laughing and waving, and marching off.'

*

Two weeks later a tragedy occurred that nursing staff always dread, and which usually happens so quickly that nothing can be done to prevent it.

Mrs Merton never wanted to be a trouble to anyone. She was not consumed by fierce independence as some people are, but with self-effacing humility. 'You girls have got people more sick than me with my rheumatics to look after. I can manage fine. I'll not be bothering you,' she would say.

I knew that it was not really safe for Mrs Merton to walk alone, but the alternative would have been to confine her to bed with cot sides around her. This was bad for a patient, both mentally and physically. It deprived them of self-respect and dignity, and was often the start of an almost infantile dependence on the nurses, which frequently hastened the end, quite apart from the fact that it usually caused acute unhappiness. I have seen patients rattling their cot sides in impotent rage and frustration, shouting or weeping, which can have a terrible effect on the morale of other patients in the ward. If the disturbance got too much, I have seen narcotics being given to quieten the patient. This is bad medicine, and bad nursing.

I decided that Mrs Merton should be at liberty to wander around as much as she wanted. In retrospect, this was the wrong clinical decision, but so often in medicine decisions have to be taken, and it is not until later that one can say if they were right or wrong.

One afternoon, Mrs Merton was going into the day room for tea when the diseased bone of her femur snapped. She fell and shattered her pelvis and was taken to the orthopaedics department at the Royal Free for surgery. The femur was pinned and plastered without too much trouble, even though the bone was riddled with cancer, but the fractured pelvis was another matter. It was diseased and shattered in several places, and bits of jagged bone threatened to penetrate her internal organs. The surgeons did what they could, but the result was that the pelvic bone did not mend, and the external wound never healed, as the stitches could not hold the muscle together. Suppuration started around the surface, but it must have been spreading beneath the muscle, because suddenly the whole wound opened up, exposing bone, tendons, ligaments, and muscle, all sticky with pus. The wound was so deep and so extensive that you could get your hand into it.

We did our best. We gave antibiotics to try to reduce the infection and the fever. We packed the wound with flavine gauze and antibiotic powders. We were able to supply one of the new electronic air beds which kept the left side of her body free from bedsores – she had to be nursed on her side all the time because the hip was shattered from the iliac crest in front to the coccyx at the base of the spine. Fortunately, the surgeons had inserted an in-dwelling catheter into her bladder whilst she was in theatre, so we did not have the nightmare of dealing with the normal urination of a patient in her condition.

The one thing we were able to do which really did help Mrs Merton was give her the Brompton Cocktail regularly. In spite of the seriousness of the wound, Mrs Merton was surprisingly unaware of its extent, because she could not see it. She knew that something was wrong with her hip, because nurses came at frequent intervals to change the dressings, but she could not turn her frail old body to look at it. She knew that her right leg was in plaster, and we supposed that she thought this was the full extent of her injuries. Incidentally, the plastered leg had to be adjusted, and it was one of the most unnerving things I have ever seen because the exposed bone and ligaments of the pelvis moved as we repositioned the leg. It was a job I always did myself, with the help of a nurse, and I insisted that when I was not on duty, an experienced staff nurse should do it. This was a task that could not be left to a couple of inexperienced student nurses.

What is it that we need at the end of life? Peace and love are the words that spring to mind. Weeks, or months, of gradual decline usually precede death, but then, very often, something intangible happens. It is as though body, mind and soul have been tuned differently, like tuning down a string of a violin or cello, so that the vibrations that create the inner resonances of the instrument are altered, and the quality of sound is different. I can find no other way of describing these subtle changes that occur before death takes over. A skin change, something different in the eyes, a weariness of movements, a quieting of the mind – there are many subtle alterations that can be seen, and they are very real. And then the end is usually fairly swift. 'Let me bide, dears,' my grandfather had said to his daughters a few days before his death. 'I want for nothing.' And they allowed him to die quietly. Most dying people seem to feel the same – the Angel of Death brings peace. Harassing a dying person to return to the life they have already left is a pointless exercise, and in many instances, cruel.

Love is not something that we receive in proportion to our merits; love is a gift of God. And I like to think that ensuring peace at the end of the day is an act of love on the part of the nursing staff. St Paul, in his Letter to the Corinthians, said that Faith, Hope and Love are the greatest of God's gifts. I suspect that most doctors and nurses will say that faith does not play a great part in tranquillity at the hour of death, because few people mention religion or ask to see a priest. But who are we to judge? None of us knows what is going on in the mind of a dying man or woman, especially if that person is beyond articulate speech. Faith is a private matter, usually held deep within a person, quite impossible to recognise or understand if you have no faith yourself.

There are many reports from people who have returned from a near-death experience, and they are all remarkably similar. Testimonies come from every part of the world, and in all periods of history. Without exception they speak of a profound sense of well-being, and overwhelming feelings of peace and calm. Some people have said they felt safety and comfort, and loving arms enfolding them. A woman has said she felt as though she was drowning in a deep green sea, and the depths contained an inexpressible joy and fullness of life that pulsed more strongly than it had ever done in ordinary life. Many have likened the sensation to lying on the surface of dark, smooth waters, and of being gently supported. Some people have spoken of having no will of their own, but a feeling of weakness and trust and languorous ease.

There are also many reports of an enveloping darkness in which a light is shining. Some speak of a longing to reach that light, others of being led gently towards it. One man spoke of a feeling that he was floating between a black sky and a black sea, between which a phosphorescent light shone. A long tunnel of velvety darkness, with a light shining at the end of it, seems to be the common link. There are also reports of beautiful music, often choirs or strings – but no tune that can be named.

These near-death experiences are well documented and the similarities are striking. No one has ever reported fear or horror associated with a near-death experience, and the absence of such reports is strong evidence that the beatific claims are valid.

Biochemists tell us that the feelings of well-being are due to endomorphs, a morphine-like substance secreted by the body in time of need. Areas of the brain secrete endomorph molecules that bind to nerve endings, and the effect is to alter sensory awareness. They tell us that the light is nothing more than the hypothalamus generating electrical sparks into the brain. The chemical activities in the body that induce a feeling of peace and light at the hour of death have nothing to do with God, they tell us, and everything to do with biochemistry.

I grant the integrity of scientists and the validity of their research, but I have seen enough of life and death to suspect that this is not the whole story. There must be more to the strange species we call humanity than biochemical reactions. If there is a God, then perhaps the brain was created to release endomorphs, and the hypothalamus to release light at time of death, for the peace and comfort of the dying.

We will never know what awaits us after death. But we *do* know, because many people have returned to tell us, that the gentle hand of love guides us through the passage that leads from life into death.

Mrs Merton's sister was her only living relative. I wrote to her twice, but received no reply and feared that Mrs Merton would be alone when she died. I told the nurses that we must therefore give her special love and care. On the space given for next-of-kin was also the name of Lady Tarrant, a former employer. So I telephoned the number given. The response was immediate. 'Harriet Merton, you tell me, dying? I did not even know that she was ill! I will come tomorrow, and I will inform my sons and my daughter. They will want to know.'

Had I told the nurses that Mrs Merton needed our love because she was alone in the world? I could not have been more wrong. Mrs Merton was surrounded by love.

Lady Tarrant told me that Mrs Merton had been nanny to her three children and had been given absolute charge of them when she was abroad with her husband. When the children grew up, Mrs Merton had been retained as housekeeper. The whole family loved her, and her devotion to the family had always been well beyond what was expected of a paid servant. Lady Tarrant spent about half an hour with Mrs Merton, who afterwards said, 'My Lady has been such a support to me in life. She was always so good, so kind. I've been blessed.'

It wasn't until the sons and the daughter came that we saw the extent of their love. They were distraught, especially the youngest, Jason, a man of about thirty-five who was well dressed, competent, affluent. No one would have expected him to break down in my office – but he did. Nanny Merton meant almost as much to him as his own mother. Was she really going to die? Could nothing be done? I assured him nothing would cure her – the sarcoma had been spreading slowly, and now the bones had broken, which usually caused the malignancy to spread faster through the lymph system and the bloodstream. He broke down and wept. I told him to spend as much time as he could with his childhood nanny, because she had, we estimated, only a week or two of life left, and the presence of those who loved her would be precious.

The older brother came with his wife. Mrs Merton was surrounded by pineapples, peaches and grapes, none of which she could not eat. When the orchids arrived, she murmured 'how pretty' and drifted off to sleep again. But when their sister arrived with her children, who had picked a bunch of forget-me-nots from the garden, Mrs Merton stretched out a frail hand and briefly returned to the world of the living.

'Forget-me-not eyes . . . Never forget my Bert, my lad. Smiling and waving and marching off,' she murmured. The children didn't understand. How could they?

Before going off duty that evening, I went into the side ward to see Mrs Merton. It was quiet in there. Time had never seemed so measureless, silence had never seemed so intense as it did while I was feeling her pulse, feeling the slow, ever slower pulse of mortality.

A nurse had put the orchids on the windowsill, and placed the forget-me-nots in a small vase on the bed table where she could see them. Mrs Merton sensed my presence and opened her eyes. 'I will soon be going to my Bert,' she murmured, looking at the vase. 'He's waiting for me, I know. Waiting, my dear lad.'

'I'm sure he is. I have not the slightest doubt he will be there to greet you,' I said.

Slowly she turned her eyes from the spring flowers to meet mine. 'One thing bothers me, though,' she said softly.

I leaned closer. 'What is it? Surely nothing can bother you?'

She made an enormous effort to speak. 'Sister, do you think he will know me? My hair was chestnut brown when he went marching off. He loved my hair. Now it's all grey. Do you think he will still love me?'

Close to tears, I said very slowly, 'Mrs Merton, nothing can change love. You know that, don't you?' She nodded her head. 'He is waiting for you, and he loves you. For him, you have not changed.'

A little moan of contentment was her response, and she glanced again at the forget-me-nots. Her lips moved, but her words could not be heard. Then she closed her eyes, and did not open them again.

I telephoned the younger son, Jason, and told him that Mrs Merton would probably die that night. He arrived at about 11 o'clock and sat with her through many watchful hours, and she died as the dawn of a new day was breaking.

None of us knows whether there is life after death, but the simplicity and beauty of Mrs Merton's faith is something I have seen many, many times. It was not necessarily a religious faith – God, the Church, Heaven, were never mentioned. Mrs Merton's faith was grounded in love. And God, we are taught, is love.

THE ADVANCE DIRECTIVE

Mrs Cunningham. The name was on the admission list for the day. Ovarian cancer, total hysterectomy at the Royal Free, and referred for radium treatment to the Marie Curie Hospital. The name rang a bell, and I remembered old Mrs Cunningham and the perpetual feud with her daughter – but was it the same person as the lady I had known when I was a junior student nurse?

Mrs Cunningham had had a minor operation, for varicose veins, I seemed to remember, the stripping of which in those days necessitated a fortnight in a hospital bed and a fortnight's convalescence. Such a lengthy stay in hospital enabled patients and nurses to get to know each other, and she invited me to her home after her discharge. She was a very interesting lady, and also amusing in a la-di-da kind of way. Her husband had been in the diplomatic service and she had travelled all over the world with him. She had a sardonic humour and her comments were witty and pithy, and mostly directed against her long-suffering daughter, Evelyn.

Evelyn was a lady of about forty, a professional, with a first-class degree from Cambridge and a worn out expression, the latter acquired, no doubt, from her daily commute between Henley-on-Thames and London. Why they lived together, when they clearly hated each other, I could never make out. They would have been better off living apart, but they clung to each other with the horrible force of a lifetime's habit. What had happened to Mr Cunningham I never discovered. They were both extremely reticent about him, but I gained the impression, rightly or wrongly, that he had disappeared with somebody else's wife and a large sum of money.

One way or another, the two ladies were very hard up. They

lived in a huge house in the best part of Henley-on-Thames, with a vast garden terraced down to the river, where they had a boathouse, but no boat. The house and garden were far too big for just the two of them, but they were too proud to give it up and move to something more suitable. And so they struggled on, Mrs Cunningham keeping house and tending the garden, which was really beyond her, and Evelyn earning the money, which just about kept body and soul together.

Mrs Cunningham had been all over India, Ceylon and North Africa with her husband, and as I had never been beyond the shores of England and was longing to hear about 'those far away places with strange sounding names', I cultivated her friendship. At the time she seemed to me very old, being sixty-two, but she had obviously had a very lively and adventurous life. In Morocco, at a time when all Moslem women were heavily veiled, she had dressed as one of them, and gone into the souks alone, something that few English women would dare to do, she told me.

'It was the time of the French Protectorate, you know.'

No, I didn't know. What did 'Protectorate' mean?

'It really means domination. "What is it worth to you, if I don't blow up your country?"'

'That sounds dreadful.'

'It's common enough. All powerful countries do it, expanding their empires. But it wasn't all bad. The French did a lot for Morocco, and a lot for me, indirectly, because it meant that I could converse with the women in the markets in French.'

'Tell me about it, please. I'm dying to hear.'

'Well, you have to get used to being woken up in the middle of the night by the muezzins' calls to prayer, cried out from the mosques.'

'The whatzzins?'

'The muezzins, the callers.'

'What sort of call?'

'A noise like animals howling. It's their religion. I can't go along with it, myself. All religions are a lot of cant, in my opinion.'

She sniffed scornfully.

'And you have to get used to never seeing a woman. I was about the only woman in the streets. If the women left their riads at all, they had to do so in groups, for mutual protection, I suppose, though I must say I was always alone, and none of the men molested me.'

'What is a riad?'

'An enclosed dwelling. It's a kind of central courtyard with the dwelling areas all around it. I always thought this arrangement was a way of keeping the women locked up, but the men reckoned it was to protect them. There's a very fine line to be drawn between protection and domination, you know.'

'Tell me about the men.'

'Well, they go around in these djellabas – long gowns with pointed hoods. Half of them look like Jesus Christ, and the other half look like Judas. I don't think I ever spoke to a man unless my husband was present. Women couldn't.'

'Why not?'

'Oh, I don't know. Religion, perhaps. I wasn't going to risk it. I wandered around alone and spoke to the women, but I thought I might be publicly stoned if I spoke to a man.'

'Oh, surely not!'

'Well, perhaps not. Perhaps I exaggerate. But I assure you, a woman could be stoned to death for adultery. Religion again! Let's go out into the garden, dear. The sun's come out, and you can help me to weed the rockery. It's not often I get help. Evelyn won't so much as lift a fork or a trowel.'

I reckoned that Evelyn probably did quite enough, earning the money, but kept my thoughts to myself.

Whilst we weeded, Mrs Cunningham continued:

'The women did all the work in Morocco, as far as I could judge. "Women and donkeys always go heavy laden", and by God, did they! Massive loads on their backs, and miles to walk. And if the woman had a baby on her back, the load would be carried on her head. Very often a strong young lad, a boy of fourteen or so, would walk beside her, carrying nothing. Though I must say a man would push a barrow or a truck. But he would never be seen carrying anything. He would lose face with the other men, you see.'

'You were going to tell me about the markets.'

'Ah yes. The souks. Fascinating. You would never see the likes here. Produce, food, animals, carpets, jewellery, ornaments – thousands of things brought in from miles around by donkey, and laid out on the sun-baked earth. Piles of fruit, fish, vegetables, meat, just stacked up on the ground. Great mounds of rice or lentils piled on a sack and weighed out by the bucket full. Meat, offal, lights, liver, brains laid on a sack, and swarming with flies, and the water seller going up and down, ringing his bell. Oh, it was wonderful! Here, for once, the women were in command, because they were the buyers. The men were the sellers, and in any economy the purchaser has the upper hand. I could have watched them for hours – the men wheedling and whining, the women firm and controlled. And the women always won.'

She leaned back on her heels and gazed up at the trees. 'Oh, I've had a great life. I don't know of any other European woman who dared to go alone into the souks, but I did. The colours, the smell of the spices, and the donkeys, the sun, and always the High Atlas mountains, snow-covered, in the distance.'

It sounded dreamy to me. I wanted to burst out of the constraint of my nurse's training and take the first boat to Morocco. The very name of the country inspired dreams. But Mrs Cunningham was continuing:

'The women had their fun, though, in the hammams.'

'What's that?'

'The public bathhouse; hot, wet and steamy. You lie naked on the stone floor, heated from underneath by wood fires, and a bath attendant throws a bucket of water over you and starts rubbing you with soap and a rough cloth – to stimulate the follicles, they say. But, believe me, that's not all it stimulates, I can tell you! All those women laughing and massaging each other! What happens in the men's hammams doesn't bear thinking of. Crowds of men and boys rubbing each other! Boys from the age of seven or eight –

just think. There's a dandelion there. Look! Try and get it out, will you?'

I had done enough weeding with my grandfather to know how to attack a dandelion.

'Good girl. You've got the root. That's more than Evelyn could have done.'

She chuckled a throaty laugh.

'Poor Evelyn. What she needs is a good slide around in a hammam. She's like a dried up bit of old soap – she needs a good rubbing and lathering in all that steam to soften her up a bit.'

She chuckled again, and I thought of poor Evelyn on the 5.30 from Paddington, returning to her clever and scornful mother and a few hours of guarded conversation and mutual backbiting.

But I liked Mrs Cunningham. It's funny how you can see real nastiness in some people, especially in their relationships with others, and like them just the same. She was different, and I felt flattered that she seemed to enjoy my company.

She invited me to her house one Saturday afternoon, but when I arrived it was clear that she had forgotten, because she had gone to stay with her son, James, for the weekend, and Evelyn was there alone. I felt embarrassed and said I would go, but Evelyn pressed me to stay.

'I suppose you've been hearing all about the souks and the hammams and the veiled women?' she said.

'Yes. Isn't it fascinating?'

'It probably is the first time you hear it, but when you get the same old stories over and over again, you can grow tired of them. Has she got to the one about the camel trek across the desert yet?'

'No.'

'She will. And the one about the time she wandered into a brothel by mistake?'

'Wow! A brothel! That's interesting. What happened?'

'She'll tell you. Nothing can be more boring than an old woman who lives constantly in the past.'

'She's had an interesting life.'

'Yes, but she's a scorpion when you get to know her. She drove my dear father into the arms of another woman, that's for sure.'

I began to feel uncomfortable; getting involved in this female feud was something to avoid. I changed the subject.

'She seems to have a lot of dislike for religion.'

'Oh yes. She is a very enlightened woman, in that respect. My father was an atheist – or is, perhaps I should say. My brother and I were brought up non-believers. Really, it is the only rational way to think. Religion has had its day. I don't know that any intelligent person can believe all that nonsense about virgin births and rising from the dead.'

I did not know how to answer. I was very young and impressionable. I had been brought up as a Christian, and had attended Sunday School, which entailed a lot of bible study, but I don't think I was very committed. To hear this older woman, who was a Cambridge graduate, make such a statement shook me.

'We are members of the British Humanist Society,' she continued.

'What's that?'

'We believe that men and women are on this earth to do their best for one another, to act with goodness and kindness and justice for the common good. There is no divine intervention – that is just the wishful thinking of weaker minds.' She glanced at me, and smiled a faintly superior smile. 'I suppose you were brought up to believe that old business about God the Father, God the Son, etc.?'

'Well, I suppose I was.'

I hadn't heard anyone talk like that before, and it disturbed me.

'Darwin proved conclusively that there is no God who made Man. Mankind has evolved over millions of years from the animal world. It's all biology, not theology. Man made God from his imagination.' She laughed derisively. 'Anyway, after the last war, what is there to believe? Nearly two thousand years of Christianity – "love thy neighbour as thyself" – and what did it produce? The German concentration camps.'

She had struck home. Nothing has ever horrified me as much as the newsreel pictures of the Belsen and Auschwitz victims which were first shown in British cinemas in 1945, and which I saw when I was ten years old.

'I hadn't thought of it like that.'

'That's because you were indoctrinated when you were a child. You need to be more of a free thinker.'

I felt ashamed. I didn't know that I was indoctrinated. It was a horrid word, I thought. I wanted to be a free thinker.

'You must take some of the newsletters of the Humanist Association. That will open up your mind. Now, let's have a cup of tea before you go, and some cake. My mother is a good cook, I'll say that much for her.'

I tucked into cake and biscuits, then cycled back to the hospital with a comfortably full stomach, but uncomfortable thoughts.

The next time I visited Mrs Cunningham, she was studying a document received from the British Humanist Association entitled *The Right to Die*.

Abruptly she said, 'I have signed an advance directive, instructing that, if I become ill, and the illness is incurable, I request voluntary euthanasia. I have placed a copy of this document with my son, my daughter, my doctor and my lawyer.' She looked thoroughly pleased with herself.

I had heard of euthanasia, but had not given it much thought. In the course of my work I had seen people die and had thought a good deal about death, but it had never occurred to me that we, in the medical professions, could actually put someone down as you would a dog.

'It makes absolute sense. I don't want to suffer needlessly. When my time comes I want my life to end swiftly and painlessly.'

'That's what everyone wants,' I said.

'Yes, and it's everyone's right – or should be. The law needs changing, and we Humanists are trying to bring it up in Parliament. Anyway, I have signed this directive. I consider it the only rational thing to do. I have discussed it with James and with Evelyn, and they both agree.'

'What does your doctor say?'

'He won't commit himself. He says it would probably cause more trouble than it alleviates. But he respects my wish to die with dignity.'

'Dignity? Wherever did you get that idea from? Death is not dignified, any more than birth is.'

'Well, that's the expression the Euthanasia Society has adopted.'

'The people who run your society don't know what they are talking about! No one dies with dignity. That only happens in the cinema when someone says a sad farewell, then his head falls sideways and he dies. It doesn't happen in real life, I can assure you. Films either make death look romantic, or horrific. It's neither.'

I giggled as only teenage girls can giggle.

'I don't think you are taking this seriously enough,' Mrs Cunningham said severely. 'Thoughtless girl. When my time comes, I want an easy death. I want to be able to go to sleep, like having an injection before an operation. You don't feel a thing. When death begins to overtake me, and bungles the process of dying, I shall want a competent doctor to assist nature and make a good clean job of it.'

'It all sounds too easy to me.'

'I have always been in control of my own life, and I intend to be in control of my death.'

That had been almost ten years before, and when Mrs Cunningham was admitted to the Marie Curie Hospital I honestly didn't recognise her: an old lady, very bent, with sparse straggly hair and a wild look about her. After surgery, she had spent a fortnight in a convalescent home to build her up and improve her strength before the radium treatment, but, nonetheless, she was so thin that every bone in her body stuck out. Her eyes were sunken, and her grey-white skin was drawn tightly over her high cheekbones, making her nose and ears look huge. Her lips were without colour and pinched tightly together above a pointed chin. No, I would not have known her; but she recognised me.

'You're the child I used to know in Reading, aren't you?'

'Yes, I am,' I said with sudden recognition.

'A stupid girl, I remember. What are you doing here?'

'I'm the ward sister.'

I held out my arm to assist her as she walked. She pushed it aside.

'Leave me alone – there's nothing wrong with me. Ward sister, you say? That doesn't sound too good. I dare say you are as ignorant now as you were then.'

She reached the empty bed that had been kept for her.

'What do you mean by putting me here? I expected a private room. I'm not staying here with a lot of stupid old people!'

She glared angrily around her at the other patients.

I explained that the side rooms were for people who were very sick, and that people like her, who could get about, and were improving, were always nursed in the main ward. She looked at me steadily.

'You mean I must be improving, or I wouldn't be here?'

'Yes, that is correct.'

'Tell Evelyn that.'

'Certainly, if you wish me to.'

'Of course I wish you to! I wouldn't have said it if I didn't mean it. And tell my son, James, also. I told them both I was getting better, but they wouldn't believe me. Fools, the pair of them.'

This didn't look good, by any standards. I had known Mrs Cunningham as an active, strong-minded woman in her early sixties, with a sharp tongue and an independent spirit, but I certainly had not expected this would develop into such venom as she grew old. In our profession we often meet people whose bewilderment and frustration in the face of illness leads to anger, but this was excessive, and I did not like to think of the effect it would have on the other women in the ward.

The Chief came to see her that afternoon, and I accompanied him. She glared at us both.

'About time, too. I don't like to be kept waiting. Well? What are you going to do for me?'

He did not say too much, but examined her abdomen, and the scar from the operation, which was healing well.

'We are going to take blood for tests.'

'That's not going to help me. I want proper treatment.'

'We cannot start until we have the results.'

'And how long will that be?'

'A few days.'

'A few days! That's preposterous. I want treatment at once.'

'We will give you tablets to prepare your body for the radium treatment.'

'That's something, I suppose. Why am I here at all? That's what I want to know. I had a hysterectomy. Thousands of women have hysterectomies, then they go home and get on with life. Why do I have to come to the Marie Curie Hospital for radium? It makes no sense.'

This was always the difficult, nay, *impossible*, question to answer. At that time everyone knew that radium was given to reduce a growth, and most people think of a growth as cancer. But this need not always be so. Many growths are benign, many are encapsulated, and even a malignant growth can be reduced to a size of no importance. The Chief explained this to her, and said that surgery had removed the growth, and that the radium, which was the most advanced medical treatment of the day, would minimise the risk of it spreading to other parts of her body. She would probably have six treatments, which might be extended to ten, depending on the response of her body, which would be determined by her physical condition and blood tests. He chose his words carefully.

'That's what I wanted to hear.' Mrs Cunningham's sunken eyes glared at the Chief. Her thin lips spat out the words, 'Advanced medical treatment.'

'Yes. You will get the most up-to-date treatment that is available. This hospital is at the forefront of research, and our success rate is high.'

'You must tell my son and daughter that. A high success rate – that's what they need to know. Fools, the pair of them. What do they know about advanced medical treatment? Nothing! Not a thing.'

She gave a contemptuous grunt, with a curl of the lips, and repeated, 'They know nothing.'

The Chief and I returned to the office.

'I think she is going to be a difficult patient to handle,' he said. 'There's something malign eating away inside her – and I don't mean the cancer. There is something else on her mind.'

I told him that I had known Mrs Cunningham ten years previously, and that she had struck me as a highly intelligent woman – strong minded, independent, and humorous. He made no comment.

Two days later her son James came to see her. Halfway through the visiting hours she called loudly to one of the nurses, 'Take him away! I won't have him here. Get him out of here.'

I was busy checking drugs received from the dispensary, and ordering more, but when I heard the angry, raised voice, I went to see what was going on. Poor James, looking embarrassed, was leaving the ward.

'Don't come back. And tell that interfering sister of yours I don't want to see her, either,' his mother's voice shouted as he left.

'What on earth is all this about?' I said as he passed. 'Please come to the office with me. Your mother has been angry and aggressive ever since she was admitted.'

We sat down.

'Now what was said? Why this outburst?' I enquired.

'I simply told her that I thought she should not have any more treatment, and that the time had come when she should accept the inevitable, and die with dignity.'

Oh dear, I thought, so was this the origin of the fear and anger? 'Please go on,' I said.

'Well, it's perfectly obvious that she is dying. The cancer is spreading. She doesn't need more treatment. She just wants an easy way out. We all do.'

'Yes, I know. You are quite right,' I said, encouraging him to go on.

'I reminded her that she had signed an advance directive years ago, and had renewed it annually.'

'That's interesting. Please tell me more.'

'She has been an active member of the British Humanist Society – we are all members, the whole family – and voluntary euthanasia is high on their agenda.'

'Euthanasia is illegal,' I reminded him.

'Yes, I know, but an advance directive saying that no more medical treatment should be given after a certain point, is not. It is perfectly within her legal rights to refuse further treatment.'

'It is. But at what point do we begin withholding medical treatment?'

'Now, of course. She is not going to get better. Anyone can see that. She's had a good life, and she's a good old age. The time has come to lay it down.'

'But your mother does not see herself as being at the end of life.'

'I can't understand it. She was always so clear-sighted, so positive in her convictions. She knows quite well that treatment beyond the point of no return can frequently cause more suffering than the original disease. But now, she won't accept it, and gets furious with me and humiliates me in public. She had a blazing row with Evelyn on this subject a few weeks ago. Evie told me about it, but I thought it was just another mother and daughter row. They're always getting at each other, you know. Well, I'm damned sure I'm not coming in to visit her again, only to be shouted at.'

He spoke in an aggrieved tone, and stood up to go.

I told him that his mother was angry because she was afraid, and that she would probably get over it. I expressed the hope that he and Evelyn would both visit, because everyone needs the family to be there at the end of life.

Immediately after visiting hour had finished, Mrs Cunningham called me over.

'Get the consultant,' she demanded, 'I must speak to him. Get him at once.'

I explained that a consultant is not on call at a moment's notice, but that I would ask him to come as soon as he was free.

She exploded with rage, and was very insulting to me, and to the medical hierarchy in general. She was creating a scene, and this was having a bad effect on the other women in the ward. I began to think that we might have to put her in a side ward after all.

'Well, don't let my son or daughter in. That's an order,' she shouted.

The Chief came after supper, and I told him of the afternoon's events. He sat, tapping his watch, before he spoke.

'The Euthanasia Society has gained in influence as medical knowledge has been able to prolong life which, it must be said, is not always a good life. I will speak to her, and I would like you to be with me, as a witness, if nothing else. We cannot have this conversation in the middle of the ward, so ask her to come here, please.'

Mrs Cunningham came to the office. I could see as she walked that her son was absolutely right, and that she was a dying woman.

She confronted the Chief even before she sat down.

'Don't you listen to my son or my daughter. They'll tell you not to let me have any more treatment. They hate me. They want to get rid of me, especially Evelyn.'

She blurted it out, hardly pausing for breath.

'There's nothing wrong with me. I'm as strong as I ever was, but they want me out of the way. Don't you listen to them.'

She jabbed her stick in the air to emphasise her words.

The Chief said that he would always listen first to the wishes of a patient.

'But what if I can't express myself? Then they will sneak in and twist your mind. They are very persuasive, and not to be trusted. I don't trust doctors; they are all as bad as each other. I've signed up. They will use it. That's what you want, the whole damned lot of you. I know what you're up to. You can't fool me.'

She was becoming irrational. Evidently this business of an advance directive had been playing on her mind to such an extent that she couldn't think straight.

The Chief explained that an advance directive had no legal validity whatsoever, and was certainly not binding on the medical profession; but either she did not hear him, or could not take it in.

'The best treatment is what I demand. Forget James and Evelyn. They are ignorant, prejudiced, stupid . . .' She rambled on, repeating herself, contradicting herself. We listened to her tirade, and the Chief again told her that she would have the best treatment available. Unconvinced, but unable to say more, she returned to her bed.

From then on, Mrs Cunningham's whole existence became paralysed by fear. Her fear of death amounted almost to madness, and an overwhelming feeling of helplessness rushed in upon her. She was lost; she panicked; she prayed to a God she did not believe in; she lost control; she screamed for advanced medical treatment, and railed that treatment was being withheld because James and Evelyn had influenced the doctors. Craven fear had roused her whole mental machinery to a state of agitation that had taken away all fatigue, all possibility of sleep, all sense of self-respect. It was a distress impossible to soothe. Drugs could have helped her, but if we went near her with a syringe she screamed uncontrollably that it was all part of the plan to do her in. She was beside herself with terror, and this reduced her to a jabbering wreck, devoid of all self-control and dignity.

We had to move her to a side ward, because of the effect she was having on other patients. She shouted that she knew why we had put her there; it was because of hospital secrecy. She knew what we were up to; all doctors were rogues and nurses were hand in glove with them. She demanded to see her lawyer, the police, her Member of Parliament. Her mind was obsessed, and nothing could divert it.

The laboratory report on the blood tests returned. Widespread metastases of the cancer were evident. The radium treatment should be started, but the Chief hesitated, because with the malignancy circulating through her entire body via the venous and lymphatic systems, it would probably be ineffective and would be distressing to her for no benefit gained. But she became hysterical and screamed that we were *deliberately* withholding the treatment she had been promised, and which it was her right to receive. So the Chief ordered a low dose, by way of a placebo. But when she was wheeled on a trolley to the treatment rooms, her fear became uncontrollable. In those days the radium treatment was carried out in a huge machine, into which the patient was wheeled, and the machine closed. She got halfway in, and then panicked. She shouted that we were putting her into a coffin to dispatch her while she was still alive. She thrashed about, and beat the sides, screaming for release. All the radiographers could do was return her to the ward.

Poor lady. She was so weak, and she was dying, but fear possessed her and filled her failing body with an agitation that allowed her no rest, day or night. She was suspicious of everyone, and the room seemed reduced in size by her wakeful, watchful eyes. It was pitiful to see, and impossible to calm. She would take no drugs, not even sleeping pills, and then she accused us of withholding essential treatment.

Illness is a revelation; one sees things one has never seen before. We saw, in Mrs Cunningham, a manic fear of death, which was not fear of cancer, because she did not believe she had it. Her fear was that death would be forced upon her because that was what she had always said she wanted. Day by day, hour by hour, she anticipated it, and the waiting nearly drove her mad. In fact, I think it *did* drive her mad.

Illness can also bring a flowering of love between people. That is one of the reasons why nursing is such a wonderful profession – we see these things. But for poor Mrs Cunningham, love was denied her at the end. She was convinced that her son and daughter were going to implement the advance directive that she had signed and re-signed. The idea was nonsense, of course, everyone knew that, but you cannot reason with obsession.

Evelyn came to the hospital several times, but her mother would not see her, and told the staff to 'drive her away'. True to his word, James did not come again, but I have memories of Evelyn's sad face as I took her final gifts of flowers and a bed jacket, and told her that she could not be admitted. The reconciliation between mother and daughter, which would have eased Mrs Cunningham's last days and consoled Evelyn in her bereavement, was denied them both.

Mrs Cunningham's mind and body could not withstand so much tension. The frenzied activity wore her out. She could no longer shout and scream, but she sobbed out of a sense of injury and injustice. She called upon God and wailed for mercy. Her terrified state of mind pursued her into her sleep and dreams, for the night nurse reported that she often woke in the night with a dreadful start and wept convulsively.

Mercifully, it did not last too long. Gradually, her mind became clouded, as it usually does as death approaches. Movement, speech, perhaps even thought, required more effort than she could command. Her breathing, circulation, and metabolism slowed down. Death overtook her, and calmed her, and, at the end, she learned that there was nothing to fear.

'Hope is not the conviction that something will turn out well, but the certainty that something makes sense, regardless of how it turns out.'

— *Vaclav Havel, playwright and President of the Czech Republic, 1993–2003*

THE BROOM CUPBOARD

The greater one's experience of death, the more cautious one becomes in making a pronouncement. The ways in which people face death are as different as the ways in which we all live.

Perhaps I should qualify this statement. The last ten to thirty hours before death are very much the same; a semi-awareness of space and time and people takes over, leading into a different level of existence, accompanied by peace and tranquillity. If left undisturbed, death is not an agony. It is the earlier period, the weeks or months, or even years of illness or ageing that are so different.

Mr Anderson was consultant to a firm of international financiers. He was a very successful man, confident, self-contained, a person who needed very little amusement or even warmth – his work was enough, and filled most of his time and his thoughts. For relaxation he liked to go long-distance trekking in mountain ranges, sleeping in wooden huts and scrambling over rocks and riverbeds. It was a total change from his business life, and kept him fit. His private life was less successful. He had married a pretty girl whom he thought he loved, mainly because it seemed the right thing to do, but he had no idea how to handle women, and his wife soon left him for another man. He was not particularly upset, and enjoyed the freedom of a bachelor's life.

He had never had a day's illness, and prided himself on keeping fit through his walking, a sensible diet, no smoking and moderate alcohol intake. He had no time for some of his business colleagues who ate and drank too much, smoked like chimneys, went everywhere by car or taxi and then complained about feeling out of shape. 'What do they expect?' he said to himself.

When he developed stomach pains and felt sick, he was slightly offended – it shouldn't be happening, he thought, so for a week he cut out rich meats and fats from his diet and ate only salads. Things seemed to improve, and he was satisfied that he had nipped the problem in the bud. But a week or two later the nausea returned, along with heartburn. He had heard of something called a hiatus hernia, but lots of people get hernias of one sort or another, so he was not particularly worried. He felt well in other ways, work was busy and he was planning his first trek in the foothills of the Himalayas. Life was too full and too interesting to bother about a little heartburn.

But things did not improve, and so, a month later, he went to see his doctor, who examined him, and found an unexplained lump in the upper abdomen. He said that another medical opinion should be obtained, and advised a gastro-enterologist at the Royal Free Hospital.

Mr Anderson was indignant.

'But I'm busy! There's a lot of work on, and I'm going to the Himalayas trekking in ten weeks' time.'

The doctor replied that they must get him into good shape for the trip, and wrote his referral letter.

At the Royal Free, Mr Anderson was taken to theatre for a routine laparotomy with exploration, and possibly a partial gas-trectomy (there were no electronic scans in those days). In theatre, the surgeon opened him up, took one horrified look at an intract-able growth of carcinogenic material, involving the stomach and duodenum, and stitched him up again. He looked despairingly at the theatre staff: 'How can one tell a man of forty-five that he has inoperable cancer and has only a few weeks to live?'

No one answered. Everyone knew how great was the respons-ibility of telling – if they decided to tell at all. Sometimes, it is better to maintain the illusion of recovery; sometimes, it is better to tell the truth. But how is one to know what is best for a particular patient? The strong-minded person who says 'I want the absolute truth,' can be the one who goes to pieces when told. But the truth can be received by another calmly, and in unexpected ways may bring resolution to life. One can never be sure, and usually it is better to let the patient take the lead. Only then can you get an inkling of what he or she wants to hear. Even so, you can be wrong, because people deceive themselves. A dying man rarely looks death in the face until the end. In the early stages of terminal illness, he might have a shrewd idea of what is going on, but usually, at that point, he doesn't want to *know*.

Mr Anderson was not told directly that he had cancer so advanced that it was inoperable. He was simply told that six weeks of radium therapy would be beneficial. He entered the Marie Curie feeling well, and was by far the most active and alert of our patients. He appeared scornful of the other men, and complained about not having a private room.

'It is bad enough that I have no privacy. But it is intolerable that I do not have the use of a telephone.'

I said that we had a pay phone for patients' use.

'Pay phone!' he spat out in disgust. 'You mean I will have to put pennies in every time I need to make a phone call?'

I said I would discuss the matter with Matron. At Marie Curie we had a policy of keeping our patients happy, as far as possible, especially if we knew their days were numbered. Matron frequently went to great lengths to oblige, and she discussed the matter fully with Mr Anderson. It transpired that what he really wanted was the use of an office from which he could continue to manage his business enterprises with the help of his secretary.

Matron swallowed hard. This was something quite new to her experience. A hospital is a hospital, not an office block, she might have said – but she didn't. He was a dying man, and who could refuse such a request? There was a broom cupboard on the first floor that was little used, would he care to look at it? Together they examined it, and Mr Anderson said it would suit him if it could be cleaned out, and a desk found. Matron did not think a spare desk was available, so he said he would have one supplied, and would also pay for a telephone to be installed. It was surprising how quickly the broom cupboard was converted into a small but adequate office. The secretary, a smart young man, immaculately suited, arrived with a car load of files and folders, and within two days Mr Anderson was at work. We never knew what business he was engaged in, but it was most unusual and the nursing staff was very impressed.

Matron's arrangement was highly beneficial to Mr Anderson, because it kept his mind occupied and his energies engaged. Sickness usually dominates the thoughts of a patient with cancer, but too much preoccupation with illness can have a destructive effect on the mind, and knowing what can happen frequently becomes self-fulfilling. Today, people who are ill will spend hours surfing the internet to find out all they can about their illness – but this isn't always a good thing.

Although Mr Anderson had not been told of his condition, he was an intelligent and thoughtful man, and he must have known that radium was given for cancer. We anticipated that he would start asking questions. One day, during a routine ward round, he said to the Chief: 'I am due to go trekking in the Himalayas in six weeks' time. Do you think I will be fit by then?'

The Chief hedged. 'That sounds pretty strenuous.'

'Yes, it will be. But it will do me good. I need a bit of fresh air and exercise.'

'I think you should find something less demanding – walking in the Wye Valley or the Cotswolds, for example.'

'I see. I will think about it,' he replied. He picked up his book again and appeared to be reading; but I knew that he was watching us as we continued the ward round.

It was not the first time I had had the feeling of being watched. Several times I had seen him observing the nurses as they went about their work, and wondered if he fancied one of them.

One day, he said abruptly: 'I have been watching you and your nurses.'

'Yes, I know, and I have wondered why.'

'You don't miss much.'

'Nor do you, it seems. But why?'

'Because I can't understand how you, any of you, can do it.'

'Because we are trained to.'

'But why start the training in the first place? From what I can see, nursing is such a filthy, disgusting job. Why should anyone want to do it, especially a pretty young girl – and some of your nurses are very young and very pretty.'

Such a statement gave me a bit of a jolt. I had never thought of nursing the sick as filthy or disgusting.

'I can't agree with you. Admittedly we deal with the clinical indignities and intimacies that sickness entails but—'

'That's what I mean. Some of these old men ...' he glanced around him fastidiously '... are in such a revolting state that I wonder how anyone can go near them, let alone do the work that you girls have to do.'

I tried to explain that each man was a person with a life, loves, dreams, hopes and beliefs, and that the illness imposed on them did not alter that in any way; in fact, illness intensified it.

'I've never seen anything like it,' he said thoughtfully.

'No. Few people even think of what illness can lead to.'

As soon as I had said the words, I wished I had not done so. I did not want him to identify himself with the 'revolting state', as he had put it, of some of the men around him. People never see themselves reaching the terminal stage of illness.

'I'm damned sure I couldn't do it,' Mr Anderson said emphatically.

An incident occurred in the hospital, and, for a while, everyone in our small, enclosed world was talking about it. Matron was a sweet, trusting soul who saw no harm in anyone. When a gentleman called at the hospital and announced that he was a representative of the British Patients' Benevolent Fund and that the society wanted to offer the Marie Curie Hospital a television for the benefit of the patients, she fell for it. A charming conversation over coffee and biscuits followed and the gentleman was shown around the hospital, which he assured her was a most heart-warming experience. A suitable location for the television was selected, and the gentleman said that the cost of installation would be ten pounds – a very large sum of money in those days, far more than an average week's pay.

Matron wrote out a cheque to the Patients' Benevolent Fund, but the gentleman requested cash, because he said he would have to pay the electricians in cash. She swallowed that one also, and went to her petty cash box and handed over ten pound notes. They parted with great goodwill on both sides, and the television and electricians were promised to arrive that same afternoon. One need say no more. Matron had many fine qualities, but spotting a con man at three paces was not one of them.

The patients had all been told of the kind offer and those that were well enough were very excited. Televisions were expensive items in the 1960s, and few of our patients had even seen one. The afternoon wore on. Several patients and nurses eagerly looked out of the front windows, and Matron was a-twitter with expectation. But the minutes ticked by, then the hours, and no electricians or television set arrived. Five o'clock came, then five thirty, and still nothing.

'Perhaps they will come tomorrow,' said a hopeful voice.

'Not a chance. He's got his ten pounds. We won't be seeing him again,' said a realist.

'It is disgusting,' said Mr Anderson, 'I despise such a man. Tell Matron that I will buy a television for the hospital, and pay for the aerial to be installed. I can enjoy it for a while, and when I am gone it will remain for the enjoyment of others.'

This was a very unexpected and generous offer, but I wondered about his use of the words 'when I am gone'. It sounded as though he knew he was going to die.

Cancer can overwhelm the body with frightening speed. Although the radium treatment was probably reducing the growth in the abdomen, we could not tell to what extent without performing another laparotomy exploration. Mr Anderson was losing weight rapidly. He was a spare man, with strong musculature, but within a few weeks he became pathetically thin. He found swallowing more difficult, and waves of nausea frequently beset him after a meal. We gave him anti-emetics, which helped a little, but one day, as he drank the mixture, he said to the nurse, 'This is not going to improve me, is it?'

'Oh yes,' she said brightly, 'we wouldn't give it to you if it wasn't.'

'There is only one thing that is going to help me,' he said, 'and that is work. My secretary is coming at two o'clock and I must go to my broom cupboard.' He grinned at the girl.

Mr Anderson always dressed in a suit to go to his office. We thought at first it was an affectation to assert his superiority over the other patients, who usually wore dressing gowns, but as time went on we realised that it was to preserve his self-respect and sense of dignity. As he lost weight, the jacket hung loosely on his thin shoulders, and he had to make new holes in his belt to keep his trousers up.

Excepting the days when he had radium therapy, Mr Anderson went to work. He even went on the day following treatment, when we usually advised patients to stay in bed because they often felt very ill. He would struggle out of bed, and one could see him trying to control the nausea and dizziness flooding his head, as he shaved and dressed. He usually returned to the ward about lunchtime, looking somewhat better. Obviously, the work was doing him good.

Pain is associated with cancer, and as the growth encroached further into the stomach and duodenum, Mr Anderson's discomfort increased. Pain is something we cannot measure. No one can tell when the level passes from inconvenient to severe, to unbearable, and we all have different pain thresholds. Mr Anderson's was probably getting to the severe stage – we could tell by the look in his eye, by the intake of breath and biting of his lip, by a slight moan that escaped as he bent over to try to ease the abdomen. But he would not take any painkillers. He had tried the Brompton Cocktail on a couple of occasions, but it had made him so sick he would not take it again, and he adamantly refused any injections.

Putting on his suit was such a struggle that particular morning.

I could see the effort it was costing him and he gave a little gasp as he leaned over to tie his shoelaces. He remained bent in that position for some time, and when he sat up, his face was grey.

'You really must have some analgesics,' I said to him.

'No, I can't. I've got to keep my head clear.'

'Then why not stay in bed for the day?'

'I am expecting some important telephone calls this morning.'

'Your secretary will be coming. Can't he take them?'

'No. I have to make crucial decisions. No one else can do it. And then there will be a lot of follow-up work.'

'Surely it cannot be so important that it can't wait until tomorrow?'

'It cannot wait. A great deal of money is at stake.'

I gasped, almost unable to believe what I had heard. Money, of all things! What on earth would he do with more money on the brink of eternity? A man obsessed with money has never appealed to me, but because I saw him wince in pain I said gently: 'You might be feeling better tomorrow.'

'I will *not* be feeling better tomorrow, Sister, and you know that as well as I do.'

Our eyes met, and, for the first time, I knew that he knew he was dying. The game of 'let's pretend' was over. I was greatly relieved.

'So you know, then?'

'Of course I know!' he said savagely. 'Radium is given for cancer. Do you think I'm a fool?'

'Do you want to talk about it?'

'Yes, but not now. I have work to do. We can talk later. The only question I really want answered is, how long have I got?'

'That is impossible to answer. Accuracy can never be assured.'

'Weeks or months?'

'No one can say. It depends on so many things.'

'Then I will continue to act as though it is weeks, and I have work to do. You could oblige me by helping me to my feet, Sister.'

I helped him to stand up, and watched with sorrow and admiration as he straightened his back, gritting his teeth as he did so.

People with abdominal pain find it eases them to bend over slightly. But not Mr Anderson – he was determined to stand straight, and he walked firmly to the door and along the corridor towards his broom cupboard.

It is generally assumed that doctors know all there is to know about death, and that, if a patient is to be told that his condition is incurable, it is the doctor's prerogative. In my experience, this idea is overstated, because most of the time doctors are not on the wards, whereas nurses and carers are.

During the time when I was a probationer student nurse in Reading, I was working on a male medical ward. I carried out simple duties such as washing the locker tops, and was at the bedside of a man who was very ill. He grabbed my wrist, and with fierce intensity barked: 'Have I got a growth, Nurse?'

Startled I said, 'Yes.'

'Thank you,' he croaked. 'No one would tell me. Am I going to die?'

'I don't know,' I said truthfully.

'But what do you think?'

'I honestly don't know. No one knows.'

'Thank you, Nurse.'

He sank back on the pillows and sighed. It might have been a sigh of relief or despair. One could not tell.

I did not dwell on the incident, and it certainly did not occur to me that I had done anything wrong, until a few days later when Sister called me to her office.

'Did you tell Mr S that he has a growth?'

I probably looked blank, but said, 'Well, he asked me, so I said yes.'

'Nurse, you are still in your probationary period. I must report this to Matron.'

The same morning I was called to Matron Aldwinkle's office. The conversation I had had with the ward sister was repeated, but I added, 'Well, what could I say if he asked me? I couldn't say "no, you haven't got a growth" when I knew that he had.'

'You should have told him to speak to the doctor.'

'But he had seen the consultant and the other doctors that morning. It was just after the ward round.'

'Nurse, we do not tell a patient directly that he has a malignancy. Most patients cannot accept it.'

'But what are we to do if we are asked?'

Matron struggled to find the right words.

'I know it can be very difficult, but you have to think quickly. Something like "I don't know" or "it has not yet been diagnosed" would be suitable.'

'But it *had* been diagnosed. And I *did* know.'

'You have to understand, Nurse, that we cannot simply blurt out the truth.'

'If I had told a lie, I'm sure he would have seen it in my face. I'm no good at lying. I've tried it before, and my face always gives me away.'

Matron appeared to be slightly exasperated. 'You have to learn to be more sensitive to a patient's needs. Well, I am going to move you to another ward. I do not think you should continue on Victoria Ward at present. I have confidence that you will learn, and improve. You may go, Nurse.'

It would probably surprise many doctors to know how frequently very junior nurses are confronted with a dilemma such as the one described. It occurs because nurses are so much closer to patients than doctors are, a situation that doctors have cultivated, creating a barrier between themselves and their patients. Often, most hospital patients are in awe of doctors, especially consultants, and feel they cannot engage in a conversation with one of these superior beings. But they are not in awe of nurses, who are with them all the time, and therefore more accessible. Indeed, since the changes in the nursing profession, requiring nurses to be college-trained rather than ward-trained as my generation was, patients don't have much contact with student nurses. So when a frightened patient asks, 'Have I got a growth?', the person most likely to be approached is a care assistant or an auxiliary, one of the many people who do the most basic and intimate of nursing duties for helpless patients. Someone close to them is what people need, someone who is on their own level, not too high-and-mighty, but approachable. And carers are nearly always women. On the whole, they are kindly, compassionate and humble. They work for the lowest of low wages, and are completely taken for granted by hospital managers. But they are the women to whom fear-ridden patients will often turn, for assurance, consolation and comfort at the time of death.

On that day, Mr Anderson returned to the ward a couple of hours later than usual, and sank into bed, exhausted. I was furious that he had over-stretched himself in that silly office, and resolved to have a word with the Chief.

Throughout the afternoon Mr Anderson slept, sometimes wincing in pain – we could see him curling up his body in an attempt to ease it – but still he slept on. He stirred as we were doing the six o'clock drug round, and sat up looking refreshed. Suppers were served at seven o'clock, and he ate without nausea or discomfort. I began to revise my opinion about the office work he was doing.

After supper is usually a good time to talk to people. The ward is quiet, the day's activities are stilled, the light is changing, and the human heart and mind seem to change with it. Mr Anderson was sitting up in bed, watching the sun sink behind the trees. It was a reddish sunset, with bands of fluffy pink clouds. Mr Anderson appeared relaxed, and I thought, with a leap of the heart, that perhaps the radium might effect a complete cure. Spontaneous recovery from cancer *is* possible, and whilst no one can explain what happens, I have seen it.

It can be a bit awkward talking to someone in the middle of a hospital ward. You have to sit close, and talk very softly. It is no good asking a patient to come to the office; that is too formal, and very often the person is tongue-tied in such a situation. No, the bedside is usually the right place, and the right moment can only be judged by intuition. I pulled the curtains around his bed and sat on the edge. He moved his legs over so that I could sit more comfortably, which was encouraging, because it indicated that I was welcome.

'It's a lovely evening,' I said, 'a lovely sunset.'

'Beautiful. I would like to go on to the balcony to see it better, but I can't be bothered to make the effort just now.'

'I could help you.'

He smiled. 'No, it's not worth it. The sun will be gone by the time we get there.'

'You are looking very much brighter this evening.'

'Well, I did a good morning's work. Excellent, in fact.'

'It obviously does you good. I thought it had tired you too much, but I was wrong.'

'I have always needed to exert myself – it's just the way I'm made. If I could get rid of this damned cancer by sheer will power and exertion, I would do so.'

'You are having radium treatment, that will limit the growth. And a positive outlook, such as yours, will help a great deal. We don't think you will be able to go trekking in the Himalayas, but Wales, or the Wye Valley, as the Chief suggested, could be possible.'

'That's encouraging. I will hold on to that one, Sister. The Wye – a bit of rough canoeing, wonderful, and some climbing – oh, I'd love that.'

'Perhaps you should cancel your Himalayan trek and concentrate your thoughts on the Wye Valley.'

'Why not? I will get my secretary to order the maps from Stanford's tomorrow.'

His eyes sparkled with eagerness, and as I looked at the wasted muscles that could not find the energy to step on to the balcony to see the sunset, I pondered the phenomenon of hope.

Hope is the one thing that people never lose, and even though they may know that they are dying, hope never deserts them. Most people hope for a new breakthrough in medical research, a new drug, a new treatment, a miracle cure, and we have to encourage this, however unrealistic it may be. But hope does not preclude an acceptance of death, and it can come in many forms.

Most doctors believe that they must never allow a patient to give up hope of a cure. The implication of this is that the medical profession is the single source of hope. This is too narrow a definition. Hope is an abstract concept, and is by no means confined to physical cure. Hope means something different to each one of us. Hope to see a daughter married, or a grandchild born, can keep life buoyant and content for weeks, or even months, beyond the realistic expectations of a medical prognosis. Many people, knowing they have cancer, have done the most extraordinary things: run marathons, cycled halfway round the globe, written books, taken degrees. Hope, directed towards an achievement, is the driving spirit, and makes the future endurable. Belief in an afterlife is also hope.

'The Wye Valley will be lovely in a few weeks' time with the spring coming,' said Mr Anderson dreamily. 'You know, when I first suspected I had cancer, I simply did not believe it. They've got it wrong, I thought. I had always been healthy, and led a healthy life. I couldn't have cancer, not at my age. I thought it must be a misdiagnosis and I was furious with the doctors.'

'Did anyone tell you?'

'No. Lies, half lies, evasions, silences – that's all I ever got. It's an insult to one's intelligence.'

'How did you discover?'

'When I came here – I knew what radium treatment is for.'

I was silent. It was so obvious, so irrefutable.

'And no one has talked to you about it until now?'

'No. Far from dispelling my fears, the lies and evasions only added to my certainty.'

'How did you react?'

'When I saw the fearful condition of some of the other men in the ward, I decided that I must kill myself. I never want to get to that stage. Never.'

'Suicide is not easy,' I said.

'No, it's not. And you know something? I don't think I have the guts. There is a window upstairs, thirty feet up, with concrete underneath. For many days I thought "I could do it today, there's no one around. A quick jump and it will all be over." But each day

I hesitated – "Not now. This afternoon perhaps, or tomorrow." And then I realised I just didn't have the guts.'

'It's not a question of guts,' I said, 'most suicides are associated with mental illness, and you don't strike me as being mentally ill. You're a realist.'

'I like to think so. But I cannot face the reality of the last stages of this pitiless disease. If I get to that stage I will want someone to polish me off.'

I didn't say that nobody realises they are getting to that stage, because by that time they are incapable of recognising it. Instead I said:

'You are having radium now. The side effects can be very severe, which is why you feel so ill and exhausted. But you must believe me, it *is* destroying the cancer cells in your body.'

'I do believe you. That's what keeps me going. I feel ghastly, but I have a mental picture of the cancer cells being bombarded with radium and giving up. It's a battle. Them or me. And I intend to win.'

'That's the spirit,' I said, enthusiastically.

'It's a fight to the death and I am a realist – you said that yourself. I have always had to fight, from my early childhood, and I always win.'

Some people are like that – failure is never a possibility – but I said, 'You would make it easier for yourself if you rested more.'

'I don't want anything to be "easier",' he said scornfully. 'Life is not easy – never has been. I don't go for the easy option.'

The night nurses were coming on duty. I had to go. He squeezed my hand.

'I'm glad we had this talk. I feel better for it.'

'And I'm glad too. I must tell the Chief about it when I see him.'

I slipped off the edge of the bed.

'I hope you have a good night. What about some sleeping tablets?'

He shook his head.

★

The following morning, when I came on duty at eight o'clock, he was up and dressed in his suit. He looked very thin, but smart. He had taken no breakfast, but had asked for strong coffee. I was not happy about this, and questioned him.

'Don't fuss me,' he said. 'I have work to do, and I must keep my head clear.'

It was the same response he always gave to the idea of analgesics, and was the changeless resolve of a very determined man.

Mr Anderson spent longer each day in his broom cupboard. The pattern became regular, and how he found the strength to work as he did we never knew. His nights were not restful because of the pain, but he always rose at 6 a.m., bathed and shaved and dressed, although the effort required was enormous. He went to his office at about 7 a.m. and returned to the ward at two, looking half dead with exhaustion. We did not know what he was doing, but something seemed to have taken possession of him, and was driving him on.

I told the Chief about our conversation, and he was not really surprised. He talked with Mr Anderson, who was nearing the sixth week of his treatment, and they agreed that he should then take a holiday and return to the Marie Curie for check-ups two or three months later.

The day of his discharge was quite emotional. We had all grown to respect him so much that his rather aloof ways did not matter; they were just part of his character. He tied up the loose ends in his office and asked Matron if it could be left undisturbed, because he might need it later, to which request she readily agreed. We knew that he was going walking and climbing, but from the way he looked, that would require a miracle. He was so painfully thin, his legs and shoulders had no muscle at all, and his face looked haggard.

'Do look after yourself, you might fall or something,' a nurse said as he was leaving. He gave her a roguish grin, irresistible to women.

'Now what have I got to lose?' he replied. 'Tell me that.'

She couldn't reply, but said: 'We are going to miss you.'

'You're a sweet girl. You all are, and I have grown very fond of you.'

He kissed a couple of the girls, and then turned to Matron. He hesitated for a fraction of a second – the navy blue uniform, the silver buckle, the high collar, the white cuffs, the frilly cap, were a touch intimidating for any man. Would he, wouldn't he? He did. Cheered on by the nurses he kissed Matron, who blushed as pink as a peony.

Mr Anderson returned looking a lot better. He was tanned from the fresh air and sunshine, and although he had not noticeably gained weight, his muscles were stronger. He told us that he had started his walking with a paltry five miles a day, which was exhausting, but day by day he improved on this until he could manage twenty miles without too much fatigue.

'And what about the rough canoeing?' I enquired.

'That also. It was a great help, having lost so much weight. You need to be light to shoot the rapids of the Wye.'

'Wasn't it dangerous?' asked a nurse.

'Yes, but that's half the fun. And if you've got nothing to lose but a life that's on borrowed time, you can do anything. I took far more risks than anyone else. It was great.'

He laughed in a devil-may-care way. 'Now I've got to get back to work. There is a good deal to be completed still.'

Blood and serum tests were taken, and a series of X-rays. The Chief was so impressed by the apparent reduction in the size of the growth, and especially in the improvement in the patient's general health, that he thought we could risk a further series of radium treatments. Normally, one has to limit the radiation because the effects on the body are so debilitating.

Mr Anderson was re-admitted, and his previous working pattern resumed. The effects of the radium were quickly evident, and the poor man became very weak and ill, but still he carried on going to his broom cupboard. It was pathetic, yet inspiring. There was no point in telling him to rest more; he took no notice.

The Chief had decided on a ten-week course of radium, which was longer than is usually ordered, and could easily kill a person, but they had discussed it, and Mr Anderson had declared that, by sheer strength of will, he would overcome the side effects. He was determined to go fell running in Cumbria, and the Chief felt sure he could manage this, although it is notoriously difficult and dangerous.

During the next two years Mr Anderson worked like a man possessed, in his city office during the months after he had been discharged, and in the broom cupboard when he was in hospital. He never let up. Work was punctuated by strenuous holidays – he walked the 190 miles of the Pennines in seven days; he climbed the Welsh mountains, including Mount Snowdon; he went frequently to Scotland, determined to climb each of the Munros and the Cairngorms. He did more in two years than the majority of us will do in a lifetime.

And it was not the cancer that killed Mr Anderson. It was the Cairngorms. In the mountain ranges, the weather can change from sunshine to blizzards in a few hours. Mysterious things can happen on those remote heights; perhaps he saw a beckoning hand, or heard a beguiling voice, luring him towards danger. 'There's nothing to lose,' was always his spur. He had flirted with Death for so long that he almost loved Her. As he fell in the snow, and his body temperature dropped, his senses would have become numb and easeful rest would have seduced him to a sleep from which he did not waken. He had not wanted to die in a hospital bed, and the cold and the snow had saved him . . .

The mystery of what had been going on in the broom cupboard was later revealed. Through a combination of hard work, speculation and professional expertise Mr Anderson had accumulated millions of pounds. Every penny of it was left to Cancer Research.

POOR VAN GOGH

What poor Van Gogh needed
was a little pill,
or perhaps not that pill
but a different little pill,
or perhaps a different one again
for a month, for a year, for life,
or perhaps a combination
of little pills, try this one, try that one,
try that one and another together,
lots of little pills perhaps he needed,
a thousand pounds' worth,
ten thousand pounds' worth,
half a million pounds' worth
given the research costs
and the cost of Public Relations
and the expectations of shareholders,

then poor Vincent could have
given up painting masterpieces
and vanished without trace
into old age.

— *David Hart*
From *Running Out* (Five Seasons Press, 2006)

SOCIAL ATTITUDES TO DEATH

Most people die in hospitals and not at home any more. This seems to be largely expected, and it feeds our fear. We shy away from closeness to a dying person, and from seeing the body, and, even if the relatives are there, in the hospital at the time, the body will be quickly whisked away and never seen again. Many people have no contact, before, during or after the event.

Yet basic, primitive and stark, hidden behind a curtain, death remains, and human imagination cannot resist it. We need to take a little peek now and then, and so we lift a corner of the curtain to get that frisson mingled with fear. The media know this and feed our desire by showing violent death in all its detail. The producers seem determined to show the most horrifying and bloody pictures. And this is as much as most people see, or want to see, of death.

Some producers have tried to show, realistically, on television how people die, and, on a couple of occasions, have actually filmed a man whilst he is dying. I am not sure whether this is helpful or not. It certainly shows that dying is not a time of physical pain or mental distress, but of peace and quietness. This is probably reassuring to some people. But, on the other hand, it is only a 'virtual reality'. But perhaps that is what people want. The idea of filming a man dying quietly in his bed so that viewers can get an impression of what goes on is no doubt praiseworthy, but, of reality, they will see virtually nothing.

Only those who have been close to the dying and seen death in all its awesome mystery can get a glimpse of what it is about – and even then only a glimpse. The whole picture includes a spiritual dimension. God is not in the churches, or the mosques or synagogues. He resides not in temples and minarets. God is not the possession of priests or rabbis or mullahs. God is at the deathbed, tenderly drawing the living soul from the dying body. God is in the grief and suffering of those who are left behind, who catch a glimpse, perhaps for a few fleeting seconds, of what life and death are all about.

Reality is not to be found in a television screen. The closeness to real death means, inevitably, closeness to our mortality and questions about the divine. Perhaps this is too much to take. If we can find no spirituality in life, death is an uncomfortable reminder of a missing dimension.

We have to go to a very different society and mingle with a people closer to nature to see a more realistic approach to death. In southern Morocco, in 2007, I was invited by a young Moslem woman to take tea with her family in her home. We entered a hole in the wall and went down a long, dark passage towards a dim light and into a tiny kitchen. There was a central place for a wood fire on the floor, and a hole in the ceiling let out the smoke and also let in the daylight. We went from the kitchen to a large room, about thirty feet by twenty. A beautiful carpet lay on the mud floor, and around the walls cushions were scattered on the floor for seating. High windows let in the daylight and oil lamps stood on low tables. Silk hangings adorned the high walls. The room was both elegant and beautiful. There was no upstairs, so this one space, plus kitchen, was home for the entire family. Other women and children came in, eager to see the stranger in their midst. The lady of the house, in good French, invited me to sit down whilst she made the tea. The cushions were very low, and I was apprehensive about sitting down in case I made an exhibition of myself trying to get up again! Seeing what at first I thought were some higher cushions I walked towards them. The lady must have read my mind or, if not, it is as well she spoke when she did.

'That is my grandmother. She is nearly a hundred years old. She is near the end of her life, and Allah will come for her soon.'

A woman was cooking, another feeding a baby, children were running around, and an old woman was dying. This is the realistic acceptance of death. The children will take it in their stride, as children always do, and as they grow up they will look upon death as a natural part of life. They had probably seen birth in that room and, without being told, had absorbed the fact that birth, life and death are all part of the whole.

But *we* cannot see this. We are too busy 'getting and spending'. The hush and momentary time-stop of the deathbed plays no part in the rush and perpetual motion of our busy lives. 'Death? What is it to us? We want to live, live, live – don't be morbid. We want sex, fun, sensations – don't be a bore. We want money, careers, possessions – don't be a drag. Friends, relationships, travel – these are the things we want. Death doesn't come into it. Go away!'

Each of us is going to die, whether we like it or not, but it only hinders acceptance of the fact if we never come near it. If we could see the infinite variety of emotions, insights, experiences and delight in little things that are granted to people as they approach the end, if we knew how human understanding and love can grow and flower in the last stages of life, if we witnessed the peace and tranquillity that is given to us in the last hours before death, we would be less afraid.

The Berber children saw the tranquillity of death in that sun-baked room in Morocco. But we seem to think that our children should be shielded from it. 'He is too young to be told. It would upset him,' I have heard. And on another occasion, ironically from a professed atheist, 'We didn't know what to tell her, so we said that Granny has gone away to live with the angels in the sky.' This sort of over-protection is misplaced. Another generation will grow up, remote from reality, and they, in turn, will want no contact with death or the dying. Parents who think they are shielding their children from something unpleasant are ensuring that, when their own time comes, they will be left to die alone.

Yet children are increasingly exposed to violent death on film, television and computer games. They have a morbid fascination for horror and many are allowed unrestricted access to these sources, so they are able to see people carving each other up, and inflicting unimaginable suffering. And this is the generation of children whose parents imagine they are too tender to be exposed to natural death. What an irony!

Many years ago Anthony Bloom, Metropolitan Archbishop of the Russian Orthodox Church in England, played an important role in my life. He said that, when he first came to this country, the thing that horrified him the most was the attitude to death that he encountered. As a Russian, he came from a nation and a church where death was a normal part of life, something we all have to face, something known, seen and accepted. But, in this country, he was shocked to find that death was almost regarded as an indecency, provoking the most profound embarrassment, and certainly not a subject to be talked about. To his surprise and dismay, he found that meaningful contact with death was comparatively rare.

He said that he visited an English family where a much-loved grandmother had died at home. The family was grieving, but the children were not around. He asked where they were, and was told that they had been sent away because they should not see 'that sort of thing'. In surprise he asked, 'But why not?' It was the father's turn to be shocked. He said it was quite unthinkable. The children knew what death was because they had seen it when a rabbit had been killed and half eaten by dogs in the garden, and they had been terribly upset. He and his wife had agreed that they must be sent away because they might have wandered into Granny's room while she was dying or, which would have been far more upsetting for them, when she was actually dead. Such a possibility could not be countenanced.

Did these parents really mean to leave their children with the idea that their grandmother was now like the dead rabbit, savaged by dogs? Children are highly imaginative. They would have sensed that something was wrong in the looks passing between adults, the hushed voices, the unfinished sentences – the 'not in front of the children'. Or worse, they might have been told silly lies about their grandmother's condition, which they would neither believe nor understand. Finally, to be sent away at a time of family crisis would have alarmed and frightened them. Their imaginations would have been inflamed, and they might have invented all sorts of lurid tales about the thing that was happening to Granny that was so terrible they were not allowed to see it.

In being kept away, they were denied seeing the true mystery and nobility of death, which any child can understand. They were not allowed to see their grandmother's slow decline, nor see her lying quiet and still, nor feel the aura of calm and peace, in fact, holiness, that surrounds the newly dead. They were left to invent their own frightening stories.

And when they returned home, Granny would be gone, with no last days in which to tell her they loved her, no chance to say goodbye, no time to adjust, no funeral – just gone.

David Hackett, consultant cardiologist, is the clinical editor of this book. His wife, Penny, is a nurse and the family is Irish. I was sitting one fine spring morning in their big kitchen with its wide windows overlooking the gently rolling fields and woods of Hertfordshire, talking about this book. It was half term and the children were home from school.

He said, 'When my mother-in-law died in 2005, in Ireland, she was laid out in the front room, which was the custom. Family and neighbours came in to pay their respects and to say goodbye. My children came, too, to see and to touch their grandmother. I don't think it upset them.'

I turned to the two children. 'Did you find it scary, seeing your dead grandmother?'

The boy, aged about thirteen, gave me one of those teenage looks that suggests, 'Here's another silly grown-up asking silly questions!' The girl, two years older, spoke: 'Well, no ... no, not really ... just ...' She shrugged, then after a moment's thought: 'Just sort of ordinary. She looked ... well ... sort of asleep. Sort of ... peaceful, like.'

She looked towards her brother and he nodded, 'Hmm, yeah,' and carried on chewing his toast – I like a man of few words!

Obviously neither of them had been upset, much less traumatised, as some people might predict.

I was having lunch with an old friend, Mark. We were talking about my forthcoming book and he suddenly said:

'My mother died in 1950 and we children were never told.'

They learned, many years later, that their mother, Julia, had developed phlebitis, apparently after the birth of her fourth baby. A clot had dislodged itself, travelled in the bloodstream, and blocked a pulmonary artery, and this had killed her.

Mark was nine at the time. His brother Robert was six and their sister Marian was four and a half. There was also a baby called Fiona, who was about a year old. They are now in their sixties and I have spoken to them all recently.

Both men told me that they could remember an ambulance coming to the house and taking their mother away. Some time afterwards (they cannot remember how long) family friends took the two boys on holiday, to the seaside. It was during this period, they have since concluded, that their mother died and the funeral must have taken place. At the end of the holiday their father joined them, and took them home to a house with no mummy.

Mark said, 'It was very quiet, very bleak, and we didn't understand why.'

Robert said, 'There was a sort of black hole that we couldn't talk about. No one said we were not allowed to, but you know how children pick up messages. We just knew that it was something the grown-ups wouldn't approve of us talking about.'

I said, 'Didn't you ask questions?'

They had received vague, woolly answers, such as 'Mummy's gone to Heaven.' Later, one of the boys asked where Marian was, and was told that she had gone to stay with Grandma.

Marian tells me she remembers it very clearly as a time of great unhappiness. Her grandmother was rather a remote figure. She says, 'I was lonely, bewildered, wondering all the time why I was there and not at home. Daddy came to see me from time to time, and then he went away again. But he never brought mummy, and

I didn't know why. I thought perhaps I had been naughty and she didn't want to see me.'

After about six months or more her father came and took her home. Apparently she ran around the house looking in every room, calling out, 'Where's Mummy? Where is she?' Her father said, 'Mummy's gone to Heaven.' She responded, 'Well, where's Heaven? How did she get there? Did you take her? Why don't you go and get her back?'

Eventually, she became aware, as her brothers had earlier, that it was something you just didn't ask questions about.

Childhood grief is beyond my competence to discuss, but other writers have spoken about the loss of a mother being devastating to development. Fears and fantasies, depression, endless searching, low self-esteem, low achievement in school, a solitary child who cannot form friendships – these and many more psychological disturbances have all been discussed. Feelings of guilt and self-reproach also come into it.

Mark said to me, 'I felt that it was all my fault, and I couldn't admit it to Robert and Marian. You see, I was the eldest, and I was a "naughty boy". I was always doing something that "upset" my mother. And I thought I must have done something really bad, and she had got so upset that she had gone away and wouldn't come back, and so I was to blame.'

Marian said, 'While I was with Granny I thought I was being punished for something I had done wrong.' At the time she was only four years old.

'The death of a mother is devastating for any child,' added Robert, 'but I am sure that the silence made it ten times worse for us.'

But I was forgetting; Julia left four children, not just three. What had happened to baby Fiona, from whom the older three were separated? She had been looked after by an aunt and uncle, and eventually they adopted her into their family.

Fiona told me that she was too young to remember the time of Julia's death, and grew up in her adoptive family thinking that Mark, Marian and Robert were her cousins. Fiona understood this was considered to be the best solution, as she was so young. She did remember being told the story of Julia who had died, but did not relate it to herself.

'So when did you find out?' I asked.

'When I was twenty-one and needed access to a full birth certificate for a visa. For years, I felt constrained about discussing the past; it is only since my parents have died that I have felt free to talk about it.'

During that memorable lunch with Mark, he said, 'I can see now that I have been searching for something all my life and never found it.' The moment was deeply sad, and I did not know what to say.

The social taboo surrounding death is deep-seated, and it is most unhealthy. How has it developed? How has it sneaked up on us? The Victorians and Edwardians used to wallow in their death scenes and funerals. Why has the pendulum swung so far the other way, so that a death is neither seen nor mentioned?

I have a theory (which deserves further research) that it started after the First World War (1914–1918) when eight and a half million young men worldwide died in battle, when twenty-one million were maimed or mutilated and when upwards of forty million died in the flu epidemic of 1918. And the carnage didn't end there. The bloodiest century in history killed up to half a billion men, women and children. Everyone was so sickened by death and loss and grieving that perhaps they just couldn't take any more. So they turned their backs, and thus started the climate of denial that inhibits us to this day.

Man was made for Joy & Woe;
And when this we rightly know
Thro' the world we safely go.
Joy & Woe are woven fine,
A Clothing for the Soul divine;
Under every grief & pine
Runs a joy with silken twine.

— William Blake, *Auguries of Innocence*

GRIEF

Cycling in south-west Ireland has been one of the loveliest experiences of my later years. The further south and the further west you go, the more remote it becomes. Hills and sky and clouds blend into the blue-grey distance. Gullies, streams and rivulets meander down to the ever-present sea. Lochs, still and grey as the granite of the hills, lie secretive and cold as ice. Cycling – meandering, really – on unmapped roads you pass through tiny villages of about fifty houses, hamlets each containing no more than four or five buildings, or remote dwellings set into a hillside, almost indistinguishable from the hill.

I recall once, passing a church. It was quite small, and in no way beautiful, but the church in its setting, with the graveyard all around it, and the hills, multi-coloured in the changing light, was so arresting that I had to stop, just to sit and gaze.

As I looked, the door of the church opened and a priest, wearing full Roman Catholic vestments, emerged. He made his way solemnly down a gravel path to the graveyard. He was followed by an acolyte, bearing the cross; followed by eight small boys in white cassocks; followed by two larger boys holding candles; followed by another acolyte, swinging his censer from side to side; followed by yet another acolyte, carrying the book of service; followed by a coffin, carried by eight men wearing black; followed by an elderly woman in darkest black, and veiled; followed by eight or ten younger men and women, all in black, with their children carrying flowers; followed by about a hundred men, women and children in everyday clothes, most of them carrying flowers.

The procession made its way down the path to a newly dug grave, covered by three trestle boards upon which the coffin was placed. The people gathered around the grave – the immediate family stood closest to the priest and his acolytes, the others scattered further away. The priest read the office of burial, responses were made, a hymn was sung, and the trestle boards were removed. As the coffin was lowered into the earth, the priest sprinkled holy water on it, and many people threw in flowers. Two men with shovels came forward and heaved the soil on to the coffin. Everyone stood silently, and, when the job was done, they laid their wreaths on the new grave. People gathered around the widow and her family, and the whole entourage made its way towards the church hall. At which point, I slipped away.

You've got to hand it to the Catholics – they sure know how to do a funeral!

But what do *we* get in this age of fast foods, faster living and instant entertainment? Twenty minutes in the aseptic atmosphere of a crematorium, piped music, electronically moved doors and curtains, a speech prepared by a stranger, ever present morticians, discreetly keeping things ticking over and on time. When the coffin slides out of sight, they ensure that the mourners are quickly led away, orderly, neatly, to make room for the next funeral party which is waiting outside. This is but a mockery of a funeral, as far as I am concerned. And who loses out? Not the dead; it is of no interest to them. But it is important for those who are left behind – those who grieve. They are the ones for whom the banishment of ritual can be so damaging.

Human beings need ritual; we need sacraments and symbols and ceremonies. We need the bell that tolls a solemn note, and a prescribed formality fitting for the occasion. We need somewhere to lay the flowers or tokens of remembrance. It does not have to be a burial; a cremation is just as good – better, in some ways. It is the solemn ritual before and after that is so important.

Nothing is more shattering than the death of a child, and often the parents never get over it. Early in 2008 I was shopping in our local high street when I suddenly became aware that everyone was looking behind me. I turned around and saw the approach of two magnificent white horses, drawing a carriage. Their dressage was white, and beautiful white and silver plumes adorned their heads.

The coachman wore silver grey. As the white and silver carriage drew closer, then passed us, we saw that it was not a carriage, but a beautiful glass bier, upon which lay a tiny white coffin about three feet long adorned with white lilies. The bier was followed by four funeral cars with blackened windows. The contrast was startling – shining white for the dead child and blackest black for the parents and those who mourned. The greater the grief, the greater the need for ritual.

Everyone in the street stood quite still whilst the cortège slowly passed on its way to the church at the end of the road. The parents must have seen (though we could not see them) the people standing quietly in the street, and I hope that the respect we showed was of some comfort to them. I looked around the crowd and was impressed by the solemnity on all the faces. That experience was what I would call community ritual, something I had not seen for years.

Community ritual has largely been stripped away, and I doubt if the majority of young people would know what I am talking about. Social life used to stop for a funeral, as everybody paused in their daily affairs out of respect for the dead.

I remember well the death of my grandmother, when I was about twelve. She had a heart attack at home and died in her husband's arms. Her body was laid out by the local handywoman, who was also the local midwife, and placed in an open coffin in the main room for friends and neighbours to come in and pay their respects. This was common practice. It may seem gruesome now, but in those days practically everyone felt it was right and fitting to go to the house with the purpose of seeing the body. They would stand quietly beside the open coffin, offer some suitable words of condolence to the bereaved, and perhaps reflect for a few minutes on life and death and their own mortality (nothing concentrates the mind so powerfully as the sight of a dead body). This is still practised on state occasions and on the death of royalty. It is a practice that is also routine in the Orthodox Church.

On the day of my grandmother's funeral, the street was quiet. Every house had the curtains drawn and neighbours stood in their doorways as the funeral procession passed on its way to the church. Shopkeepers closed their shops for a while, and this ritual greatly helped my grandfather. I know, because he told me so. 'She was treated with proper respect,' he said. Afterwards, he did not have to hide his grief because neighbours understood and gathered round to support him. He lived alone for twelve years after her death, but was never lonely.

For many years afterwards the whole family gathered at Grandad's house on her birthday and took flowers to her grave. I remember my uncles and aunts, a noisy bunch, joking their way through the woods to her graveside, where we all sang her favourite hymn. Then we all walked back to the house for a party. For my grandfather, this continued family ritual was just as important as the rituals at the time of her death.

Bereavement can be a devastating event. Dark clouds seem to cover the face of the earth. Reality evaporates and movement is suspended. An abyss of despair seems but a step away. The experience is very much eased if you have had the time to prepare for it, but there is no preparation for sudden or violent death and the shock that comes with it. The distress can be so traumatic it can lead to illness, and if the relative has to go to the mortuary to identify the body, particularly if it has been mutilated, the trauma can go on for years. There is always the question, 'Why? Why did God allow it? There can be no God if such a thing can happen.' Rage, hatred, and bitterness can burn or corrode, and often there is anger. Usually, God has to take all the blame, even from people who don't believe in Him. Depression can follow, and years of professional counselling may be necessary. If true clinical depression develops, anti-depressant and psychiatric drugs are often prescribed: but this is not always the best way of treating a severe response to a life event.

In bereavement, only time – occasionally years of time – can heal and allow the person to start living again. It is a time of emotional crisis, and the greatest need is for companionship – not all the while, just someone to be there from time to time to listen, talk, occasionally to hold a hand, or even to take over for a while. But sadly most people, especially elderly widows, find themselves isolated and edged out of society if they have no man to accompany them. Most of us are so screwed up about death that we cannot even bring ourselves to *talk* to someone in mourning and the feeling of abandonment compounds the loneliness that inevitably follows the loss of a life partner or loved one.

Consequently, the bereaved will often try to hide their grief in a number of ways. They try to be cheerful and pretend everything is all right when, really, they are breaking apart inside and only want to cry and cry. Suppressing grief is a recipe for disaster and many people who act in this way suffer physical or mental ill-health at a later date.

Society has changed so much in the last fifty years. Families are smaller and move about more, communities barely exist – a group of strangers thrown together cannot be described as a community. Counsellors take the place of friends and neighbours, and bereavement groups replace communities. These are vitally important, and some have described them as lifesavers – 'I don't think I would be alive now if it had not been for my counsellor'. All hospices, NHS hospitals, most local councils, and most churches run bereavement groups in which people can sit and talk about their loved ones – and simply talking about the departed is frequently all that is needed. Such groups are important, because someone who has already suffered and recovered from a devastating loss can communicate meaningfully with others in the same position.

To be present at the time of death can be one of the most important moments in life. To see those last, awesome minutes of transition from life into death can only be described as a spiritual experience. And then afterwards, when the body lies still, one gets the strange feeling that the person has simply gone away, as though he has said, 'I'm just going into the other room. I'll leave that thing there while I'm gone; I won't be needing it.' It's a very odd experience – the body is there, but the person has gone. No one would say, 'I *am* a body'; we say, 'I *have* a body'. So what, therefore, is the 'I'? The

'I' or perhaps 'me' has just stepped into the other room. It is a strange feeling, and I can't describe it in any other way. Another thing that is strange is that the body left behind looks smaller, quite a lot smaller, than the living person. The face looks the same, but calm and relaxed, wrinkles and worry lines are smoothed, and a feeling of serenity pervades the entire room. But the person, the 'I', has gone.

It also greatly helps the process of mourning to see the body after death, and preferably to assist in the laying out. Nurses used to do the job when I was young girl, and we always asked the relatives if they wanted to help. Nurses don't do it any more, but anyone can ask the morticians if they can assist, and they will not be refused, even though it would be unusual these days. Respectful laying-out is all part of the ritual to which a dead person is entitled. Handling a dead body is not a repugnant or frightening experience and, somehow, it helps to accept the fact that the soul of that person has gone if you treat the body with reverence and respect before it is finally disposed of by cremation or burial.

The husband of one of my dearest friends died in hospital of lung cancer, but she was with him most of the time in the last few weeks. She told me, 'I was with him, and I could see that he was going to die, so I pulled the curtains round and lay on the bed beside him. I took him in my arms (he weighed almost nothing, he was so thin) and whispered to him and kissed him. He knew I was there. Then he just stopped breathing, but I didn't move. I stayed there with him until he was quite cold. Then I got up and went to one of the nurses and told them that he had gone. The nurse came to check, and touched him.

'"But he's quite cold," she said. "When did he die?"

'"It was at half past two – I know because I looked at my watch."

'"But you should have come and called one of the staff; it's nearly four o'clock now," the nurse said.

'"No, I wanted to be alone with him, quietly, lovingly, giving him time for his soul to leave his body."

'"This is most unusual," remarked the nurse, and gave me a very funny look. But I didn't care what anyone thought. I knew that he was safely on his way to wherever we go after we die, and I left the hospital, happy.'

Counsellors tell me that, increasingly, they encounter guilt associated with grief in bereavement. This is often because most people die in hospitals and not at home, and those left behind feel they have let the loved one down. They feel a sense of shame that he or she died alone, in the care of strangers. In my own life, I know that I still feel guilty, after thirty years, that my poor mother died alone, even though I also know that I was forcibly prevented by a couple of strong orderlies from entering the resuscitation room in which she died. In contrast, in 1996, my mother-in-law died at home in her daughter's arms, and she described this as a beautiful, peaceful death. My sister-in-law was very close to her mother, but her bereavement has been eased by the knowledge that she did her duty, with love, right to the end. When talking about it, she repeatedly uses the word 'beautiful'.

Many hospitals, and all hospices, now try to offer support to enable people to die at home. Support for the relatives, I mean, because it is not always easy, especially if the last stages of illness are prolonged. To be able to die at home is what most people want and, if it is possible, close relatives want it also. There have been many attempts to reverse the national trend towards a hospitalised death in recent years, such as the National End of Life Care Programme, the Liverpool Care Pathway, the Gold Standard for the Care of the Dying. Every hospital trust now has such a policy in place.

Charles, an old friend of mine, died at home in December 2005. His wife, Dorothy, was with him.

Talking with a widow shortly after her husband's death can be a moving experience. There is no pretence, no effort to make an impression, just the loss and the depth of memories. Sentences are broken, disjointed, started and not finished. Thoughts are random. I will use Dorothy's own words as I wrote them down:

'He had prostate cancer twelve years ago, but recovered, and was active till nearly the end ... but in July I could see that he was going down in health ... he had no pain ... it was a big effort for him to do anything ... no pain ... just weariness ... he didn't realise at the time that he was dying ... the pain only started on Sunday ... perhaps the cancer had come back ... I don't know ... the Macmillan nurses came and he had morphine patches ... slow release, you know ... very good, very effective ... on Thursday he was worse, and he said "I think I am dying" ... I said, "Don't worry, I am with you and will stay with you" ... but on Friday he was bright and breezy ... until the last day he went to the lavatory by himself, with a Zimmer frame, you know ... and he shaved himself ... his hand was steady ... the weather was beautiful, really beautiful ... he went to the window and looked at the sun on the garden and said, "The world has never seemed more beautiful ... I want to take a photograph, and you can remember our last days" ... I fetched his camera, and he took five pictures ... I have them here ... they are beautiful ... then he went back to bed ... he never got up again ... he knew he was dying ... he had said many times, "If I have to go into hospital I will find a way of killing myself" ... I had already promised him that he would not, because I would look after him ... the doctor came that day and said he would probably live another two or three weeks but I said no, he is dying ... I can see it in his eyes ... Friday night he wanted no supper, and he wouldn't drink, either ... it was a terrible struggle to get him to take even a few sips of water ... I could see by his eyes he was going, and I called the children ... I have a son, three daughters and six grandchildren ... One of them said she would stay with him during the night, whilst I got some sleep ... at three o'clock she woke me up and said, "He is dying, you are right, his breathing is very slow, he is going" ... I held him, saying over and over again, "Go in peace, don't worry, you are safe, go in peace" ... I kept saying these things all the time ... he heard me and understood ... he knew he was dying ... his breathing was getting slower ... slowly, slowly, he went away ... After that I didn't leave him ... he was not conscious, but I kept saying, "Go in peace, my love, don't worry, everything is all right, go in peace" ... and slowly, slowly, he went away ... and his breathing stopped at eleven thirty in the morning ... it was a beautiful day, the sun was streaming through the window ... it was a beautiful death, too ... we laid him out ... a day or two later I found a note in the drawer of the cupboard beside his bed ... it read, "I hope the love I have for you will linger on and support you through the last years which I had so longed to share with you ... " (She showed me the note, written in spindly, shaking handwriting.) ... he must have written that for me a few days before he died ... so you see, he knew he was dying ... we were married fifty-two years ... it was a perfect ending ... I am not sad ... lonely, yes, but not sad.'

Then Dorothy told me that one of her daughters arrived with her son, a boy of thirteen, after the death had occurred. The boy said, 'I want to go into the bedroom to be with Grandfather for a while. Don't come in, any of you. I just want to be by myself, alone with him.' He shut the door, and ten minutes later, quietly and solemnly, came out. But he never said a word about his thoughts and feelings.

That boy showed a maturity and wisdom beyond his years. He faced up to death in the only way that is meaningful – by being close to it. It was an act of love, but also an act of sound common sense, which some instinct told him was necessary. He voluntarily drew close to death, and was not afraid, an experience that will stay with him as he grows and matures.

The last words of the last monastic office of the day are, 'Lord, grant us a quiet night and a perfect end.' It is something that we can all pray for, but it is something that we can in no way command, because, at the end we are entirely dependent on the love and goodness of others.

The turning point in many lives is bereavement. Many have channelled their grief into activities for public benefit, and this has helped them transform bad into good. For example: Philip Lawrence, headmaster, was murdered outside his school in 1995, while trying to defend one of his pupils from an attack by a gang from another school. His widow set up an award scheme for good citizenship by young people, and works towards this aim.

In 1863, after her four-year-old daughter fell downstairs and broke her neck, Josephine Butler started working with young girls dragged into prostitution, and her lifelong work led to the repeal of the Contagious Diseases Act in 1886. There have been many examples of courageous and life-changing activities of lasting value inspired by the trauma of bereavement.

Facing death induces us to see life through new eyes; our perspective is altered, sometimes profoundly. Most of us live a headlong existence, so we are too busy to question the meaning of life. Suddenly all is changed, all our values are open to question and doubt. Even those who are non-believers begin to search for answers to questions like, 'What is the meaning of life?' 'Why are we here?' 'What is life?' 'What is death?' Bereavement leads some of us to think that there must be more to life than that which is concrete and visible, and we find there is a larger, deeper purpose than we had ever suspected. For some, asking these questions, even though there can be no positive answers, can transform their whole way of living.

STROKE

Mrs Doherty's life, for many years, had been perfect, she told all her friends and neighbours. 'Who could ask for more at my age? I'm in good health, I am independent, I am always busy, but can go on holiday whenever I want. Above all, I see my grandchildren all the time. I miss my dear husband very much, but Jamie has been very good to me since his father died.'

James and Tessa Doherty had three children aged between six and sixteen at the time of this story. They had a large house and garden, and when Jamie's mother was widowed, they suggested she should come and live with them; but Mrs Doherty valued her independence and did not want to relinquish it. However, a few years later, the house adjoining the bottom of their garden came on to the market and Jamie suggested that they should buy it for his mother. He pointed out that she would have complete privacy and independence, but also be close to her family as she grew older. Mrs Doherty inspected the house, and hesitated. She loved the home she had shared with her husband for forty years, in which they had brought up three children, but she knew that it was too big for one person; she was getting older and would have to move at some stage. The children ran around the empty house with her, full of excitement. 'You'll be coming to live near us, Granny. Lovely!'

'I'm not so sure,' she replied cautiously. 'Let me think about it.'

'Please,' they chorused. 'Please, Granny.'

'Don't pressure me,' she said.

What tipped the balance of her indecision was the remark of one of the boys:

'Daddy can cut a hole in the fence, and make a gate, then we can come and see you whenever we want to.'

That did it. Any woman would have been foolish to refuse. In due course her large house was sold, the new one bought, and the move accomplished. It was total success from every point of view. She had a small but comfortable home, a small garden which she valued, and complete independence. Jamie duly removed a section of fence between the two properties, and a gate was installed, which was always left open. Not only the children, but the dog, ran freely from one house to the other.

Mothers-in-law can frequently be a pain to their daughters-in-law. But Tessa had no such complaint. In fact, she valued her mother-in-law's proximity, help and company. She was expecting her fourth baby and was feeling more tired than she had in the other pregnancies. The three children, all under ten, were a handful. The summer holidays came, and Tessa was in the last weeks of pregnancy; it was hot, and half the time she was exhausted. The fact that she could send the children down the garden to Granny was a great relief to her. 'I don't know how I would manage without you,' she said. But what she valued most, she realised, was the fact that her mother-in-law never criticised and never interfered. She was helpful, but neither demanding nor domineering. Jamie was delighted. After all, the whole idea had been his in the first place. He congratulated himself on a good plan well executed.

The eldest sibling in the Doherty family, Priscilla, was a successful accountant who lived in Durham with her husband and children. She maintained a good relationship with Jamie, although they did not see each other all that often. Their sister, Maggie, was a freelance journalist for women's magazines, and a writer of romantic short stories. She had struggled to hit the big time, but had never quite managed it. She was unmarried, but had had a succession of men, each of whom she maintained she loved, and whom her mother hoped would prove to be 'Mr Right'. But something always happened, and the relationship broke down.

Maggie loved her mother and her brother and sister deeply. They were her anchor in life. She also loved her nephew and nieces as if they were her own and she was a great favourite with all of them, because she was fun, she was lively, and she was full of bright ideas about interesting things to do and places to go to. They loved listening to her stories, and boasted to their school friends about their auntie who was a writer. When she was 'between jobs' she always went to stay with Jamie or Priscilla and enjoyed their family life. It reminded her of her own childhood.

Maggie had been her father's favourite, and she missed him dreadfully. There was an ache in her heart that would not go away, and she knew that he had been the man of her life, and that there would probably be no one to replace him. 'But at least I've got my brother and sister, and Mummy,' she thought (though she was over forty she still clung to the childhood 'Mummy'). And when the brittle existence of a freelancer overwhelmed her, she turned to her mother for comfort. She had been deeply unhappy when the old house was sold. With it, she felt, were sold all her associations with the past.

The Women's Institute does not immediately conjure up pictures of fast and furious living. But it is not everyone who wants a frenetic lifestyle, and certainly not Mrs Doherty. 'I leave that to the young,' she would say, as she watched her sixteen-year-old granddaughter spend the entire day beautifying herself to go out with her boyfriend to a party. 'The party doesn't start until ten o'clock – it won't end until the small hours of the morning. Bliss!' sighed the girl.

'You enjoy yourself, dear. I've got cakes to make for the WI jumble sale in the church hall this afternoon and I must get on.'

'Boring,' said her granddaughter with a pitying sigh. 'Poor Granny!' and she flitted off.

'Boring? Not a bit of it,' thought Mrs Doherty, as she sieved the flour and rubbed in the butter. Her life was as full and rich as the cake she was making. Each week she spent an afternoon at the local hospice helping with the mobile library; an afternoon at the hostel for battered women, listening to horrifying stories of violence and abuse; a morning at the primary school helping the slow readers group. She was the backbone of the flower arranging ladies at the church; second contralto in the local choir; a reader to the blind; a collector for Christian Aid; and a tea lady for the local cricket club, not to mention a full-time grandmother to four lively children, the eldest of whom had just informed her that her life was boring.

The local branch of the WI went from strength to strength when Mrs Doherty took over the chair. She threw herself into the task and, with real flair, organised the members into doing things they had never imagined, such as a sponsored cycle ride for grandmothers, a visit to a shipbuilders, a trip in an air balloon. Day trips to cathedrals and stately homes are old hat, she thought, so what about an outing to a metal foundry, an RAF base, a lifeboat station? For three years the Women's Institute fizzed under Mrs Doherty's competent guidance.

The ladies were enjoying a guided tour through the sewers of London. They had to wear special clothing, boots and hats. After an explanation of the safety precautions, with some trepidation they set off. The guide related the history of the sewers, how raw sewage had been dumped directly into the Thames until the mid-Victorian era, when London was awash with effluvia. The fear of cholera breeding in stagnant cesspits was very real.

One of the ladies muttered, 'I think I'm going to be sick.'

The guide was unsympathetic. 'It's the methane gas,' he explained. 'It's quite a pleasant smell when you get used to it.'

The group continued on their way, the guide telling them about Bazalgette and his visionary ideas for the construction of a new sewage system for London. He was describing the struggle the engineer had to get his plans approved, when Mrs Doherty muttered, 'I feel funny,' and leaned heavily on the woman beside her.

'It's only the methane,' called the guide. 'Please try to keep up at the back there. We don't want anyone to get lost.' Mrs Doherty couldn't keep up. She leaned more heavily. Two women tried to support her, but couldn't. Her voice was slurred. 'I'm so sorry. I don't know what's happened. I feel fu ... fu ... fu ...' and she slid to the ground.

Mrs Doherty had suffered a stroke.

The difficulty of getting the unconscious woman out of the sewer was considerable. Two ladies tried to carry her, but the slippery surface of the tunnel made it impossible. Others said they would go to get help, but the guide assured them they would get lost if they tried. With great courage and strength, he hoisted Mrs Doherty across his shoulders and carried her the half mile to the exit shaft. One of the ladies was supporting her head, and several times the guide slipped and nearly went over, but not quite, and he did not drop Mrs Doherty. 'It was a nightmare,' the ladies said afterwards. The journey, the bumping, and the length of time taken probably added to the injury sustained after the initial stroke.

A DANGEROUS SUBJECT

'Stroke' is a good word. It is much better than medical words. There is no warning, no time to prepare when a stroke brings you down. Strokes can vary in severity from mild and transient, to catastrophic with permanent injury. They are caused by one of three things: thrombosis, embolism or haemorrhage, in order of severity.

Thrombosis is caused by the hardening and narrowing of the cerebral arteries, which can give rise to both chronic and acute changes in the oxygen supply to the brain. Blockages in the tiny cerebral arteries are associated with a slow, progressive disturbance of cerebral functions, punctuated at intervals by seizures or attacks, called transient ischaemic attacks (TIA) or mini-strokes. Stroke due to thrombosis is less common, nowadays, because of the early diagnosis of high blood pressure and hardened arteries, and drug treatments available to rectify these conditions.

An embolus is something floating freely in the circulatory system. Several things such as air or fat or necrotic material from a tumour are possible emboli, but the most common is a blood clot. Our blood gets thicker, and flows more sluggishly, with an irregular pulse, as we grow older, and clots are liable to form. When an embolus reaches an artery too narrow to allow it to pass, it becomes lodged, and the tissue beyond it is no longer fed with oxygen and will die. These blockages can occur in any part of the body, but if one of the cerebral arteries is blocked, the result will be a stroke. The severity can be mild or severe, and this will depend on the position in the brain and the size of the area affected. The incidence of a stroke due to an embolus has been greatly reduced by preventive measures – drugs such as Warfarin, which thin the blood, and those which reduce high blood pressure.

A stroke caused by haemorrhage cannot be foreseen and, there-fore, cannot be prevented. It is due to the rupture of a weak spot in a cerebral artery. We all have weak patches in our blood vessels and they normally cause no trouble. But just as the strength of a chain is in its weakest link, so it is with blood vessels. Under tension, the weakest link will snap. In certain circumstances, the weak spot of an artery will burst and blood will escape into the surrounding area of the body. This can occur in any artery, in any part of the body, and the site of the haemorrhage will determine the severity of the damage. If it ruptures in the cranium, it causes a stroke. It can occur at any age and is quite unpredictable.

I was a ward sister at the Elizabeth Garrett Anderson Hospital for Women in London when Mrs Doherty was admitted. She was in a deep coma, and her skin was colourless and cold, although covered with perspiration. Her temperature, blood pressure, pulse and respiration were subnormal. We did not think she would live for long – such a severe stroke was usually terminal. The houseman who attended whilst we admitted the patient, said much the same as I had been thinking: 'The kindest thing would be to let her die quietly. However, I must do a lumbar puncture to diagnose the cause.' This she did, revealing abundant blood in the spinal fluid, which was diagnostic of a cerebral haemorrhage.

We contacted the next of kin. Jamie left work at once and came to the hospital, but Priscilla was in Durham, and Maggie was on an assignment. The consultant surgeon, Miss Jenner, explained to Jamie that the prognosis was uncertain, but that a craniotomy could be performed to open the skull and suck out the blood and fluids that had collected and would be causing pressure inside the cranium. It might also be possible, she said, to locate the origin of the bleeding and tie it off.

Jamie looked alarmed, and Miss Jenner explained that opening the cranium is not all that difficult, and trephining the skull had been performed since pre-Roman days, and that sucking out the blood is not a lengthy business and would certainly relieve pressure on the brain, which was essential if Mrs Doherty was to stand any chance of recovery. (Miss Jenner was a general surgeon. What she suggested was not brain surgery, for which a specialist brain surgeon would have been required. Also, a general surgeon in the 1960s had a far wider role than today.)

Jamie was asked to give consent for the operation. He hesitated. 'I am not sure that she would want it. She wouldn't want to be debilitated, I am quite sure of that. She is eighty-two, she has had a full and active life, and to go, while she is still getting about and enjoying herself, is what she would want.'

His words raised an element of doubt in Miss Jenner's mind. 'This is always a difficult moment, probably the hardest you will ever have to face. To treat or not to treat. To leave well alone, or to intervene. But I assure you, that if we do not operate quickly your mother will die later today.'

Poor Jamie. What a situation! And the decision was on his shoulders. His instinct said 'leave well alone', but he couldn't bring himself to say it. He needed help. 'I must speak to my sister. I will ring her office; please God let her be there.'

He went and telephoned Priscilla, who was at her desk. He explained what had happened, and what the consultant had said. Priscilla was unequivocal and immediate in her response. 'She must be operated upon. You must sign the consent form. We cannot morally, or even lawfully, as far as I know, withhold from her the chance to survive.'

Jamie did not hesitate to give his consent for operation.

He remained in the hospital, and spoke again at length to Priscilla, who said that she could not come to London until the work she was engaged in had been concluded. She did not want to pass it to her junior, and, as there was nothing she could usefully do in London, she would remain. Jamie contacted his other sister, who sobbed uncontrollably when she heard the news. 'Darling Mummy, my poor darling. I'll come at once.'

The day dragged on, and the hours hung heavily for Jamie. His mother had looked ghastly when he saw her. She had appeared to be dead, but obviously was not, because she was taking in great noisy, sucking breaths, horrible to listen to. At the same time, the competent matter-of-fact attitude of the hospital staff had reassured him. She would be all right; she was a tough old bird, he told himself.

The operation was done under general anaesthetic. The cranium was opened, and blood and serum sucked out, but the source of the bleed could not be found. X-rays were taken from every angle, but were inconclusive. Clinical signs suggested that the bleed was in the left side of the brain, but natural clotting had halted the flow. No further probing would have been appropriate, and so the piece of skull bone was replaced, and the wound sutured. Mrs Doherty was returned to the ward.

We had prepared a side ward to receive her and she was lifted on to the bed. Her breathing was quieter, but very slow, and in other ways she looked worse than before, because her head had been shaved. The bandages on her skull were deeply bloodstained, because there are numerous small vessels on the scalp, and they bleed profusely. Two draining filaments had been left *in situ*, and were sticking out. She was attached to two drips, one blood, one saline, and a laryngeal airway for continuous oxygen. Frankly, she looked barely human.

Nurses are accustomed to these things, and we were neither surprised nor alarmed, but Jamie was still in the hospital, and wanted to see his mother. He could not be refused. Miss Jenner had already told him of the operative procedures, and said that when the nurses had made his mother comfortable he could be admitted.

I went to the visitor's room myself, because I wanted to prepare him. I knew that the sight of a patient after cranial surgery can be a terrible shock. We were talking together, when suddenly the door flew open and a woman burst in, her hair dishevelled, her eyes swollen and her face red and blotchy.

'Where's Mummy?' she cried, 'I must see her. She needs me.'

Jamie introduced his sister Maggie.

'It's been a terrible journey. I've had four changes of train, and nothing to eat all day – but I've brought these flowers for her. I know she likes roses; they are her favourite flower. She will love them . . .' She started to cry, and pulled out a wet handkerchief.

I told her that her mother had returned from the operating theatre only an hour earlier.

'An operation? You didn't tell me about an operation, Jamie,' she said accusingly. 'What operation?'

I said that it had been necessary to open her mother's skull to suck out the blood.

'Blood! You opened her skull! Oooh, Mummy!'

Jamie took hold of his sister and explained, quietly and sensibly, what had been done. He and I exchanged glances and I could read his thoughts – was Maggie in any fit state to see her mother? But we could not refuse her.

We went to the side ward. I told Maggie that we must be quiet, and not disturb her mother. We entered the ward and stood silently by the bed for a moment or two. Then Maggie said, 'But where's Mummy?'

What a dreadful moment for any ward sister. I bit my lip and said softly, 'Here. This is your mother.'

'No, it's not. Do you think I don't know my own mother? This must be the wrong room. Where is she?'

'No. It's not the wrong room. This *is* your mother.'

I could feel the panic rising in the woman beside me.

'But it can't be . . . that's not Mummy!' Her voice was trembling. 'I don't believe you. You're lying. You must be!' With every word there was a rise in decibels. Jamie took hold of her.

'Maggie, come away. This is no place for you. Come with me.'

Firmly he led her out of the side ward. Hysterical screams could be heard echoing down the corridor.

Brother and sister left the hospital. Jamie telephoned at 10 p.m., and the night sister told him that his mother's condition was stable, and that he should ring in the morning.

Jamie came to see his mother each day. He did not stay for long, because there was nothing he could do. His mother was unconscious, but there was no deterioration in her condition. Maggie did not come to the hospital, but her telephone calls were so frequent that I had to instruct the main switchboard to limit her calls to the ward to two a day.

I spoke to Priscilla in Durham, on the telephone. Her voice had a very clipped accent, pleasant to listen to, but somewhat intimidating. She sounded like the sort of woman who would assume she was in the right and brook no contradiction. There was not a lot that I could say, beyond what she had already heard from Jamie, that their mother's condition was stable. She said she would remain in Durham.

About a week later, Mrs Doherty showed signs of regaining consciousness, first by the twitching of the legs and then restlessness which became extreme. Her pupils, which had been tightly closed, responded to light. Grunting was heard, and slurred attempts at speech. Jamie sat by the bedside for some time, holding her hand, and she obviously knew who he was and took comfort from his presence. Maggie came, but she cried so much it would have been better if she had not come at all.

Mrs Doherty gained consciousness and began to understand what was going on around her. She responded well to questions and instructions from the staff, such as 'Can you raise your left arm? Can you raise your forefinger?', but she was severely hemi-plegic. She could not move the right side of her body at all, her right eye and her mouth and tongue slumped heavily to the right, and she could not speak. Several times she tried, but the sound was quite incomprehensible. Tears gathered in her eyes as she desperately tried to make herself understood.

Nursing her was difficult – but it always is with a patient in such a condition – and took a great deal of our time. We moved her every two hours, repositioning her limbs and treating pressure areas. We removed the naso-gastric tube, cleaned her mouth, and raised her into a semi-recumbent posture. We spoon-fed her with semi-solid feeds, but she found swallowing difficult, and the food frequently trickled out of her mouth. If any fluid went into her trachea, she started choking, and it had to be sucked out. The physiotherapist came daily, treating the paralysed limbs. The stitches and drainage tubes were removed from her scalp, and we put a little white cap on her head, which made her look more feminine.

Maggie informed her clients that she would be taking a break and would be living in her mother's house for an indefinite period. She had become reconciled to her mother's condition, and came in daily, sitting with her for long periods of time, talking to her about her life, her boyfriends, her plans for the future. Should she give up freelancing? But what would she do instead? Her mother could make no response.

Maggie chatted on, and she discovered what many people learn – that a hemiplegic, speechless person loves to be talked to as though nothing is wrong, and no verbal response is expected. Maggie talked about her father, and days in the old house when they were all little, about the tree house in the garden, and picnics in the summer by the stream, and 'Do you remember, Mummy, when we thought a bull was coming for us, but it was only a cow which had strayed?' She chatted endlessly, and the happiness it gave to both of them was beyond measure.

One day she said: 'Priscilla is coming tomorrow to see you. She won't stay with Jamie or me – she insists on staying in a hotel. I'm scared of Priscilla, Mummy, aren't you? She's so cold and stiff and correct and I'm sure she disapproves of me. But every time she looks at me in that way I think of when she was a little girl and we went to a birthday party and she put on roller skates and was wobbling and slipping all over the place. She wet her knickers, and when we sat down for tea she left a big wet patch on the cushion of the lady's nice chair. That makes me feel better and I think, "Well, you weren't always perfect, Miss Perfect".'

They both laughed, and saliva trickled from the side of her mother's mouth. Maggie tenderly wiped it away, and kissed her mother. She whispered, 'We've had such fun, haven't we, Mummy darling, and we'll have fun again when you come out of hospital. I'll always be there to look after you.'

Priscilla arrived the following day. She was tall, slim and dignified. Her features were composed as though nothing could ruffle her, and her nostrils were very close and narrow, which made her appear to be sniffing slightly all the time, an effect intensified when she pursed her lips and raised her eyebrows.

In spite of her apparent composure, Priscilla was very tense and ill at ease. A hospital was quite outside her experience; she was no longer in control. Before she had even seen her mother, she asked to speak with the consultant. I said that Miss Jenner was in theatre all morning, and had a clinic in the afternoon, and that I did not expect to see her on the ward that day. Her nostrils contracted and she said in a clipped, precise voice, 'Please inform Miss Jenner that I am residing in London for a limited period and that I request an interview at her earliest convenience.' I said that I would do so, and did she wish to see her mother? She replied, 'Yes, of course.'

I led her to the side ward. Two nurses were there. They had washed Mrs Doherty and changed her nightie and managed to get her out of bed to sit her in a chair. One of them was on her knees on the floor, adjusting Mrs Doherty's feet to rest on a footstool; the other was tying a bib round her neck to catch the saliva as and when it dripped. Her body slumped to the right, in spite of the pillows they had placed to try to keep her upright, and she looked up as best she could by moving her head and raising her left eye a fraction. She obviously recognised her daughter, because a gurgling sound came from her throat and she moved her left arm in greeting.

Priscilla did not say a word. I opened the window a little, and one of the nurses looked at me questioningly. Should they attempt to give Mrs Doherty her morning drink? We understood each other without a word being said – this woman was undoubtedly intimidating, and would probably be critical. To attempt to give a drink to her mother, even from a feeding cup, would probably be repellent to her. No morning drink. Not yet, anyway.

One of the nurses placed a chair beside Mrs Doherty. I asked Priscilla if she would like a cup of coffee, but she shook her head. She still had not spoken. We left the room and shut the door.

Five minutes later she came out and asked to see me. The confidence, the assumption of superiority, had been knocked out of her.

'This is a bad business, Sister.'

'Your mother has had a severe stroke, which is always distressing to see.'

'I was not aware it would be as bad as this.'

I refrained from saying that she did not look nearly as bad as she had a fortnight earlier. Instead, I said, 'Your mother is making progress as well as can be expected.'

She turned suddenly, almost angrily. 'But she cannot speak!'

'No.'

'She can only make gurgling noises.'

'The side of her brain controlling speech has been affected.'

'Well, what are you going to do about it?' she demanded.

'There is very little we can do, apart from physiotherapy, to encourage the healing powers of nature.'

'Healing powers of nature! Is that *all* you are doing? There must be some drugs she can have. What about all the miracles of modern medicine we hear so much about?'

I thought how the miracles of modern medicine can prevent someone dying from a stroke, but cannot restore the loss of speech nor the loss of muscular control that are its legacy.

'I must see the consultant. I must discuss what can be done about this distressing situation.'

I was explaining again that Miss Jenner was not expected on the ward until the following day, when I heard a familiar voice in the corridor. 'Excuse me a moment,' I said, and went out. It was Miss Jenner.

'Hello, Sister. We closed theatre earlier than expected, so I thought I would just pop down to see how Miss Patterson is getting on. Perhaps that drain can come out. And if you can find a cup of coffee, that would be nice.'

I told her that Priscilla, Mrs Doherty's eldest daughter, was in the office and wanted to speak to her.

'I'll see Miss Patterson first, then have a chat with her.'

A little later, before we parted for lunch, I caught up with Miss Jenner, and she told me what Priscilla had said. 'She seems to think that we can restore her mother's speech and movement by drugs. It astonishes me, the ignorance of the most fundamental medical facts that intelligent, well-informed people sometimes display.'

'Very true,' I laughed.

'She seems to think that because we have not already done so, we are being negligent, and have missed an obvious point.' She shrugged her shoulders despairingly. 'I don't know what she thinks we should be doing, but she is demanding another medical opinion.'

'And will you get one?'

'Well, I shall have to get a geriatrician's assessment for her mother. She can't stay here indefinitely. This is an acute surgical ward. She will have to go to the geriatric ward. That will give her daughter the second opinion she requires.'

Miss Jenner sighed deeply. She was a lady in her fifties, about twenty years older than I was.

'It used to be so much easier in the old days. When I was a medical student it was not expected that anyone would survive a massive cerebral haemorrhage. All the medical textbooks, all the lecturers, informed us that death would result within a few hours, or at most a few days.'

'I doubt if anyone would say that now.'

'Oh no!' Miss Jenner said emphatically. 'No one would dare to say such a thing. They would be in serious trouble. It is a very dangerous subject.'

Miss Jenner left, and I sat very still at my desk, my mind going back about twelve years. Miss Jenner had used exactly the same words that Matron Aldwinkle had used when I was a student nurse – 'This is a dangerous subject.'

A FAMILY DIVIDED

The geriatrician came to assess Mrs Doherty and advised a rehabilitation centre. Miss Jenner said that the patient could not remain for long on the acute ward, and asked if a bed could be found on the geriatric ward until rehabilitation. It was not easy – there were too many patients and too few beds available. The consultants both knew the difficulties. 'We'll ask the medics. They have more of a turnover than we do.' The medical registrar came to see Mrs Doherty and said that a patient with colitis would be discharged at the end of the week and a bed could be available.

Miss Jenner saw Priscilla and told her that two specialist opinions had been sought and that her mother would be transferred to a medical ward for treatment for the aftermath of a stroke. Following on from this, her mother would go to a rehabilitation centre. The woman seemed satisfied with this and said, 'I will reside in London until next week, and then I must return to Durham.' Then she said, very formally: 'On behalf of my family I would like to thank you, Miss Jenner, for saving my mother's life. You obviously acted with great skill.'

She turned to leave and had to pass her mother's door. She put her hand on the handle, and paused. One could almost feel the indecision going on in her mind, her sense of duty telling her she should go in, yet opposing that, her fear of seeing her mother, of not knowing what to do or say. She half turned the handle, then released it, and started to walk away. At that moment Maggie came round the corner with an armful of flowers.

'Priscilla! You old stick! You didn't tell us you were coming in this morning. How is she?'

Priscilla hesitated before answering. She looked exceedingly discomfited, and then said truthfully, 'There is no change.'

'But is she awake? Was she glad to see you?'

Priscilla could not answer. Her nostrils closed to narrow slits and her shoulders tensed.

'Priscilla!' Maggie was furious. 'You are impossible. You came here to see the doctor, not to see Mummy. How could you?'

'Don't make a scene here in the corridor, with everyone listening.'

'I don't care if the whole world can hear me! Dear Mummy, lying there ill, and you don't want to see her.'

'Stop this behaviour. We will go in together.'

She opened the door, and they entered. The staff nurse and I looked at each other.

'Wow, that was a near thing!' she said. 'We don't want them fighting here in the corridor. You see it all in this life, don't you, Sister?'

I could only agree.

We had a busy morning. There were five cases for theatre. That meant preps and pre-meds, calling the porters, arranging for nurses to escort patients to theatre and, afterwards, back to the ward, post-ops to be received and cared for, and student nurses to be taught the details of post-operative nursing. I was thankful to have a very good staff nurse, who was highly experienced and loved the drama and excitement of an acute surgical ward. She was indispensable on such a morning.

We had almost forgotten about Mrs Doherty when suddenly Maggie came screaming out of the side ward. 'Sister, Sister, come quickly. Something's happened.'

The staff nurse was there before me. She said, as I entered, 'I think it's another stroke. I've called the doctor, but of course our team is in theatre. One of the medics will come.'

One look was enough to confirm Staff's assessment. Mrs Doherty had slithered from her chair, and was slumped on the floor. Her eyes were wide open, but her pupils had receded upwards, and only the whites were showing. Her mouth, hanging to the right side, was open, and copious frothy fluid poured from it.

Maggie was sobbing and holding her mother in her arms. Priscilla was leaning against the wall, her face as white as a sheet. She was struggling to control her breathing, and her eyes were staring horrified at her mother.

'My God, we are going to have two strokes on our hands, if we are not careful,' I thought, and went over to her.

'Would you please go to the office and ring your brother, Jamie? Tell him to come, because this looks serious.' Giving someone in a state of shock a job to do is usually the best way of dealing with the situation.

I whispered to a nurse, 'Go and ask the ward maid to make some strong coffee for that lady. She's going to need it. Then prepare a lumbar puncture trolley.'

Two porters were just entering the ward to take the next patient to theatre. It was fortuitous. I called them in to help us lift Mrs Doherty on to the bed and shortly afterwards the medical registrar arrived. She said, 'We must sedate to stop these muscular spasms, then I will do a lumbar puncture.' I said that the trolley was ready. We turned the patient, and doctor inserted the long needle between the third and fourth lumbar vertebrae. The fluid draining out was heavily bloodstained. 'We can assume another haemorrhage. This patient belongs to your team, not ours. She must be seen by Miss Jenner.'

Maggie was in the room – she refused to leave her mother – and asked how long that would be. I said that Miss Jenner was in theatre and the list was due to finish at 1 p.m. It was then 12 noon. Mrs Doherty was deeply unconscious, breathing noisily and very slowly. Her pulse and blood pressure were very low. I thought, *This is it. She won't survive this one*, and said to Maggie, 'We must keep your mother very quiet. I am sure you will want to stay with her.' She nodded tearfully.

In the office, Priscilla was looking a bit better. She said that her brother Jamie was on his way and that they would see Miss Jenner together.

Jamie arrived at about 12.30. Theatre closed slightly ahead of time, and Miss Jenner came straight to the ward, still in her theatre clothes. I accompanied her into Mrs Doherty's room and Jamie and Priscilla joined us.

Miss Jenner examined her patient and said exactly what the registrar had said: 'A second cerebral haemorrhage has occurred.' She said no more. Maggie sat by the window, crying quietly. Priscilla stood by the door, looking tense. Jamie stared at them both, and said:

'I don't think any further treatment should be attempted.'

Maggie sobbed quietly. 'But she will die, Jamie,' she said in a tiny voice.

'She will, and it will be for the best.'

'How can you say that? For the best! What a wicked thing to say. Our darling Mummy!' Her voice was rising.

The accusation stung. 'I'm not wicked. I'm being realistic.'

'I hate you. Realistic! At such a time!'

'Don't create another scene, Maggie,' interrupted Priscilla.

'You cold fish,' she shouted. 'I suppose *you* want Mummy to die also – then you won't have to come and see her. Is that it?'

'I decline to answer. You are getting hysterical again.'

'I'd rather be hysterical than cold and heartless like you two.'

Miss Jenner and I looked at one another. This was not the time or the place for a family row. Miss Jenner turned to Maggie and said gently: 'Your brother is probably right. The time has come to let go, and allow your mother to die in peace.'

Maggie looked up with unspeakable anguish.

'Let go? She is all I have. She was getting on so well – almost talking to me. I was beginning to understand what she was saying, and she understood every word I said.'

Maggie sobbed quietly into a wet handkerchief, and Jamie gave her his, and put his arm around her. No one spoke for a moment, and between sobs she continued, 'I've been getting the downstairs room ready for her – it's all so pretty, just as she would want it.' She looked up at Miss Jenner. 'Is there nothing you can do?'

Miss Jenner did not answer. The silence in the room was tense. The sound of stertorous breathing from Mrs Doherty seemed unusually loud.

Then Priscilla spoke. 'Is there anything you can do to relieve my mother's condition, Miss Jenner?' Her voice was precise, and demanded an answer.

'I could do another cranial exploration,' she said quietly.

'Then it must be done.'

'No,' said Jamie, 'I *won't* allow it. She has gone through enough already.'

'It *must* be done,' Priscilla retorted.

'Why? In God's name, why?'

'Because it *can* be done,' Priscilla said.

'I do not advise it,' said Miss Jenner. 'I cannot be confident that she will survive a second operation.'

'There you are, Priscilla,' Jamie said, 'Medical advice is against operation.'

Priscilla ignored him, and spoke to Miss Jenner.

'Will she survive without operation?'

'It is unlikely. In fact, I must answer no, she will not.'

'When is her demise likely to occur?'

'That is more difficult to predict.'

'Days? Weeks?'

'Oh no, not weeks. Maybe later today, or during the night.'

Maggie screamed, 'No, oh no, no, *please*!'

'So the balance in favour of survival is to operate?'

'Yes, it is.'

'Then it must be done.'

Jamie confronted his elder sister. 'I don't agree, and I will not give my consent to operation.'

'Your consent will not be necessary. I will give mine.'

Maggie jumped up, her tears stopped, her face hopeful.

'Oh Priscilla, you're wonderful. Can it be done, Miss Jenner? Can you save Mummy?'

'I cannot guarantee it.'

'But you can try, can't you? And I will look after her when she leaves hospital. I *want* to look after her.'

Jamie was exasperated. 'You just want something to fill your empty life.'

'Don't be so beastly. You just want her out of the way.'

Miss Jenner interrupted. 'Please. You can settle your differences elsewhere.'

Jamie looked furious. 'I don't want her "out of the way", as you put it. I just want what is best for her.'

'And you think it's best for her to die? You ... you ...'

She turned to Miss Jenner. 'Please, oh please try.'

'I cannot guarantee a successful outcome, and therefore I am reluctant to operate,' the surgeon said.

'What is the balance in favour?' asked Priscilla.

'I would say about fifty–fifty. Not more.'

'Then it must be attempted.'

'No,' said Jamie, 'It would be going too far. Why are you so keen on a second operation, Priscilla, when it is against medical advice?'

'I am not "keen", as you put it. I merely say that if an operation can relieve the pressure on her brain and save our mother's life, then it must be done. To do nothing, and allow her to die, would show indifference or negligence, which I cannot allow.'

'Priscilla, you are so sensible. We must do all we can for Mummy.' Maggie turned to Miss Jenner. 'Don't listen to Jamie. He doesn't understand. We can't just allow Mummy to die.'

Miss Jenner replied, 'Your mother is going to die anyway. An operation will only delay death.'

'That's what I've been trying to say, Maggie, only you won't listen. And it's the reason why I don't think it should be attempted. We must do what's best for her. I appeal to you, Miss Jenner.'

'Be quiet, Jamie. Don't listen to him, Miss Jenner.' Maggie was sobbing again. 'Mummy could get better. It's quite possible. She has been improving every day this week. I have seen it. She can nearly talk – at least, I can understand her, even if you can't. We must do all we can for her.'

Priscilla spoke again. 'If a second operation holds any chance of survival, then it must be done. I cannot have it on my conscience that, when my mother was seriously ill, I stood by and did nothing. I am not even sure about the *legal* rectitude of non-intervention.'

Jamie, tight-lipped, said, 'I think you are wrong, both of you. It will only impose more suffering on her.'

Priscilla said, stiffly, 'I am confident the hospital staff will be able to reduce any suffering to the minimum. It is a simple matter: if a life can be saved, it must be saved, and a fifty per cent chance of survival is worth taking. She has been a good mother to us all, and we owe it to her.'

She turned to Miss Jenner and me.

'I want it recorded that I request a second operation on my mother, to relieve the congestion on her brain. If you will get a consent for operation form, I will sign it now.'

I glanced at Miss Jenner and she nodded her head. I went to the office and returned with the necessary form and filled it in, ready for signature. Miss Jenner did not say a word, but left the room. Priscilla and Maggie signed, Jamie refused to do so.

When I returned to the office, Miss Jenner was sitting with her head in her hands. Poor woman – she had had a full morning in theatre, had another clinic in the afternoon – endless responsibilities – and now this. She looked drained.

'There is something formidable about that woman. She is relentless in her logic, but she is wrong, in my opinion. Logic is a bad master. She may be right legally, but she is wrong morally and ethically. I'm sure of that.'

'Her last words sounded like a threat,' I said.

'They were.'

'Can anyone threaten a consultant? Surely a consultant's opinion must be respected?'

She laughed, pulled off her theatre cap, and ran her fingers through her hair.

'Not any more. Medicine is changing fast. Professional expertise and experience are no longer enough. Now we have the law breathing down our necks.'

'That doesn't sound too promising for medicine.'

'No it is not. But you heard her words – "if it can be done, it must be done". I don't agree – I think it is a question of balance and restraint, but if it came to a court of law, my professional opinion would count for very little.'

'A court of law?' I exclaimed in alarm.

'Perhaps not a civil court, but the BMA have their own tribunals, and they have unlimited power to make or break a doctor's career.'

'Surely you don't think Priscilla would sue you, or anything like that?'

'No, I don't, it would be out of character. But her sister might. She is a very emotional woman who is clinging to her mother and won't let her go. She wouldn't listen to her brother Jamie, nor to me, because we would not say what she wanted to hear. If her mother dies today or tomorrow, which is possible, Maggie will blame me, and say that the death could have been prevented, but that I refused to operate. It would only require a letter to the BMA suggesting that I have been negligent in my professional duties . . .' Her voice trailed off.

'And what then?' I ventured after a minute. I could see she was deep in thought.

'What then? Suspension on full pay whilst enquiries are made. Endless statements, investigations into my professional competence.'

'That can't be in doubt.'

'I'm not so sure. Past record may count for something, but it is no defence. At a BMA tribunal, how could I stand up and say, "I thought we should let the old lady die"?'

Put like that, it sounded both callous and unprofessional. Miss Jenner laughed bitterly.

'And even if I didn't use those words exactly, you can be sure the press would.' She heard my exclamation of surprise and indignation. 'Oh yes! The press would be there all right. The tabloids love that sort of thing. They would drag me through the gutter, given half a chance. I can just see the headlines, "Consultant Surgeon says *let the old people die*". I, and the hospital, would be named and shamed.'

Miss Jenner let out a long shuddering sigh.

'My local paper would make it front-page headlines. They've

got nothing much else to report – apart from the occasional "flasher" on the common! It would really be big news for them. And that's where I live, and do my shopping, and take my dog for a walk.'

Her voice was nearly breaking.

'I hate to think of it all. Even if my decision was vindicated by the BMA, the damage would have been done.'

She looked up, and her face looked ten years older.

'Against my better judgement, I will have to operate. I have no choice. Instruct Theatre Sister to prepare for a trephine, will you please? And I will speak to the anaesthetist.'

She stood up, looking more resolute.

'I must go and speak to the relatives first.'

'What about lunch?' I said 'You have had nothing.'

'There's no time. I'll eat later.'

'You'll need something inside you. I'll get the ward maid to prepare a sandwich and coffee for you.'

'Thanks. That sounds nice. I'll go and see them now, then have a bite.'

The operation was successful. The bleed was less serious than before, and had been attended to more quickly than the first stroke. A small bleeding point was located and tied off. Free blood and serum were sucked from the cranium, a clot removed, and the patient returned to the ward. Nursing procedures were as before, and Mrs Doherty regained consciousness within three days.

Maggie was overjoyed and spent most of each day with her mother. Before returning to Durham, Priscilla called at the hospital a couple of times and expressed her satisfaction. Jamie also came to see his mother each day. He looked at her paralysed limbs, and listened to her gurgling attempts at speech, and murmured 'I hope to God this never happens to me.'

Mrs Doherty remained on the ward for three weeks, and then was transferred directly to a rehabilitation centre. For a month she received physiotherapy, ultrasound, passive movement of the limbs, swimming sessions, and many of the exercises that attempt to restore strength to wasted muscle. A speech therapist helped her with jaw and tongue movements, vowel sounds and consonants.

It had been ten weeks since the first stroke and a measure of improvement was undoubtedly seen, so Mrs Doherty returned home with Maggie to care for her.

All went well to begin with. The old lady was obviously pleased to be home, and Maggie was full of enthusiasm and happiness. The children came in to see their Granny, expecting her to be the same, or very nearly. But when they saw an old, old woman, who looked nothing like the grandmother they remembered, slumped in a chair, her face fallen to one side, one eye closed, saliva trickling out of the corner of her drooping mouth, they backed off, afraid. She saw their alarm, and tried to smile and hold out a hand in greeting. But when she tried to say, 'Hello darlings, I've come home,' it sounded like 'Ga ga wa wa ga'. The youngest one ran away in terror, and the eldest girl murmured to herself, 'Oh, how dreadful.'

People paralysed from a stroke are usually fully aware of what is said, and what is going on around them, and Mrs Doherty wept, great tears that she could not wipe away running down her face.

Maggie did her best. But she had completely underestimated the difficulties involved, which, even for a professional nurse, can be daunting. A district nurse came in for four hours a week, but Mrs Doherty required twenty-four-hour nursing every day, and the only person to do it was Maggie. Feeding, drinking, washing, bathing, help with dressing – all had to be attended to. Soiled underwear and bed linen had to be changed frequently, and even though a bathroom and lavatory, specially designed for invalid use, had been built on to the ground floor room, Maggie found that getting her mother on and off the lavatory was a monstrous task. Mrs Doherty tried desperately to help herself, but early one morning, when she'd managed to get out of bed, her Zimmer frame was just a little too far away, and, in trying to reach it, she slipped and fell, and lay on the floor, wet and cold, for several hours.

Another thing Maggie had not expected was the boredom. Each

day was the same – a struggle with physical necessities, until Maggie felt she could scream. Although Mrs Doherty's speech had improved to the point where she could say a few words, she could not carry on a conversation, and her attempts to do so frequently led to tears of frustration. In the end Maggie gave up trying to speak to her mother. In the winter, when the days grew dark and wet, Maggie wondered how much more she could take.

Mrs Doherty made heroic efforts to do things on her own. She was not a woman who wanted to be a burden to her daughter. She did the exercises advised by the physiotherapist, but progress towards mobility was minimal. Had she been twenty years younger, it might have been different, but she was simply too old to build up new muscular strengths. Every little thing was a labour for her to achieve; frequently, she wept uncontrollably.

Jamie came to see his mother each day, but did not stay for long. It was difficult to communicate and conversation was confined to banalities. He could see the strain imposed on Maggie, and though they both thought often of the scene in the hospital, and Miss Jenner's rejected advice, neither of them ever mentioned it.

One day Jamie said to his sister, 'You need a holiday. You can't carry on like this. You'll crack up.'

Maggie burst into tears. 'If only I could. But I don't see how I can leave her.'

'Tessa and I could take over.'

'I don't think you could. She needs someone with her all the time. You have to go to work, and I doubt if Tessa would do all that I do.'

'Then she'll have to go into a nursing home for a while. I will make enquiries and arrange something. You must have a break.'

'That would be wonderful. Thank you, Jamie.'

He could see her depression and was concerned. Everything about her, her clothes, her hair, her face, her nails, was neglected. Even her body language was so unlike the Maggie they had always known.

'Do you think you'll ever go back to writing?'

'Oh, I don't know. Can't see it, somehow. I had a letter from one of my magazines today, telling me that they were taking me off their books. That's bad news.'

Jamie didn't say anything but arranged for a nursing home to take his mother. It was not easy, because of his mother's incapacity. Most nursing homes wanted old people who needed no nursing, he discovered. He found one, eventually, who said they would take her for two weeks, providing she was not incontinent. Jamie assured them that she was not, but would require help in getting to a lavatory, or a bedpan. The expense was colossal, but Priscilla agreed to help pay.

Mrs Doherty was terrified when she was told that she was going to a nursing home for a fortnight. She couldn't express herself but kept saying 'No, no, no,' and shaking her head and crying. She managed to formulate the words 'Let me stay here', and then added, 'Please, please, oh please,' but no one took any notice. When two men came with a special recumbent chair in which to carry her, she resisted with all the puny strength she could muster – but they took her anyway.

The stress of being moved, and the mental agitation, the new surroundings, strangers taking care of her – it was all too much for the old lady, and she went rapidly downhill in the nursing home. She would not eat or drink, she made no effort to move, but lay inert in her bed. Her time, at long last, had come, and Mrs Doherty died five days later.

A man
half bent over on the sofa, eyes down, asleep or awake.
An assistant puts a mug of tea in his hand
but he can't hold it or isn't ready, she puts it gently
on the sideboard next to him, With the cup shakily
in his hand now (I am watching) he raises it slowly
to his ... But where to go? The cup goes to his glasses,
almost touches them, then slowly down again, up again,
this time halfway to his mouth. The cup (I am watching)
is on the sideboard again. A biscuit has been put
into his hand. Using both hands shaking, and with
tiny movements he tries (I am watching) to break
the biscuit. With a small piece of it he tries to find
his mouth. He fails and lowers his hand again
very slowly. His left hand holds the biscuit half away.
His right hand has gone right down past his knees.
It comes up again. He achieves breaking the biscuit
again and with his right hand reaches his mouth
with a tiny piece (I am watching) and gets it in.
Now he has found the cup of tea on the sideboard
and holding it in his right hand he is drinking from it
very slowly, all the while his head down ...
He tries to stand
and very slowly turns and is soon
heaped about the end
of the sofa, his weight greater than his power to shift it.
Two assistants help him up and sit him back on the sofa.
One says 'Stay there'. But he wants to move, so they
help him up and he walks or is walked across the room
and into an armchair. One of the assistants pulls out

the footrest which tips the chair back. (I find myself
swaying). She puts the stool under the footrest
to support it. She adjusts the head rest, pats his chest
and says, 'There,
have a rest.
He closes his eyes
and is still.

— *David Hart*

This poem and that on page 145 by David Hart were written when he was Poet in Residence at the South Birmingham Mental Health Trust, 2000–01. *A man half bent over* was originally written in an Older Adults Assessment Ward as it occurred, very very slowly, the version here being newly made. At the annual conference of the Royal College of Psychiatrists at the Queen Elizabeth II Conference Centre, a Van Gogh self-portrait reproduced as a poster for PR purposes by a drug company led to the writing of *Poor Van Gogh*. The whole sequence of residency poems with commentary was included in David Hart's *Running Out* (Five Seasons Press, 2006).

DEMENTIA

The reality of an ageing population is that many of us will end up in residential care in our final years. Taking only the figures for dementia, one in four people over the age of eighty now suffers from progressive dementia of the Alzheimer's type, and from ninety onwards that figure rises to one in three. At the time of writing, there are more people over sixty-five in the UK than there are children under sixteen. This is recognised as one of the most serious social problems of the twenty-first century. Who is going to look after these hosts of demented old people? Who will be there when we die?

Dementia is probably the one thing that people over the age of sixty-five dread more than anything else. It must first be said that to see this progressive decline is almost always worse for the immediate family than for the sufferer, who is usually unaware of what is happening.

There are many types of dementia; Alzheimer's is the most common, but there are others. Confusion mimics dementia, and misdiagnosis is often made. Confusion can arise from all sorts of things – the death of a spouse or a partner, or of close relatives or friends; new surroundings, new faces – we can all suffer, at any age, from confusion. It is not confined to the elderly by any means.

Seventy per cent of all people in care homes are confused, probably because the life they have known for seventy or eighty years has come to an end, and now they are surrounded by strangers. On top of this, depression may be part of the trouble, arising from being in a care home in the first place. Often the person is grappling with the grief of bereavement, and loneliness, and the feelings of being useless and worthless contribute. The treatment is friendship, love, care, sympathy, understanding – all the qualities that generosity of the human spirit can give, and little else. Drugs and other medications have a small part to play, but if a misdiagnosis of dementia has been made, drugs can add to the confusion and deepen depression.

True Alzheimer's disease is quite another matter. It is not confined to the elderly, but can start early in life. It is an identifiable disease, of unknown cause, of no known cure, and progressive until death occurs. There is no telling whom it is going to strike, but as our life span increases, the risk of dementia increases.

The symptoms of Alzheimer's dementia start with frontal lobe forgetfulness of events, names, places, mixing up times, places, people, which is not difficult to live with and, in fact, can be quite endearing.

But Alzheimer's disease will lead to other things, such as personality changes, aggression, destructive behaviour, dirtiness, random accusations and anger, and dangerous or obscene behaviour. We now recognise these as symptoms of the disease. Physical changes also occur – blindness, apparent deafness, inability to chew or swallow, inertia, muscular weakness or paralysis. Those who retain muscular strength can sometimes develop excessive walking habits – they walk from morning to night, never stopping until they fall exhausted. We are kind to these people, now – former generations of doctors and nurses kept them in chains.

The family can usually cope with these, and other manifestations of Alzheimer's. It can be very difficult, but with day-to-day help from professional carers, they manage, inspired by love, respect and pity for the person affected. The condition is irreversible, but the patient can live for years before the degradation of the final stages occurs.

It is when Alzheimer's reaches these stages that institutional care becomes necessary. The patient is helpless, can neither speak, eat, swallow, spit, nor cough. The body is unable to hold itself upright, the head rolls sideways or forwards on the frail neck, which cannot support the weight. The mouth hangs open and saliva dribbles out continuously. Not infrequently the muscles, instead of becoming limp, develop rigidity, and the body is twisted backwards into grotesque shapes that cannot be moved. Either way, the patient has to be strapped to a chair, and will also be doubly incontinent. The sufferer knows nothing and no one, and has reached the stage rather nastily known as a 'vegetative state'. It is as near to death as anyone can be, and most people would say, 'I would rather be dead'. Yet today, people can live like this for years.

In my days of nursing, patients seldom reached this state, because they died first from one of many possible causes: heart or kidney failure, bronchitis, pneumonia, septicaemia caused by bedsores, starvation because they could not swallow, choking because food or fluid entered the lungs and they could not cough. Pneumonia was the usual release. We called it 'the old man's friend'. Life-saving treatments were fewer than are available to us today, but also, and perhaps more importantly, medical people had far more autonomy. We were not hemmed in by bureaucracy and endless rules and guidelines. A doctor and the ward sisters could agree that treatment should not be given to a specific patient under specific circumstances, and this decision would not be questioned. Today, fear of litigation inhibits all decision-making.

In his outstanding book *How We Die*, Sherwin B Nuland tells the moving story of his friend Philip Whiting's descent over six years into the extremes of Alzheimer's.

> ... Phil became totally incontinent but was quite unaware of it. Although fully conscious, he simply had no idea of what had happened. Urine soaking his clothes and smeared some-times with his faeces, he would have to be undressed to clean off the filth that profaned the pittance of humanness still left to him ...
>
> And through it all, he never stopped walking. He walked obsessively, constantly, every moment the ward personnel let him ... Even when he was so weak that he could barely stand, somehow he found the strength to walk back and forth, back and forth, around the confines of the ward ... Once seated, the frail body bent sideways because Phil didn't

have the strength to hold himself up any longer. The nurses had to tie him in lest he topple to the floor. And even then, his feet never stopped moving . . .

During his final month of life, Phil had to be tied into bed at night to prevent him from getting up to resume his incessant walking. On the evening of January 29, 1990, in the sixth year of his illness, puffing breathlessly from the effort of one of his fast, forced marches, he stumbled into his chair and fell to the ground, pulseless. When the paramedics arrived a few minutes later, they tried CPR [cardio-pulmonary resuscitation] to no avail and sped him to the hospital, which was right next door. The emergency room doctor pronounced him dead of ventricular fibrillation leading to cardiac arrest . . . *

The Methodist Homes for the Aged is an excellent, non-profit-making charity, and takes a high percentage of patients with Alzheimer's who require twenty-four-hour care. The carers work cheerfully, motivated by a sense of vocation and duty. The Methodists have a specific policy for care of the dying, set out in their booklet *The Final Lap*. The teaching is based on acceptance of death as a fact of life, and the need to prepare for its coming, and I was discussing this with a chaplain for one of the Methodist Homes. All of their chaplains are closely involved with, but not responsible for, medical practice. Citing Nuland's description of his friend's condition and death, I posed the question, 'Would you really allow such an aggressive resuscitation attempt upon anyone in that condition?'

I expected him to say, 'No, we accept death and respect the dead.' But he didn't. He left it open by saying, 'The trouble is, it is increasingly hard to define death – the boundaries are so blurred, and we do not have in each individual Home a member of staff who is qualified to pronounce death.'

* from *How We Die*, Sherwin B Nuland, Alfred A. Knopf, New York, 1993

He sat pondering for a minute, and then continued.

'Apart from that, no Home wants to have too many deaths. You see, it is our policy to integrate the Home into the community, so that residents are not isolated. If too many coffins are seen leaving the premises, this could start fear and suspicion and gossip among people living in the area. You never know what might be said. This would be bad for the Home, and all the residents would suffer.'

As he said that, the memory of my neighbour's experience flashed through my mind. The house is large, with about ten rooms and half an acre of garden, and at the time, a young family was living in it. The wife, Ginnie, was a trained nurse who enjoyed looking after the elderly, so the family decided to open four of the rooms as a residential home. They all lived and ate together, and it was a happy arrangement. The old people enjoyed the company of the children, who in turn had the advantage of seeing and living with old age. The young husband kept chickens and geese and grew vegetables. One of the old men made it his responsibility to feed the chickens and collect the eggs. A couple of ladies helped in the kitchen.

Then misfortune struck. Within a month, two of the old people died. Police investigations followed; then the local press. Repeated interrogations reduced Ginnie to a shadow of her former self. The local paper made it a matter for front-page headlines. The coroner's verdict was that the deaths were from natural causes, and Ginnie was completely exonerated, but the two remaining residents were taken, against their will, to a registered care home, and quite a crowd gathered outside the house to watch their removal. Ginnie was distraught, because it did not end there.

The things that were said locally about Ginnie were vicious. I know, because I heard them. Matters got so bad that, eventually, the family was forced to move.

I told this story to the chaplain. He said, 'I am not surprised. It is the sort of local reaction I would have expected.'

'What do you do, then, if someone looks near to death?'

'It would depend on the circumstances, but quite probably we would send the person to hospital.'

'That's not satisfactory, is it?'

'No, but we have to be so careful, and it gets harder for us all the time. We even have people with feed-pegs coming into our Homes. So then someone has to make the decision to remove it . . .'*

His voice trailed off, and I could sense the heartbreaking difficulties that have to be faced.

A feed-peg – or gastrostomy, or jejunostomy, or other parenteral routes – is an alternative to a naso-gastric tube. It is a plastic tube inserted through the abdominal wall into the stomach and fixed in position. The purpose is to enable liquid feeds to be given directly into the stomach. A study of the care of patients in the USA with Alzheimer's, or advanced dementia due to another cause, found that fifty-five per cent of people who died of the condition, died with a feed-peg or a naso-gastric tube in place.**

In January 2010 a report on *Oral Feeding Difficulties and Dilemmas* was published by the Royal College of Physicians, together with the British Society of Gastroenterology, and endorsed, among others, by the Royal College of Nursing. This presented the results of a three-year study under the chairmanship of Dr Rodney Burnham. It reports that thousands of old people are being forced to have feeding tubes implanted in their stomachs if they need to be admitted to a nursing care home, and that this is a widespread problem, because many care homes say they will not take a patient until they have had a gastrostomy.

The report states that the practice of force-feeding old people through tubes in their stomachs is seldom necessary, is highly

* It is very difficult to remove a feed-peg because it is a life-maintaining device. It requires a major medical/legal decision and this is not easy to come by.
** Ahronheim, J C, Morrison, R S, Baskin, S A, Morris, J, Meier, D E. Treatment of the dying in the acute care hospital. Advanced dementia and metastatic cancer. *Archives of Internal Medicine*, 1996; 156: 2094–100.

invasive and should not be undertaken lightly. Critics have questioned the Royal College of Physicians' findings and pointed out that only a doctor can decide whether a person should be subjected to a gastrostomy, to which the RCP replies that there is pressure on doctors to authorise it in order to free up hospital beds by discharging patients into residential care.

Why is this practice 'widespread'? Why do nursing care homes only accept a patient with a gastrostomy? The answer is that it will take a carer fifteen to twenty minutes to spoon-feed a patient adequately, whereas it takes about two minutes to pump a semi-liquid feed into a stomach. Drugs can be administered with the same speed and efficiency. Time is money, and the advantages are obvious.

We, the general public, are responsible for this. We are paranoid about not letting anyone who cannot feed himself die quietly as nature intended. Without knowing it, we push for force-feeding of old people.

Wherever they meet, nurses talk shop. On a walking holiday in Italy I met Sandra, an American nurse from Florida. It was May 2009, and my mind was full of the book I was writing, so I mentioned it. Her face changed from mild interest to focused attention, and her voice became urgent.

'Oh my God! This book has gotta be written. We do it all the time. Hell, it's crazy. We dialyse people who are ninety-eight per cent dead. They don't know anything, can't move, can't swallow, can't talk, totally incontinent, an' we do renal dialysis, three times a week. Hell, it's just crazy.'

'Can you go on?' I asked.

'I tell you, we got a guy in our clinic at the moment with creeping paralysis – it's got a lot of new fancy names, but it's the same ol' thing, creepin' paralysis – starts in the peripheries an' creeps up through the body, an' when it gets to the lungs that's it. Or it used to be. But not any more. This guy's had it for two years, slowly, slowly losing all sensation an' control, creeping slowly up, an' it's got to his lungs. So what do we do? Eh? We bring in a respirator. At the same time he loses control of swallowing – so we pass a naso-gastric tube. It's obscene.' She had to pause before continuing and her voice became slower and sadder. 'Poor ol' guy, he was so sweet. It alters y'nursing perspective, y'know. When you're looking after someone with Alzheimer's or creepin' paralysis, you build up a real relationship, with a real person. When it gets to a respirator and artificial feeding, you're just maintaining a machine, and the person gets to be a chemical reactor. It's not the same at all.'

The sunshine suddenly seemed less bright, and the Bay of Naples less beautiful.

'Do you think profit is the motive?' I asked.

She shrugged. 'Your guess is as good as mine.'

'When will it all stop?' I enquired.

She was fierce in her reply.

'I'll tell you. It'll stop when the money runs out. When relatives have to pay for it out of their own pockets. When they can't demand that the insurance pays for it. *That's* when it will stop.'

'When the money runs out'! Great poets and writers and thinkers can express the inexpressible, and see way into the future. Samuel Beckett, in his book *Malone Dies*, published in 1951, wrote, 'There's no place in America where a man can die in peace and with some dignity, unless he lives in abject poverty.'

The possibility of extending life for long periods of time opens the door to exploitation, and I have a hunch that it's possible a good many people might be kept alive for the money they bring in.

Look at it this way. Only a small number of nursing care homes are non-profit charities, and these are mostly faith-inspired. The majority of care homes are profit-making establishments, which can be bought and sold on the open market. Some of them are public limited companies, with a board of directors whose first responsibility is to their shareholders. Care homes can be very profitable, and it is alleged that some directors lead millionaire lifestyles.

Every institution, be it something like a school or a sports club or whatever, relies on numbers to keep going. If the numbers drop, the institution becomes economically unviable. Private clinics, rest homes and nursing care homes, all of which rely on cash flow, are no different. They have to maintain a certain number of paying patients to keep going. A death represents loss of revenue. The more expensive the place, the more urgent the need to keep the beds filled.

Everyone I have tried to speak to on this matter shuts me up, or changes the subject. But body language is more eloquent than words. A sudden gasp of breath, a widening of the eyes, or tightening of the mouth, suggest that I have dared to broach a subject best avoided.

Betting has never been my obsession, but I would bet that my hunch is correct!

WHO CARES?

Half a century ago, there was no distinction between nurses and carers, because student nurses did all the work that carers now do. A young girl's nursing training started with three months' classroom induction. Then followed a full year of basic, hands-on, bedside nursing care – in other words, all the mucky work. Two more years of ward work had to be completed before State Registration. We were constantly under the strict supervision of the staff nurses, ward sisters and, ultimately, Matron – all of whom had been through the same training. It was a real apprenticeship.

But nursing was firmly stuck in the past, based on the old Nightingale tradition – docile acceptance of rigid discipline under a hierarchical system that was sacrosanct. Reform was necessary.

The Salmon Report (1966) appeared first, proposing new management principles for nursing. Some of these changes were undoubtedly needed, but I remember the shock that swept through the profession, and later the whole of society, when it was announced that the post of matron would be axed, leaving no one with overall responsibility for nursing standards.

1972 brought the Briggs Report. It proposed that nurses' courses in further education colleges should be established. However, nurses were still working long hours on the wards, and if they left, someone would have to replace them. This problem was not, and has never yet been, adequately addressed.

The Griffiths Report came next (1983), under the chairmanship of Sir Roy Griffiths, the Chief Executive of Sainsbury's, with a committee that did not include medical or nursing representation. The report recommended that management based on business models should be introduced to save the government money. According to Griffiths, there should be no difficulty in transposing the principles of commerce to the NHS. Once you let economists and accountants get their hands on things, you quickly lose sight of the original objective!

Project 2000, 1986, was the work of a new statutory body, the UK Central Council for Nurses (known as the UKCC) who, with the Royal College of Nursing, debated the training of nurses. Higher education was becoming absolutely essential. One small example will suffice to illustrate this: in my years of training we had a few hundred drugs, of which about forty or fifty were in common use. Now, medicine has hundreds of thousands of drugs in its armoury, of which about one thousand are in daily use. They all have to be known – their dosage, action, reaction, cross-reactions, allergic reactions. If I were working on the wards today, with my level of knowledge, I would be a danger to the public! A good education is essential, to degree standard.

Project 2000 aimed to bring students under the aegis of academia, thus removing their isolation from mainstream student life, and enhancing the image of nursing as an academic discipline. This, in my opinion, is a wonderful aim. Project 2000 is lengthy and wide-ranging, mostly relevant only to the professions, but the following are three of the main features of reform that are pertinent to the care of the sick and ageing:

1. To separate education from service by conferring super-numerary status on students and creating bursaries in place of training salaries.
2. To create a single register that would do away with the Enrolled Nurse grade, and to simplify the designation of first-year student nurses.
3. To establish a new clinical grade of support staff, essentially to replace junior nurses and enrolled nurses, whose function would be fulfilled by these aides.

'To separate education from service'. Herein lies the rub. Nurses need higher education, but they also need practical training in bedside nursing. A thousand and one tiny details, some so small they are barely perceptible, are involved in basic nursing care, and these details have to be learned; they are not obvious to the casual observer or to someone who thinks they could just do the job.

The second reform dealt with the proposal to do away with the State Enrolled Nurse (SEN) qualification. Nursing staff had always had assistant nurses or auxiliaries to help them. The Voluntary Aid Detachments (VADs) in the military hospitals of the First World War are just one example. Later in the century, the SEN received a training approved by the Royal College of Nursing (RCN) that was essentially the same as the first year of student nursing. The course appealed mainly to married women who had family commitments, who enjoyed nursing but did not want responsibility. I worked with several and, as a ward sister, knew that an SEN was a great asset, providing stability and continuity on a ward. Also, she was often a mother figure to nervous young students, doctors as well as nurses. But Project 2000 looked ahead to a single register of graduate nurses, in which a second grade of enrolled nurses had no part.

When I read the words 'To establish a new clinical grade of support staff,' I was unclear what this might mean, but assumed it could easily be found out. Two months later, after an exhaustive study of professional papers and government reports, after rushing around all over the country interviewing people, I am still unclear, and get the impression that everyone else is, too!

Let's start with the name or title for these support workers. My researches produced about twenty different names. When I told this to a spokesman for the RCN, he laughed: 'Over the history of the RCN we have come up with 295 different names for support staff, and there may be more.'

From the inception of Project 2000, statutory powers enabled the UKCC to phase out the apprenticeship approach in favour of more academic training. Nurses started to leave the wards, and that was when carers came in. It was the first time the word 'carer' had been used as a job description. Hitherto, they would have been called auxiliaries, assistants, or one of the 295 options. By the 1990s, the title Health Care Assistant (HCA) became accepted, and this seems likely to stick.

In my capacity as an ordinary person, or 'Everyman', seeking to get to grips with this revolution in healthcare provision, I studied a great many documents, Government Reports, professional reviews, websites and journals distributed for public information by the Care Quality Commission (CQC, formerly known as the Healthcare Review Body). Whilst the area is muddy and changing all the time, the following is taken from my researches and is accurate at the time of writing:

Question (from 'Everyman'): So who does the basic nursing these days?

Answer (information gleaned from CQC documents): Health Care Assistants.

Q: And who trains them – the RCN?

A: No. The employer, the Trusts, the NHS Training Authority, the care home, the agency or an independent hospital.

Q: What training could the Trust give, for example?

A: This can vary. Some trusts offer up to six weeks induction and training, whilst others provide two weeks of support for new Health Care Assistants.

Q: What training would a private hospital, clinic or care home give?

A: There is no national standard, and on the whole it is very little, a couple of days at most. However, all health care workers must show the Criminal Records Bureau clearance, and complete a brief induction.

Dear Heaven, it can't be true! And we had fifteen months' training in basic nursing.

I have two nieces who are health care assistants. One of them told me that she had worked with disabled children, and decided to change to geriatric nursing. She said, 'So the agency sent me on half a day's training.'

'What!' I gasped. 'You can't be serious!'

'Yes, that was it, half a day. But remember, I had had experience in caring, and I had done some home visiting, too. If I hadn't, I suppose they would have sent me for a whole day, perhaps even two.'

So it *is* true.

Induction consists of three parts, which can be completed in a morning:
1. Fire drill, conducted by a fire officer
2. Moving and handling
3. Protection of vulnerable adults.

'Moving and handling' is instruction in how to use the winches, slings, pulleys etc., required for moving or lifting an immobile or helpless patient. Some of this equipment can be very complicated, and the company that makes these gadgets supplies a video instruction on the correct use. The purpose is to protect the employers and suppliers from claims of injury to nurses or care assistants from moving or handling patients incorrectly.

'Protection of vulnerable adults' is basically looking at different kinds of abuse, such as staff bullying or manipulating patients, or thieving. It is a video documentary, made by professional actors with advice and short, acted scenes of what can be done, and what one should not do. The purpose is to protect the employer from claims of malpractice. The video takes about forty-five minutes to run.

National Vocational Qualifications (NVQs) have been available since the 1970s. They are based on national standards of practical competence in a wide range of occupations (over 1000) varying from bricklaying to hairdressing to catering.

In 1988 the Healthcare Review Body (now the CQC) examined the position of carers, and, as a result, the NVQ training was started for prospective health care assistants. This is essentially a qualification in *practical* skills, and the training is on-the-job experience. There are three levels of achievement, trained, monitored and assessed by . . .

Question (from 'Everyman'): ... by whom?

Answer (from my research): It could be that the trust has a nurse-led training, followed by supervision of practice by a qualified assessor, and then both internal and external verification by an awarding body such as the City and Guilds.

Q: What is the training for care assistants in private hospitals or clinics or in nursing care homes?

A: This will depend on the organisation. In theory, a nurse on the staff should train and monitor care assistants. But, in practice, this is unreliable because some employers will take a carer after a day's induction and there may be *no* nurse available to offer further training. There can be a wide difference between the training and supervision of care assistants in NHS hospitals and those employed privately.

Q: If the private establishment has no nurse to train potential carers, who does train them?

A: National Care Training Providers.

Q: And what training do they offer?

A: Telephone help throughout the day.

Q: So is it seriously proposed that basic nursing can be learned by telephone?

A: It is a telephone support line.

Q: Is this support line open at night?

A: No. Care assistants also have one-to-one contact with a specially trained NVQ Care Assessor.

Q: How often is one-to-one contact available?

A: By appointment, when it can be arranged.

I have mentioned my two nieces who are HCAs. The younger one is on NVQ Level 3, and her elder sister is on Level 4. I asked the younger why she did not take the Level 4 qualification. She replied: 'I don't see the point. I wouldn't earn any more.'

'But it says here in the syllabus that you would.'

'It may say that, but I wouldn't get it.'

'What do you earn now?'

'About £5.40 an hour. It might be £5.70 – I'm not sure.'

Her sister interrupted: 'I was on £5 something an hour for years and years, even after I passed Levels 2, 3 and 4; it made no difference to the pay. But now I get £8 something an hour because I have worked there for a long time. That makes a big difference.'

My nieces both work in nursing care homes, one in Reading, the other in Plymouth. I asked them why they did the work for such a pitiful wage. They replied, almost in unison, one echoing or agreeing with the other:

'Because I love it.'

'It is deeply satisfying.'

'I love knowing that I have made a difference to some old person's life who might be lonely or unhappy.'

'At the end of the day, or night as it might be, you feel you have done something worthwhile.'

'It's very rewarding work.'

I looked at them with deep respect. I have always loved them both, but had no idea of the depth of their vocational commitment and unselfishness. Sue, the older sister, is a very thoughtful and impressive woman. She is a Jehovah's Witness, which is a life-affirming religion, and she bubbles with laughter half the time, and radiates warmth, kindness and compassion, which she says, in a large part, has come from her faith. She sees it as God's commandment that she should be a Witness by working for those in need. I am sure she would work for nothing if she did not have bills to pay.

I sent this chapter to them both for approval and had a letter in reply from Sue containing the following paragraph:

I have chatted with Jayne and we are both of the same mind, that maybe we gave you an unfair description of our training, which I must make clear is always ongoing throughout our working life in the units we are employed in. There are always updates in line with CQC and care standards. We are not nurses but care assistants who provide a vital role in the physical and emotional care of the people who for one reason or another find themselves in care homes or day centres such as ours.

This is the ideal standard, expressed by two ideal care assistants, and I know it to be true; the CQC, with support and advice from the RCN, is all the time striving to improve standards through on-going training. However, the stark fact is that a huge number of people working in private hospitals, clinics and nursing care homes have no training whatsoever, and do not stay long enough in the job to benefit from the training that may be on offer.

Nursing Care Home Managers are supposed to employ only people with NVQ Level 3 qualifications. However, a survey conducted for the End of Life Care report, issued by the National Audit Office in November 2008 (p.6, sub para 15) found that fewer than five per cent of nursing care home staff had this minimum qualification. Why, then, are they employed? The reason is because the managers are desperate for staff. They must have someone to cover the varying shifts over twenty-four hours, and night duty is the hardest to get anyone for. They could not function if they insisted on this Level 3 qualification.

An NVQ seems to be the minimum qualification that is obtainable. But it can be bypassed altogether. Agencies offer a bit of training that amounts to shadowing another carer for a few hours, and this is accepted as enough for someone to get a job.

It seems to me that care assistants fall into one of three categories:
 1. Those who are wholly and selflessly dedicated.
 2. Those who enjoy looking after people, but don't want responsibility.
 3. Those who can't get any other job.

The last comment is certainly not meant in a derogatory way. A great many of those in the third group are newly arrived immigrants from middle European countries (the former communist bloc) who need a work permit to stay in the country, and who can get one by signing up to take the NVQ Healthcare at Level 1, and working in a care home. Many of these boys and girls are very good indeed, and I have met them. They are young, bursting with life and happiness, not afraid of hard work or getting their hands dirty. Also, having been brought up in a culture that does not exclude the old from family life, they are gentle and understanding.

In 2013, it will be mandatory for all newly recruited nurses to have a degree. It will not be possible to enter the nursing profession by any other door. Suddenly it is upon us – *health care assistants will be the most significant workforce in hospitals and care homes.* At present, it is estimated that there are over 700,000 practising HCAs in the UK, but, as they are not registered or regulated, the number is not really known. Their training has been insufficient, to say the very least, yet they will be the ones who do the basic bedside nursing that is the foundation of nursing care, as anyone who has suffered long-term illness or debility will tell you. It is also, for this reason, the most noble.

Doctors come and go, but nurses or care assistants are always there. All the high-tech, multi-drug paraphernalia in the world is as nothing beside the human need for human touch and contact – which is what good bedside nursing is all about.

We can prolong life for decades, and resuscitation is fast becoming the norm, and all these people will have to be looked after. The decisions are made by government think tanks, by teams of professors at the British Medical Association, by ethics committees consisting of philosophers and theologians and senior judges. But having come to their conclusions, and issued their reports, they can walk away from the problem. They don't have to do the work. The work is left to care assistants, who receive barely a living wage for work that is arduous and demanding, and for whom the strain can sometimes be insupportable.

We are a rich nation, and like all rich nations we need a sub-culture of underprivileged people to do the dirty work that we would not want to see our sons and daughters doing. Much of the work of care assistants falls into this category, and they are the ones who will look after us in our old age. It is worth remembering that, when our faculties, our senses, our mobility and our organs fail us, health care assistants will be more important to us, and have far more power over us than doctors.

Let me end this chapter by reproducing some of the NVQ introductory literature, which can be obtained online. It is addressed to prospective health care assistant candidates at the initial entry level:

NVQ Care Programme Information Pack

There are no academic qualifications needed to be a care assistant. All care assistants are expected to undergo a twelve-week induction programme *[this is frequently not observed – author's comment]*. Direct experience is not necessarily required for the job, but it is useful to have some experience in working with people. Care Assistants are in high demand and it is relatively easy to get a job. The main employers are social services, hospitals, private or NHS nursing homes and agencies.

Personal skills: Care Assistants need to have excellent inter-personal skills and the ability to work with all kinds of people in situations which can be stressful or emotionally draining. More specifically they should have:

- A friendly approach and the ability to put clients at ease, whatever their physical or social needs
- The ability to be tactful; and sensitive at all times
- A good sense of humour
- A high level of patience as shifts can be long and often stressful
- Excellent communication skills
- The ability to deal with aggressive or anxious clients
- A certain level of physical strength
- Good stamina
- The ability to stay calm under pressure
- The ability to think quickly and solve problems as they arise.

Working Conditions: Care Assistants usually work shifts, which means their hours and days of work vary from week to week, and may include night shifts or weekend work. Shifts can be long and demanding, so care assistants need to have good stamina and both physical and emotional endurance.

The contempt with which this hedonistic society looks upon simple virtues is reflected in the pay reward. We offer care assistants £11,000 a year: that is £5.70 an hour, with no guaranteed sick pay, holiday pay or maternity leave, and no guaranteed pension.

Would you, the reader, do it? Could you? Would you advise your son or daughter to become a health care assistant?

Truly, truly, I say to you, when you were young you girded yourself and walked where you would; but when you are old, you will stretch out your hands, and another will gird you, and carry you where you do not wish to go.

— *St John, ch.21, v.18*

CONGESTIVE HEART FAILURE

The year was 1968, and I was night sister of a small provincial hospital. I walked into the ward, and there he was – Dr Conrad Hyem. We recognised each other instantly, though it had been many years since the night in Poplar when we parted. No doubt we had both changed. I was a married woman in my thirties with two children. And he? Well, he was very much changed. He looked frail, sitting up in a hospital bed, breathing with difficulty, a bluish tinge around his nose and lips, and an anxious look in his eyes. The ward was quiet after the daytime bustle, and peaceful. A single light glowed above the bed of the frail old man suffering from congestive heart failure. I went over to him, sat on the edge of the bed, and took his hand. He squeezed it, and a crinkle in the corners of his eyes showed his pleasure.

'Jenny Lee,' he whispered, 'after all these years ... I have not forgotten you. How could I? And now you come to me when I am dying. You are thrice welcome. What a happy chance.' He sighed with contentment, and squeezed my hand again, such a weak little squeeze. 'A happy chance.' He looked up and smiled once more.

The effort to speak had made him breathless, and he leaned back on the pillows panting, shallow breaths, his nostrils dilated with the effort to take in more air. An oxygen cylinder was beside his bed, and I turned it on and placed the mask over his face. He breathed the life-giving gas for a few minutes, and then pushed it away. I adjusted his pillows, and he leaned back comfortably and closed his eyes. I whispered: 'I must go round the wards and see my other patients, but I will come back; be assured of that.' He nodded and smiled and patted my hand. 'Jenny Lee,' he whispered, 'a happy chance.'

★

A hospital is a lovely place to work in at night. Staff is reduced to about ten per cent of the number required during the day and there are no routine admissions or discharges, no routine surgery, no moving of patients to special departments for treatment, few telephone calls. All is quiet. I refer here to the general wards of a hospital, and *not* accident and emergency, where day can blend into night, and night is usually more hectic than day.

I went quietly around the hospital, taking the night report from each nurse in charge, seeing a patient here or there, checking a drug, adjusting some treatment, mentally noting this or that to be checked on the next night round, and then returned to the male medical ward, where I sat in the office reading Dr Hyem's notes. Congestive heart failure was the diagnosis. Long-term diabetes, for which condition I had treated him in the first place, had caused generalised atheroma of the arterial circulation (atheroma – from the Greek for 'porridge'). Just as a plumber may say, 'Your central heating won't work because the pipes are all furred up,' so it is with the circulation. The arteries become congested and the heart, which is the central pump, gets weaker and cannot work properly.

I paused in my reading to ponder what I knew of his past life, his moral strength, his suffering, his mental anguish, and his heart's grief at the loss of his wife and children in the Nazi gas chambers. 'His heart's grief' – can the heart grieve, or is it just a pumping mechanism to circulate blood and oxygen throughout the body? Is mankind just a series of reactions to chemical and biological stimuli, or are we more than that? Will we ever know? Perhaps it is better that we can never be sure.

I continued reading. Dr Hyem had had several warning attacks of angina pectoris, which can best be likened to cramp. It is painful but not fatal. For years he had been inhaling the fumes of amyl nitrite and taking digitalis, which is a very ancient extract of the foxglove plant, known to mediaeval monks, and cultivated in their herb gardens. At the same time, atheroma of the blood vessels caused sluggish blood flow, and his heart's efficiency was compromised. This led to other problems.

Oxygen is the key to animal life. If every cell in our bodies does not receive sufficient oxygen, it will die. That is what had been happening to Dr Hyem for several years. Due to lack of oxygen, the functioning of his lungs, kidneys, liver, pancreas – all his organs – was affected and their efficiency seriously diminished. This is the end result of congestive heart failure.

Eventually, Dr Hyem's labouring heart could take no more and he had collapsed in a shopping area. An ambulance was called and had brought him to hospital where we were able to treat him. In these days of high biotechnological medicine, the treatment available back then does not seem much – morphine sedation, bed rest and an oxygen tent, amyl nitrite, digitalis, heparin (an early form of clot-buster), mersaryl (an early diuretic). It may seem very little, but it was enough to pull him through, at least temporarily.

I turned to the second page of his notes, and read, 'Next of kin – none.' That was all. Dr Hyem, a Viennese Jew, living in the wrong place at the wrong time, had lost his entire family – murdered. At the end of life, all that could be recorded of these atrocities was 'Next of kin – none.'

Within a few days Dr Hyem improved. His heart rhythm had stabilised and his breathing became easier. The oedema lessened somewhat, and the cyanosis all but disappeared. He was able to get up and sit in a chair. He could walk to the lavatory. He could take a bath, with a nurse's help. He could talk without exhaustion, and even read a little. His diabetes had been thrown out of control by the attack, and the amount of insulin he had been taking for many years was no longer applicable. His urine had to be tested, and an insulin injection adjusted twice daily, otherwise he would have developed hyperglycaemia and acidosis. But, all things considered, there was a big improvement.

I was so happy to meet him again and to be able to give him my friendship and professional care. Each evening we talked, and this was when he told me a little of his personal wartime experiences. But I am sure he left much untold, things that were too painful to put into words. I expressed my surprise, once, that he was not bitter. He said: 'We have to forgive the unforgivable. But that does not mean forget. These things should be remembered. But if we do not forgive, we will poison our lives, and the lives of others, and evil will win.'

I thought of my poor Uncle Maurice, who had spent four years in the trenches in France and Flanders in the First World War, and whose whole life had been eaten away by savage hatred and resentment. He spent forty years hating mankind. Dr Hyem's philosophy of forgiveness was not only wiser, but kinder to himself.

We could talk only for short periods because, firstly, it tired him, and secondly, I was night sister, with a whole hospital in my charge and many duties to attend to. Nonetheless, I was grateful for the opportunity to get to know him better.

Sometimes he spoke of death, as my grandfather had. 'My time has come and I am content. "Everything in its season", as the prophet teaches us; "there is a time to live and a time to die".'

On another occasion he said, 'I have seen so much horrific death in the camps and I think about the spirits of the departed more and more as I draw closer to them.'

Little sentences or half sentences, here and there, built up a picture of his philosophy.

'Why did I survive? I often wonder. Why did I have to bear the perpetual pain? To die would have been easier. I'm glad my time has come at last.'

On another evening, he was reading his Hebrew prayer book when I approached his bed. He looked up, with a wry smile.

'From ancient times Jews have described death as "God's kiss". Wishful thinking on the part of a people who have suffered for two thousand years at the hands of cruel men, I think. Death is only a "kiss" if it comes naturally. What do you think, eh, Jenny Lee?' (He always called me by that name.)

One evening, he said to me, 'I know enough about the human body to know that one day, perhaps quite soon, I will have another heart attack and that will be the end of my life. I want it to be the end. I don't want anyone messing about with me, trying to pull me back from the brink.'

'It's unlikely,' I said. 'This is a small hospital. We only have a resuscitation room with two beds, and I don't think it is very well equipped. Anyway, you are seventy-eight and no one with any sense is going to try resuscitating a man of your age.'

'That's a comfort. Nonetheless, promise you won't let them do it.'

I promised, but said he should speak to the consultant and to the ward sister about his wishes. He told me that he had already done so.

These were the last words that Dr Hyem spoke to me. I went off duty at 8 a.m. During the day he suffered a massive heart attack and was not expected to live. The onset had been sudden. He was reading the morning paper and gave a cry, clutching his chest, and collapsed unconscious. It was thought that a blood clot, which is always liable to develop if the circulation is sluggish, had probably lodged itself in one of the pulmonary arteries.

Dr Hyem was treated as an emergency, with all the drugs and equipment available at the time, and he rallied.

At 8 p.m., when I went on duty, Dr Hyem was semi-conscious, but stable. If it had not been for the drug treatment and oxygen he would have died, probably within an hour or two of the infarction. However, he was close to death. I looked at him with deepest sadness. To lose an old friend is not only sad, but always tinged with regret, regret for all the little things left unsaid or unfinished. I had planned, in my mind, that, as he seemed to be getting better, and as he lived quite close to us, he could become part of our family group. I knew that my husband, an intellectual if ever there was one, would like him and be endlessly fascinated by his conversation. Perhaps my little girls would like him, too, and see him as a grandfather; this would be a source of happiness to him in his old age. All these plans – and now it was not to be.

A nurse was taking his pulse and blood pressure when I went into the ward. I told her to stay with him, and that I would return when I had completed my first night round in order to sit with him.

I completed the night round and returned to Dr Hyem, taking

with me all the hospital notes and records from my office, so that I could write them up while I was sitting there. I told each of the nurses and the night porter where I would be, if needed.

I sat behind the curtains in the dim, green-shaded light. I listened to the hushed sounds of the ward. Dr Hyem was no longer in pain. He was unconscious, or perhaps semi-conscious, and breathing slowly but deeply. His pulse was not perceptible at his wrist, but I could feel the carotid beat, very faint and irregular. His eyes were closed, and his expression peaceful.

At ten o'clock we turned him, a nurse and I, and he seemed to be faintly aware of the movement. I leaned over him and said slowly and clearly, 'Hello, Dr Hyem. It's Jenny Lee. I am here with you, and I won't go away.' He made the faintest sound to indicate that he had heard and understood. I took his hand, and his fingers moved in response. Then he sighed and drifted into sleep again, or was it unconsciousness? Where are the boundaries in these states? Later, he was beginning to feel hot, so I took a cold flannel and wiped his face, neck and chest. Again a faint sound, a sort of appreciative 'Mmm ...' on the outward breath told me that he knew I was there, and that he wanted me there.

I have always been convinced that unconsciousness, in a dying patient, is not wholly without perception or feeling, or even thought. The dying, even to the last breath, know who is with them. Perhaps they drift in and out of awareness of this world and indifference to it. Perhaps they are entering, or perceiving, another world that we cannot see. Where does life begin, and life end? Where do two worlds meet, or is it an illusion? We will never know. Birth, life, and death are mysteries and it is fitting that we should never know.

I sat with Dr Hyem for an hour or more. A telephone call came through, and briefly I went to another ward to answer a nurse's request to check a drug, but returned to my friend's bedside. He looked very peaceful, and I felt sure he would slip away before morning. The darkest hour before dawn is the time when the forces of life leave the body most frequently. After the tragedies and traumas of his life, I was glad that Dr Hyem was dying peacefully and painlessly.

At about midnight, an urgent call came from the children's ward. A baby who had been operated on for repair of a cleft palate was having breathing difficulties. I said I would come and asked a nurse to stay with Dr Hyem.

The baby was choking and turning slightly blue. The night nurse had been feeding him water, but a little must have been regurgitated into the nasal cavities, making him choke. It was alarming, but not terribly serious. Holding him head down, patting his back to encourage coughing, and sucking out the fluid, restored normal breathing fairly quickly. The baby took no harm. However, one look at the nurse told me that she was in a far worse state than the baby. She was deadly white, shaking and sobbing uncontrollably. Not long before that incident a baby had died in a nurse's arms, and the whole ward had been sad and subdued. No doubt the girl was thinking of that. She kept saying, 'I don't know what happened, Sister. I don't think I did anything wrong. Was it my fault?' I had to reassure her and told her it could have happened to anyone. I suggested she should sit quietly, cuddling the baby, for a while, and asked another nurse to bring her a cup of cocoa.

With one thing and another, I was away from the medical ward for longer than was originally expected.

OPEN HEART RESUSCITATION
(also known as Direct Manual Compression)

I returned to the male medical ward to resume my vigil with Dr Conrad Hyem.

Tread softly as you draw near to the bedside of a dying man, for the space around him is holy ground. Speak in hushed tones, with awe and reverence, as you would in a cathedral. Let not the mind engage in trivial thoughts. The awesome majesty of Death can only be met in silence.

As I approached the ward, I was aware of light and commotion coming from within, and when I entered, I saw that it was coming from Dr Hyem's bed. The curtains were drawn, but brilliant light was shining and half the men in the ward seemed to be awake.

I pulled aside the curtains and found a full-scale open-heart resuscitation being carried out by three doctors, one of whom, the registrar, had a scalpel in his hand.

Dr Hyem was lying flat on his back. His chest had been cut open on the left side, from the sternum to the lower back ribs. Blood was oozing out, and the smooth chest muscle was glistening in the bright light. Rooted to the spot, unable to breathe or make a sound of protest, I watched the registrar with a swift, easy movement slice through the pleural muscle, revealing the ribs.

'Retractor,' he demanded.

I found my voice. 'No! No! What are you doing? Stop! Stop it, I say!'

He ignored me. He inserted the retractor between two of the ribs, and turned the ratchet to open the double arms of the instrument to their full potential. I heard a rib crack.

'Stop it!' I shouted.

Perhaps he had not heard, as he continued with the ratchet, and I heard a second rib crack.

'Scissors,' he demanded.

By then I was getting close to hysteria. I took a couple of steps forward.

'What are you doing? Stop it. He's dying – can't you see that? Leave him alone.'

The doctor was cutting through the pericardium with surgical scissors. He muttered, 'Who the devil are you? Get to hell out of here.'

He inserted his hand through the open chest wound and grasped Dr Hyem's heart; then he began a series of steady, firm compressions.

There was blood all over the place, dark venous blood, black and sticky, covering the doctor's white coat, and the sheets and pillows scattered across the floor.

'It's fibrillating badly, but at least there's some movement,' he said as he continued his compressions. 'How long have we been at it?'

'Two minutes twenty,' replied one of the housemen.

'Not bad. If we keep it up, we should win. Here. You take my place. Then you will know what to do next time.'

He withdrew his hand and stepped backwards. One of the others took his place and inserted his hand through the hole in the chest wall.

'Can you feel the heart?'

The young man nodded.

'The ventricles fibrillating, like a jellyfish wriggling?'

Again the houseman nodded.

'You can? Good. Now just squeeze the lower myocardium – regular – firm – steady; one squeeze about every second. That will force the blood upwards, out of the ventricle into the upper chamber and into the circulation.'

This was obviously a teaching exercise.

The older man stood up and stretched his back. He wiped his bloody hand down his coat.

'That was good,' he said with satisfaction. 'We are winning. I can feel a pulse in the jugular.'

223

Then something spine-chilling occurred. Dr Hyem, lying flat on his back, opened his eyes and stared into the brilliant light shining directly on him. His mouth hung open, and a rasping roar was emitted from the depths of his throat. It was a ghastly noise, like the whoop or howl of an animal in agony. The sound rose to a crescendo and then stopped abruptly, and the silence that followed was almost more dreadful than the roar.

I ran around to the other side of the bed and took Dr Hyem's head and shoulders in my arms in a futile attempt to protect him. He looked at me, I swear he looked at me, and in his eyes was reproach. He had said, 'When my time comes I want it to be the end. I don't want anyone messing about with me.' I had promised that he would die peacefully, and I had let him down.

I have lived with that look of reproach all my life.

'I told you to get out of here, woman. Now clear off and don't interfere,' barked the registrar.

'I am the night sister,' I exclaimed, 'and Dr Hyem is in my care!'

'Bloody fine care you give, trying to be obstructive.'

Then to the team, 'He's coming round. Excellent. Ah! There's the porter with the machine. Splendid. Bring it over here.'

He spoke to the two younger doctors. 'Fix it up, and it can take over the massage. Now, we will want a central line through the iliac vein, and another in the subclavian, but try the iliac first, and a shot of adrenaline direct into the myocardium. Get a tracheal tube down him, and fix up the oxygen supply.'

Then again, to me: 'Look, I told you to clear off.'

'I am the night sister.'

'I don't care if you're the Queen of bloody Sheba! Get out of the way. I want to get a tracheal tube down him.'

I was pushed aside, and one of the young doctors tried to insert the catheter into the lungs. It is not an easy thing to do, and he had to make several attempts.

'Arch the neck. It will go down easier. More than that, pull the head backwards; you've got to locate the trachea. It's no good if the thing goes into his oesophagus. We don't want to oxygenate his guts.' He laughed at his own joke, and the others laughed in unison.

'Have you no respect for the dead?' I bleated, despairingly.

'He's not dead, you stupid cow. He's coming round. This has been highly successful.'

There was nothing I could do. I covered my face with my hands to hide my tears and fled to the office. The nurse whom I had left sitting with Dr Hyem only half an hour earlier came in.

'Are you all right, Sister? You look dreadful. Can I get you a cup of tea?'

I couldn't look up. 'What happened?' I moaned. 'How did this happen?'

'I was sitting with him, like you said, Sister, and he stopped breathing, and I couldn't feel a pulse, and I didn't know what to do, so I rang the emergency button.'

That was all that was needed. A young, inexperienced nurse, seeing death, possibly for the first time, and quite possibly frightened at being alone, and me, her senior, unavailable. So she had pressed the emergency button, and a resuscitation team arrived. Once started, the process could not be reversed. And, as the registrar had proudly stated, it had been highly successful.

LAZARUS

The wound in Dr Hyem's chest was sutured under local anaesthetic, the broken ribs realigned, and the chest bound, to keep them in place. We then raised him to a semi-recumbent position and changed the bed linen. Oxygen was directly entering his lungs, so his colour was good, and the cardiac machine maintained his heartbeat. Fluid was dripping into his circulation, and drugs were introduced to raise the blood pressure, to stimulate the heart muscles, and to thin the blood; antibiotics, a clot-buster and diuretics completed the cocktail.

The registrar and his team were exhilarated by their success. They had saved a life, and that's what medicine is all about. Lazarus had been raised from the dead. It was a miracle of modern medicine.

The team prepared to leave, all of them exhausted. By then it was 3 a.m., but adrenalin had been pumping through their bodies and now they were worn out. The registrar apologised for his rudeness. 'It's the tension that gets me,' he said. 'I'm not aware of it. I snap at everyone, they tell me.' He left with instructions about monitoring the cardiac, pulmonary and blood pressure responses to the machines, and the adjustments that should be made in the event of physical changes.

Dr Hyem breathed quietly all night. His pulse and blood pressure were steady. The drip dripped, the oxygen hissed, the cardiac machine hummed quietly, and the twenty or more men who had been awake during the commotion of the night fell asleep as dawn was breaking.

I had many other duties to attend to in the hospital, but stayed with Dr Hyem as much as possible, and, as I looked at him breathing quietly, I began to feel ashamed of myself. He was alive. Why should I have wished the old man dead? It was unworthy of

me; wicked even. He was alive due to the miracles of modern
medicine. Nearly twenty years had passed since I had started
nursing and everything had changed, scientific advances in drugs,
surgery, in technology. I was old-fashioned, I told myself, and must
embrace these changes.

At 6 a.m. I started my morning round of the hospital. It was still
dark, but the return of day could be felt in the air – sleepy sparrows
began to chirp, an early morning milk delivery could be heard in
the streets, the first kitchen workers were arriving. As I finished
my round, light was returning, and the fears of the night, enshrined
in all our fairy tales, were receding. Had the darkness played its
part in exaggerating the terror I had felt for Dr Hyem, I wondered?

By about 7 o'clock I had finished the morning round and was
able to return to Dr Hyem. The registrar was there before me,
checking the dials and drips, listening carefully to his patient's
heartbeat and lungs, taking a sample of blood for path lab
investigations.

'I owe you an apology,' I said, 'I doubted you.'

'No, no, not at all. It can be pretty scary, but as you can see, it
can be successful.' He held out his hand towards Dr Hyem, who
looked peaceful. 'Not every attempt turns out as good as this one.
In fact, if I'm honest, most fail. But it's worth having a go, just to
get a result like this.'

He continued with his checks and adjustments, saying as he
did so, 'New techniques for resuscitation are being pioneered in
America. Some of our teaching hospitals are using them. Stat-
istically, they are more effective. I would like to try them myself,
but we don't have the equipment here in this backwater.'

He's a good man, I thought, and a dedicated doctor. He can't
have had more than a couple of hours' sleep, but still he felt the
need to see his patient before starting the day's routine.

He patted Dr Hyem's hand. 'Well, you're doing nicely, Dad.
I'm pleased with you. We'll have you running around again in a
few days. I'm off to get some breakfast now, and I'll come in and
see you later in the day.'

As he left he said, 'I've got a morning in theatre. Tell Sister

Tovey I'll be here around lunchtime.' Then to Dr Hyem, 'Doing nicely. You're doing well. Keep it up.'

Such energy, such confidence, is invigorating.

Sister Tovey, the ward sister, to whom I gave the night report, felt differently. She was a woman about twenty years my senior and was nearing retirement. She had been nursing throughout the war, with two years spent in Egypt, receiving casualties from the fighting in North Africa, a great many of whom died for want of adequate medical attention. She was a woman of vast experience and few words.

'Dr Hyem told me he wanted no resuscitation,' she said.

'He told me that also.'

'And he told the cardiologist. I know, because I was there at the time.'

'It must be recorded on his notes, then.'

Together we looked, and there, written quite clearly on about the fourth or fifth page, were the words, 'In the event of cardiac arrest, do not resuscitate.'

'I suppose they didn't see that,' I muttered.

'More likely didn't look! These resuscitations have to be carried out at lightning speed. There's no time even to think. Just get on with it, that's the message. I don't like it. Not a bit.'

'Well, he's alive,' I said.

'What for?' she demanded.

The question seemed callous. But was it? Or was it realistic? My first doubts, momentarily dispelled by the registrar's breezy confidence, returned. I did not reply.

'What for, I say? Congestive heart failure? Renal failure? Liver failure? I must speak to the cardiologist about this. I don't like it.'

'Well, he seems to have recovered and his condition is stable. There is nothing more I can say or do. I'm worn out. I must go home and get the children off to school. Then I must go to bed.'

We parted, and my mind was in turmoil as I drove home. The events of the night were screaming in my poor tired brain. Had it been a triumph, or a tragedy? The registrar's confidence and Sister

Tovey's doubts were struggling with each other. That dreadful cry, like all the ghosts and ghouls of Hell, kept sounding in my ears. But it was probably not a conscious cry, I told myself, just the involuntary emission of residual air in the lower lungs escaping through slack vocal cords. He was alive, and his condition stable, that was the main thing. One should not drive after a night like that, when the mind is in such a state. It was surprising I did not have an accident.

The children restored my equilibrium. I defy anyone to get too serious when there are children around. Their laughter, their squabbles, their endless questions, their intense passion if a crayon or a book is lost, flying around the house to get a pair of gym shoes – all these little things brought me back to normal. We ate breakfast together, and I found, to my surprise, that I was hungry. Then there was a knock at the door, and a little friend arrived, then another, and the girls raced off together to the primary school down the road. I went to bed and slept, reflections on life and death eclipsed by the vitality of children.

Dr Hyem did not die, but he did not live, either. His heart had been in failure for a long time, and now all his vital organs began to fail too. The slow gradations of decay set in.

Failing circulation, caused by a congested heart, creates 'back pressure', affecting all the organs of the body. In Dr Hyem's case it caused congestion of the lungs, so he had great difficulty in breathing. Fluid collected in his lower lungs, creating a bubbly, rasping sound with each breath. The fluid became infected and pneumonia developed, which was treated with antibiotics.

The back-pressure from inadequate cardiac output puts added strain on the kidneys, which were struggling to excrete the body's waste products. Uraemia, or blood poisoning from renal failure, was kept at bay by intensified doses of diuretics.

Back-pressure put new strain on the liver, already grossly distended and striving to cope with the rising acidosis caused by diabetes. The pancreas, the gall bladder, the intestinal tract – all of them were congested.

Back-pressure forces fluid to leak out of the arterioles, the smallest blood vessels, into the surrounding tissues. They become waterlogged, a fluid swelling known as oedema. Ascites developed in the abdomen. Dr Hyem was totally bedridden. He sat there, day after day, with his legs, thighs, buttocks, scrotum, and belly swollen with oedema and ascites. However hard we tried, bedsores could not be prevented.

Had back-pressure affected his brain, or was it something else? Dr Hyem hardly spoke during the last weeks of his life. When he did attempt to mumble a few words, they were slurred and barely audible. His eyes were usually closed, but when open the pupils were dilated and fixed. The resuscitation, although quick, may not have been quick enough. Small areas of the brain may have been starved of oxygen and died during the minutes that had ticked by during resuscitation.

All the medical staff in the hospital took a great deal of interest in Dr Hyem, for open-heart resuscitation was a sufficient novelty in a small suburban hospital in the 1960s to attract attention. The registrar who had led the team became something of a celebrity. The staff all crowded around the bed, studied the notes, and regarded the machines and dials and drips with scientific interest. The cardiologist spoke to the lung specialist, the urologist to the gastro-enterologist, and the diabetic specialist to the dietician. They took brain scans (EEGs), heart scans (ECGs), recorded blood count and electrolyte balance (electrolytes were all the rage at the time), took X-rays of his chest, aspirated his lungs, measured his insulin levels and the mounting acidosis in his blood, changed his drugs, increased the changes, tried new drugs, changed them again and increased them again. They held special meetings to discuss the case; they could not have done more.

But, as the days stretched into weeks, the doctors visited less frequently and departed more quickly. Did they just lose interest, or had the passion for progress spent itself? Was there no more scientific or biochemical excitement to be gleaned from Dr Hyem? Doctors tend to regard a dying patient as a personal failure, and frequently withdraw if the process goes on for too long. Dr Hyem was dragging on and on. Perhaps the reality of a slow, lingering death was more than they could stomach.

The doctors made all the decisions affecting the physical condition of Dr Hyem, but they did not see the details of what this would entail: the reality and the humiliations endured by Dr Hyem were witnessed only by the nursing staff.

Daily, hourly, we treated bedsores that developed quickly because of immobility, oedema and a watery diarrhoea that poured from him in the early days. The sores quickly became great, stinking holes, which we packed with flavine but which became black around the edges from lack of blood supply. The diarrhoea cleared up, and chronic constipation replaced it, which aperients and enemas could not shift, so a nurse had to remove, manually, lumps of impacted faeces from his rectum. When I read *that* in the day report, I hoped fervently that Dr Hyem's sensitive mind had been so damaged that he was not aware of what a young nurse was doing to him.

Spoon-feeding a little semi-solid food was always difficult, and was frequently regurgitated, trickling out of the corners of his mouth, over which he had no control. The amount of food and fluids and the quantity of glucose in the drip had to be monitored all the time, and balanced against his insulin injections to control his diabetes.

His breathing was always laboured and painful to see. His cough reflex was seriously depressed and he could not bring up the sputum that collected in his lungs. A frothy exudate bubbled from his mouth sometimes. A physiotherapist came in to try to help him to cough by palpating his chest, but this caused so much pain to his broken ribs that the idea was abandoned. With stagnant, infected fluid in his lungs, his breath became foul smelling. Pleural aspiration was ordered to drain off some of the fluid and a cannula was inserted into his lower lungs, and a little watery stuff drained away. This relieved the pressure for a while, but it did not halt the accumulation. It seemed that Dr Hyem would drown in his own bodily fluids.

A catheter was in place all the time, and this avoided incontinence of urine, which would have made the bedsores worse, but it had to be changed every few days, and kept clean, which was unpleasant and possibly embarrassing for Dr Hyem. Unless we cleaned his mouth every two hours with glycerine, his tongue became so dry that the skin peeled off, and ribbons of grey, stringy stuff could be pulled from his throat.

The doctors saw none of this. Junior doctors sometimes get an idea of the suffering and humiliation that patients endure, and what nurses do, but a consultant seldom does. The more senior a doctor, the less he knows of the unpleasant details. None of this will appear in medical textbooks, which are written by academic and scientific medical experts, who spend much of their time in laboratories and libraries. Only nurses are at the bedside. And nurses don't tell.

The end came for Dr Hyem because his renal failure and long-standing diabetes could no longer be controlled, and acidosis developed over a few days, first with abdominal pain, and a decreased volume of urine. Then his blood pressure dropped and his pulse became thin and rapid, his ocular tension was low and his skin became very dry. The doctors decided not to attempt treatment, and he drifted into a diabetic coma from which he could not be roused.

Dr Hyem died peacefully, five weeks after a successful resuscitation from cardiac failure.

FAITH

I need no assurances – I am a man who is pre-occupied of his
own soul;

I do not doubt that whatever I know at a given time, there waits
for me more which I do not know.

I do not doubt but the majesty and beauty of the world is latent
in any iota of the world;

I do not doubt there are realizations I have no idea of, waiting for
me through time and through the universes – also upon this earth;

I do not doubt I am limitless, and that the universes are limitless –
in vain I try to think how limitless;

Did you think Life was so well provided for, and Death, the
purport of all Life, is not well provided for?

. . . to die is different from what anyone supposed . . .

— Fragments from *Faith Poem* and *Song of Myself* by Walt Whitman

CARDIO-PULMONARY RESUSCITATION (CPR) IN HOSPITAL

In 2008 I was visiting a friend who was in an acute medical ward of a large county hospital. I walked directly into the single room where I expected to find her, but she was not there; she had been moved to the main ward. In the bed was an old, old lady who looked as near to death as anyone I have seen. Her skin was as white as the sheets, her eyes sunken and rolled up towards her forehead; her cheeks were hollow, her mouth hung open, and her breathing came in ragged gasps. In my nursing days, we would have assessed that she had only a few hours to live and the ward sister would have instructed a nurse to sit beside her, just to hold her hand or to stroke her hair, or to whisper a few words now and then.

There was not a nurse in sight. Two gently humming machines were her only companions. Monitor pads were stuck to her arms with wires leading to one machine where lights flickered and a graph line was being traced. The other machine had wires attached that disappeared under the bedclothes. An oxygen cylinder hissed continuously, and a transparent catheter was attached to her nose with sticking plaster. A saline drip running into her arm and a urine drainage bag hanging from the bedside completed the picture.

I stood gazing at her for a couple of minutes thinking, *Poor old lady. What have you done to deserve this?* She was a total stranger to me, and I knew nothing of her medical history, but as the bed was in acute medicine, the likelihood is that she had collapsed from acute coronary failure caused by a heart attack. Someone had found her and called an ambulance, and this was the result. Nearly dead, surrounded by advanced medical technology, and not a soul around, except a stranger who had walked in by mistake.

This is what most of us can expect, unless we are very lucky. If anyone collapses, from whatever cause, at home or in a public place, the chances are that they will be taken to hospital. Only the medical team involved knows what goes on in the resuscitation room of a hospital, because lay people are excluded. When my mother died, I was pushed out and the doors were locked on the inside. There may be good reason for this, such as the risk of introducing infection into the room, but I suspect it is more because a relative may try to stop what is going on.

Sherwin B Nuland was a consultant surgeon at Yale University Hospital and teaches surgery and the history of medicine at Yale. In his remarkable book, *How We Die*, published in 1995, he has described the process of hospital resuscitation as accurately and objectively as any medical man can for the lay readership:

> Having countless times watched those teams fighting their furious skirmishes, and having often been a participant or their leader in years past, I can testify to the paradoxical partnering of human grief and grim clinical determination to win that actuates the urgencies swarming through the mind of every impassioned combatant. The tumultuous commotion of the whole reflects more than the sum of its parts, and yet the frenzied work gets done and sometimes even succeeds.
>
> As chaotic as they may appear, all resuscitations follow the same basic pattern. The patient, almost invariably unconscious because of inadequate blood flow to the brain, is quickly surrounded by a team whose mission is to pull him back from the edge by stopping his fibrillation or reversing his pulmonary oedema, or both. A breathing tube is rapidly thrust through his mouth and down into his windpipe so that oxygen under pressure can be forced in to expand his rapidly flooding lungs. If he is in fibrillation, large metal paddles are

placed on his chest and a blast of 200 joules* is fired through his heart in an attempt to stop the impotent squirming, with the expectation that a regular beat will return, as it frequently does.

If no effective beat appears, a member of the team begins a rhythmic compression of the heart by forcing the heel of his hand down into the lowest part of the breastbone at a rate of about one stroke per second. By squeezing the ventricles between the flatness of the yielding breastbone in front and the spinal column in the back, blood is forced out into the circulatory system to keep the brain and other vital organs alive. When this form of external cardiac massage is effective, a pulse can be felt as far away as the neck and groin. Although one might think otherwise, massage through an intact chest results in far better outcomes than does direct manual compression.

By this point, IVs [intra-venous drips] will have been inserted for the infusion of cardiac drugs, and wider plastic tubes called central lines are being expeditiously inserted into major veins. The various drugs inserted into the IV tubing have assorted purposes: They help to control rhythm, decrease the irritability of the myocardium, strengthen the force of its contraction, and drive excess fluid out of the lungs, to be excreted by the kidney. Every resuscitation is different. Though the general pattern is similar, every sequence, every response to massage and drugs, every heart's willingness to come back – all are different. The only certainty, whether spoken or not, is that the doctors, nurses and technicians are fighting not only death but their own uncertainties as well. In most resuscitations, those uncertainties can be narrowed down to two main questions: Are we doing the right things? And should we be doing anything at all?

* A joule is a unit of heat, energy and force – in this case electricity.

Far too often, nothing helps. Even when the correct answer to both questions is an emphatic 'yes', the fibrillation may be beyond correction, the myocardium unresponsive to the drugs, the increasingly flabby heart resistant to massage, and then the bottom falls out of the rescue attempt. When the brain has been starved of oxygen for longer than the critical two to four minutes, its injury becomes irreversible.

Actually, few people survive cardiac arrest, and even fewer among those seriously ill people who experience it in the hospital itself. Only about 15 per cent of hospitalised patients below the age of seventy and almost none of those who are older can be expected to be discharged alive, even if the CPR team somehow manages to succeed in its furious efforts.

It has probably been known for centuries, even millennia, that the heart can stop, and be restarted, although nothing was written about it for posterity. Nearly two hundred years ago, a Dr Silvester described how it could be done, by laying the patient on his back and raising the arms, to aid inhalation, then lowering the arms and pressing them against the ribs, to aid exhalation. It is not recorded whether anyone believed him in the early 1800s.

A century later, the idea was taken up by several doctors, and a similar technique described, combined with mouth-to-mouth resuscitation. This technique was included in *Scouting for Boys* by Baden-Powell, published in 1908. Few other people took it seriously, and certainly not the conservative medical profession, who always take decades to accept a new hypothesis. But, for the whole of the first fifty years of the last century, it was vaguely known that if you fished someone out of the canal, or something like that, mouth-to-mouth puffing and rubbing the chest could sometimes be effective in restoring life.

Eventually, in the 1950s, the medical profession got on to the idea, and the modern techniques of cardio-pulmonary resuscitation (CPR) were developed at the Johns Hopkins Medical Research Faculty in Baltimore, USA – although many other medical teams in other countries were working on the same theories. Within a

decade, their findings and teaching had gained widespread acceptance throughout western medicine.

Different techniques were developed and experimented with.
The open-heart resuscitation that I witnessed being applied to Dr
Hyem, was the first method adopted by the medical profession,
and its popularity lasted for around ten years. It has been replaced
by electrical impulses, or shocks, directly administered to the
heart, which are no less violent, but more effective. The giant
international drug and engineering companies started competing
with each other for the huge financial gains to be accrued from
producing ever more powerful cardiac stimulants, and manu-
facturers of surgical equipment bent all their efforts into resuscitation technology. It was big, big business.

From the 1970s onwards in the UK (earlier in America), the
intensive care unit and resuscitation became central to clinical
practice, and no hospital could afford to be without the latest
techniques and equipment. 'Crash' was all the rage. Everyone was
very gung-ho about it and cheerfully tried it on almost any dying
or dead patient. Young doctors, nurses, and technicians had to be
taught the techniques and older ones needed to practise. Pompous
old consultants and starchy old ward sisters who questioned the
technique were told to get up to date and live in the real world.
Those who warned about 'playing God' were told they
were religious fanatics and everyone would be better off without
them.

Those were exciting days to be in medicine. Anything was
possible. We could conquer death itself. Job vacancies appeared in
the *Nursing Times*: '*Be in the Front Line. Be a Life Saver. Join the
Resuscitation Team. Work in the Intensive Care Unit at – – Hospital.
Apply in writing.*' Adverts like this were quite common, and
I attended a conference where this type of wording was strongly
condemned by the RCN.

Exhilaration was in the air; but then, slowly, the demoralising
feeling sneaked up on us that something was not quite right.
Respect for the dead had been thrown out of the window.

*

The speed with which resuscitation swept through the medical profession was astonishing, and it was far too quick for it to be properly thought through. Drugs were introduced with bewildering haste – too hasty for proper trials to have been conducted. I gained the impression, in those days, that new cardio-pulmonary drugs were tried on patients, the attitude being, 'He's dead, anyway, so there's nothing to lose.' The equipment and the voltage of electricity was hit or miss because no one really knew how far to turn up the dial. Medical and paramedical staff had to master techniques that could only be learned on the job.

When I was a staff nurse at the London Hospital, we had a death on the ward. I was off duty at the time, but the next day the ward sister told me that she went behind the screens about twenty minutes after the patient had died to ensure that the eyes were closed and the chin supported, and found two young doctors trying to insert a central line into the iliac vein in the groin.

'What are you doing?' she demanded – ward sisters had a presence in those days. The young men looked up at her guiltily.

'Have you no respect for the dead?' she said contemptuously, as she covered the body with a sheet. They said nothing, and went away.

My sister Pat is a Queen's Nurse (Queen Alexandra Royal Army Nursing Corps). She trained from 1965–69, mostly in Singapore. She returned to England in 1969, to Aldershot Military Hospital, and was put straight on to night duty. The first night, she took the report and was told that if an emergency occurred she must press the AMSET button (Army Medical Services Emergency Team), but she was not shown where the emergency button was situated.

She did the usual drug round and noticed that a man was not in his bed. Thinking that he would return later, she finished the drug round, which took about half an hour. By then, he still had not returned, so she went to look for him. She couldn't get into the lavatory, and so she crouched down on the floor to peer under the door, and saw two feet sticking up. Her first thought was to press the AMSET button, but she didn't know where it was. She searched everywhere, poor girl, but still couldn't find it. So she telephoned the night sister, who called the emergency team. They came with mobile resuscitation equipment and dragged the dead man out of the lavatory.

Pat told me that he was quite cold and stiff, and must have been dead for some while, because she had done a complete drug round and then spent time searching for him, then more time searching for the AMSET button, before the team arrived. Nonetheless, with all the drugs and equipment at their disposal the team attempted to resuscitate.

Pat said, 'He was an old man, bless him, over seventy, and he was sick. I watched it all with horror, all that violence. There was no way they could get him back to life; he was quite dead, stiff and cold. But they carried on. Eventually, they gave up, of course. He had had a ruptured aortic aneurysm.' A ruptured aneurysm is not cardiac arrest, so resuscitation attempts in this situation were futile and inappropriate.

When I trained at the Royal Berkshire Hospital in the 1950s, there was no resuscitation. My niece, Joanna, trained at the same hospital twenty-five years later, and I asked her how much of it went on. She said,

'It was relentless, every day on every ward throughout the hospital. Every bed had a crash button beside it. There were half a dozen crash boxes around the ward, and the crash trolley placed centrally. If anyone died the nurses had to rush to the bed, press the crash button, detach the top and bottom of the bed, lie the patient flat with no pillows and start banging hard on the chest, pumping the sternum up and down to force a heartbeat, whilst a second nurse had to do mouth to mouth resuscitation until the crash team arrived. Then they started intensive resuscitation with drugs and electrical equipment. All nurses had to do this; it was a rule and was absolutely enforced. There was nothing we could do about it. We young nurses would ask the sisters, "Why? Why old Mrs C or why Mr S? Why is he not No Crash? He's terminally ill. He'll never get better." The sister would say, "I don't know, but we've got to do it. All I can say is don't rush, don't be in too much of a hurry to press the crash button, don't bang too hard on the sternum – if you can delay things for a few minutes, he might be able to die before the crash team can get at him."'

I told Joanna about the solemnity in a ward that had accompanied a person to their death when I was a young nurse. She said, 'Well that's all gone. When I trained it was rush, noise, panic, even shouting sometimes.'

I asked Jo what the success rate was. She thought a bit, then said, 'Very low. I can't really put a percentage on it, but very low. The trouble was that very often the body would twitch, and they thought this was a sign of life, and when the electric current hit the heart the body would really jerk – again, taken as a sign of life. But it's not, at least not necessarily. There can be a twitch, more than one, after death, which I think is part of the nervous system shutting down.' I agreed with her, and said that quite often I had seen someone die, and then, a minute or even two minutes later, suck in a great noisy gulp of air, which is called an 'agonal gasp'.

She laughed and said, 'I've seen that too; and *heard* it. It can be really scary, especially if you are a young nurse in the middle of the night, and you are not expecting it ... spooky!'

I joined her laughter and commented that medical people are known to have a black sense of humour.

'Too true. We need it,' she said.

These are just a few examples from a family of nurses to illustrate the frenzy that overtook medicine during that period of medical history. It also illustrates that medicine, like any other profession, is prone to fashions. Today, in the twenty-first century, there is more discrimination in undertaking resuscitation, but even so, the prognosis is poor. Nuland stated that only fifteen per cent of hospitalised patients below the age of seventy would survive cardiac arrest and resuscitation, and almost none over that age. That proportion has remained unchanged.

Yet, even with more selection, a lot of resuscitation goes on in hospitals. Doctors know that in most cases it will be futile, so why do they carry on doing it? The answer is two-fold. Firstly, and most importantly, for the sake of the fifteen per cent who *do* survive. The second reason is more complex. The burdens placed upon doctors and nurses by public expectations are crushing. Doctors feel blamed for every death and, driven by a combination of guilt and doubt and fear, they strive all the time to save a life. They know that if they don't make the maximum effort, and someone dies, they could be in serious trouble, which could destroy a career. The fear of litigation is ever-present.

Yet the public, and particularly the media, are so fickle that, having saved a life, doctors are then often accused of needlessly prolonging life and causing suffering. Whatever they do they will be in the wrong. Sometimes I wonder why anyone ever becomes a doctor or a nurse at all!

The heyday of resuscitation in hospitals was around 1970–95. Since then, much more restraint and discrimination has been observed. Doctors are now more ready to write a Do Not Attempt Resuscitation (DNAR) order if it is foreseen that a patient has a diagnosed condition with progressive advanced illness from which they will not recover, and for which resuscitation would be futile. Details of the General Medical Council (GMC) directive to doctors issued May 2010 can be found in Appendix I.

To discuss the prognosis with the patient is ideal, but it is often difficult, or plain impossible. Some patients are not approachable on the subject of their own death; some doctors cannot bring themselves to mention the dreaded word, and, in that case, an experienced nurse may be better. Some patients, surprisingly, have never even thought about it and say, 'I don't know – I leave it to you, Doctor.' Others say, 'I want to go when my time comes.' Everyone is different, every doctor and nurse is different, and every clinical situation is different. What is necessary, in all 'Would you want to be resuscitated?' situations, is time. Such a discussion, if handled sensitively, could take all afternoon – and who, in the busy setting of a modern hospital, has that amount of time at their disposal? Probably no one. So an informed discussion is often hurried, even rushed, or pushed aside for a day that never comes.

Everybody must think about these things and discuss them

with family, friends or carers long before a nervous young doctor tentatively raises the issue, or a lady with a clipboard comes round and says, 'I'm filling in a patient's questionnaire – do you want to be resuscitated? Shall I put a tick in the box, or not?'

At this point, it must be emphasised that resuscitation is the only medical procedure for which you have to say, quite specifically, that you do not want it. In the absence of such a refusal, resuscitation will be attempted.

What happens if the patient cannot make this decision? It used to be the law that no one could make such a decision for another person. But the Mental Capacity Act, 2009, alters that. An assessment must be made thus:

1. Can the patient understand and retain the information?
2. Can he/she weigh the risks versus benefits?
3. Can he/she rationally come to a decision?

If the answers are negative, relatives, close friends, and long-term carers can assist, or even make a decision, providing he or she does not stand to gain financially from the death of the person involved, and providing he or she is rational and reasonable.

The Reverend Mother of a convent I know well, told me that Sister K had suffered a severe cerebral haemorrhage and was taken to the local hospital where the bleeding continued. When the Reverend Mother arrived at the hospital, the staff had Sister K on a trolley, and were on the point of transferring her to the neurological surgery unit of the City Hospital several miles away. Reverend Mother, who was an experienced nurse and midwife, said, 'I could see at once she was dying, so I said to the staff nurse, "Look, she is not going to recover. Is this necessary? Can you not put her back in bed and leave her to die in peace and with dignity? I will stay with her." And they did. Sister K died peacefully and prayerfully a few hours later.'

In preparation for this book, I visited the archives of the Royal College of Nursing in Edinburgh. The archivist told me that her sister had trained in Dublin at a time when nuns ran many of the hospitals. She said that the nuns always seemed to know when someone was going to die, and they weren't afraid of death, they knew how to handle it. On the same visit, I also spoke to several nurses and care assistants. In the course of conversation, a senior cardiac nurse said, 'Death in hospital is a violent event,' and the others agreed with her.

Most emphatically, we *don't* know how to handle it. It's no good blaming the medical profession. There is a collective responsibility here. We have lost the ideal of reverence at the hour of death, and put our faith in science and technology instead. That is what has transformed the natural and peaceful ending of life into a violent event.*

* For an update, see Appendix I, Medical Aspects of Cardio-Pulmonary Resuscitation, by David Hackett, MD, FRCP, FESC.

'How people die remains in the memory of those who live on'

— *Dame Cicely Saunders*

999

Beatrice is a friend of mine. She and her husband are farmers, and I rang her to order some meat for the weekend. She told me that the family had had a very stressful time.

'My mother died nine days ago. She was seventy and had suffered a heart attack. She'd had one twelve years ago when she was only fifty-seven, but had recovered, though she had to take it easy. She knew the heart wall was thin, but she was OK.

'My sister Kelly went to her house to take her shopping, and found her dead in her chair. Kelly dialled 999. The voice that answered ordered her to lift our mother on to the floor and start resuscitation by compressing the sternum to restart her heart. Kelly obeyed. While she was carrying out the instruction she heard a crack from the ribcage. She says she will never forget that crack. Two men arrived very quickly and cut off Mum's nightdress and started work. Kelly telephoned me, and I came. It took me about twenty minutes to get there. As soon as I walked in, I could see Mum was dead – I'm a farmer, I see death all the time, and there's no mistaking it. The men were working away with their equipment. I pleaded with them, "Stop it. Can't you see she's dead?" They just replied, "We've got to. We can't stop yet." I shouted back, "Well, you won't be doing her any favours even if you do bring her back to life. Her brain will be dead by now." But they wouldn't stop. Eventually, the ambulance arrived, and then the paramedics took over.

'It was a dreadful time. My poor sister – she's in such a state of shock. She says she can't get the sound of that crack out of her head. I don't know when she will get over it.'

Beatrice was talking fast, the words tumbling out. Then she paused and spoke more slowly and thoughtfully. 'The trouble is, we'd never discussed it, never asked Mum what we should do if

246

she had another heart attack. We all knew it was possible – in fact, if I'm honest, we knew it was quite likely after the last one. But that was twelve years ago, and I suppose we had put it out of our minds. We *should* have discussed it. I think everyone should. It would have saved her, and us, from all that dreadful business. I don't like to think what my poor sister is going through. She blames herself, of course, but it wasn't her fault. I think everyone should discuss these things.'

It was a couple of months before I managed to speak to Kelly. I had asked, but perhaps she did not want to talk to me or anyone else so soon. But a couple of months later, after she had been on holiday, she felt ready to re-live that fateful morning.

Kelly told me, as Beatrice had, that she had driven to the house to take her mother shopping, and found her dead in her chair.

'She was sitting quite still and peaceful, but absolutely dead – there was no mistaking that. I reckon she had been dead for quite a long time, because she was in her nightie. When she was expecting me for our weekly shop, she would always be up and dressed by about 9 o'clock. But it was 10.30 and she was still in her nightie ... so I reckon she died before 9 o'clock.'

Her voice was very quiet, and it faltered several times as she spoke. She continued:

'I didn't know what to do ... I suppose the shock made me panic. My first thought was, *I must get help*, so I rang 999. I spoke to a man, who said, "I have ordered the ambulance crew, and until they get there you must start resuscitation." I said, "It's too late, she is blue." He said, "No, you must." I repeated, "It's much too late. She's quite dead." He ordered, "You have *got* to. Get your mother on to the floor, and do as I say. I'll talk you through it, until they arrive." I struggled to lift my mother, and told him, so he said, "You *must* get her off the chair and on to the floor." I ended up pulling her. It was an awful thing to have to do.'

I gently asked, 'Why did you do it? You don't have to do what a voice on the telephone tells you to do.'

'No, I know. But I suppose I was numb with shock ... I don't know . . .' Her voice trailed away. 'Then he said, "Start firm, hard pressure on her breast-bone, rhythmically, about two beats per second. I will count you through, start now – one, two, one two." I did . . . and then . . . I heard that crack, from her ribcage.'

She couldn't speak after that for a long time. I didn't know what to say. I think I murmured, 'You poor soul,' or something like that. Eventually she was able to carry on.

'Two men came and took over. They pushed a tube down into her windpipe and pumped in air, or perhaps it was oxygen. They cut open her nightie and wired her up to a machine, which they switched on. I couldn't bear to see her like that, on the floor, she was so modest, her nightie pulled away, and two men over her. I tried to cover up her lower parts, so she wasn't too exposed – it was silly, really – but I kept thinking how mortified she would have been.

'I went and telephoned Beatrice. There was nothing I could do. The men carried on for ages. They were talking to each other and I heard the words "an atrial response". My sister arrived, and asked them to stop, but they wouldn't. Mum's colour began to return. She had been very grey, but the pink colour was returning to her skin. Then the ambulance arrived. Two paramedics came in with more equipment. I don't know what it all was. They started injecting her feet, about one injection every few minutes, and Mum was looking much better, in fact she looked quite normal; she just wasn't breathing.

'Beatrice was getting quite upset and begged them to stop – they said they could detect a response – she shouted that it was the oxygen making her look better, and there was no response because she was dead, couldn't they see that? But they took no notice and carried on. They must have been at it for more than an hour, because it was getting on for 12 o'clock when they finally gave up.'

Kelly was so distressed, I felt that perhaps I had been tactless, and shouldn't have asked her to re-live that morning. I said something to that effect – it was hard to know what to say. But she replied, 'That's all right – I agreed to speak to you, so I will.'

'Next, the police arrived. The paramedics told them what they had done, and packed up. They covered my mother with a spare duvet cover on the floor while the police took a statement. Then they wanted another one from me, which they wrote down. After that, they did a full body examination of my mother. This has to be done in the event of an unexpected death, they told me, in case of foul play or homicide.

'The policewoman phoned the undertakers, and they arrived. They asked if we wanted to say goodbye to our mother before they took the body away. We did, of course we did, but, you know, it's not so easy when there are two police officers in the room, and pagers bleeping and voices talking, and undertakers wanting to get on with their job. So we didn't really get to say goodbye to her. The undertaker took her, and we never saw her again.

'She had to go for post-mortem, because it was an unexpected death. Even though Mum had a known heart condition, and had had a previous severe heart attack, a postmortem had to be done because she had not seen a doctor for about six months.' Apparently, if you have not seen a doctor for a fortnight before death, the law is that a post mortem must be carried out to discover the cause of death. In fact, it is very rare for any sudden death at home not to be referred to the coroner for postmortem examination.

'We were asked if we wanted to see her after the postmortem when she was back in the undertaker's parlour. But I didn't want to. I knew all the time I would be looking for the incision marks of what they had done to her. I saw the postmortem report – every part of her had been opened up and examined. I didn't want to see what they had done.

'The coroner reported the findings on autopsy:

1. Ischaemic heart disease
2. Old myocardial infarction
3. Acute myocardial ischaemia.

'The coroner said that establishing the exact time of death was always difficult, but it could reasonably be stated that death had occurred before 9 a.m. – that was one and a half hours before I found her, and before resuscitation was started.'

We talked a little about the sadness of it all, and Kelly said:

'I think she had a peaceful death – there was no sign of a struggle, or anything like that, and her face looked comfortable and happy, not anguished, as though she had been in pain or distress. By the time all that resuscitation was started she wouldn't have known, or felt the pain of those electric shocks, the tube being pushed down her throat, or the injections. In spite of what they called "an atrial response" I don't think she would have known anything about it, and felt no pain or shock.'

Then Kelly told me something that interested me greatly. She said:

'I was talking about this with an acquaintance, and she told me that her mother had died one Christmas lunchtime, and that the family called no one. The men of the family simply carried her to her room, and laid her on her bed. They did nothing, because four years previously she had suffered a heart attack and had been successfully resuscitated. After that, she was so brain-damaged that she had to be looked after constantly. The family didn't want it to happen a second time.'

I don't call it 'doing nothing'. I call it respecting the dead in an appropriate and humane way, and enabling the family to say goodbye to their mother.

I am grateful to Beatrice and her sister Kelly for their kindness in giving me this information, knowing that it was for publication. My sympathies go to them both for the troubled memories they retain. But I am sure that Kelly was right when she said that her mother died peacefully – she died quietly in her own home, in her own armchair, which is what we all hope for. It was what happened afterwards – events for which they were not responsible – that was grossly disturbing.

Beatrice's words to me, when she told me what had happened, stick in my mind. She'd said, 'The trouble was, we'd never discussed it. We didn't ask her what we should do if she had another attack.

We should have done, because we knew she had a weak heart, and it could happen any time. But we didn't. I think everyone should talk about these things.'

Beatrice is right – everyone *should* discuss these matters, and make their wishes known. But accurate knowledge of the reality of events is in short supply. Most people get their information from the media, especially television hospital dramas, which portray a fantasy world in which resuscitation is usually successful and has no side-effects. There is a lot of debate amongst medical ethics committees, which is valuable, but their efforts are hampered unless the general public knows what the real issues are. *Everyone* should have proper information about what resuscitation involves; what the initial success rate, the long-term success rate, and the possible side effects are.

Cardio-Pulmonary Resuscitation may be more carefully monitored and restrained in hospitals today, but the incidents in the community are increasing. For example, in 2010 St John's Ambulance started a national fund-raising campaign to raise money to purchase thousands of Automatic External Defibrillation (AED) machines. This is just one of the many initiatives in the community.

Anyone involved in healthcare, however loosely – police, ambulance crews, clinicians, social workers, Red Cross volunteers, care assistants, first aid workers – all are shown how to use the AED machine, and the rule is that an attempt to resuscitate *must* be made unless there is a clear and unequivocal order not to do so. This is the DNAR order (Do Not Attempt Resuscitation) commonly used in hospitals. However, in the wider community such an order is not generally available, even if it has at some time been made. A person may have a living will, but if they collapse at the shops, who is going to know?

In country areas, where a hospital may be some distance away, lay people are trained and given the equipment to resuscitate, so that they can be immediately available. These people are volunteers, called Community First Responders, and they are linked to the ambulance service. I think Kelly and Beatrice's mother must have been treated by such people at first, because two men arrived within a few minutes of Kelly's phone call, whereas it took about thirty minutes for an ambulance to get to the house, which is in the countryside.

Since the turn of the millennium, portable defibrillators have been developed and are being used in the community. They are monitored electronically, and require no training. You simply open the lid and all the instructions are clearly printed: lay the collapsed person flat on their back, expose the chest, attach the pads to the points indicated, and switch on. The machine will pick up the extent to which the heart is fibrillating. At a signal from the machine, everyone around must stand back, and a shot of electricity is directed into the heart, which will stop the heartbeat altogether, thus stopping the fibrillations. This can be repeated several times, and will usually allow the heart to restart a rhythmic beat, at least temporarily, until an ambulance arrives with trained paramedics who can administer more aggressive treatment.

These defibrillators are now available on the open market, and there is a great deal of interest and excitement about them. Supermarkets, shopping centres, sports arenas all have them. Before many years have passed, health and safety regulators will no doubt require every public place to have one. Our love affair with machinery ensures that, once it is available, it will be used – regardless of whether it is appropriate or not.

Old age is no protection, because this would be described as age discrimination, which is, of course, illegal. I can envisage an old lady, of eighty-five or more, collapsing in a church service. The churchwarden rushes to get the defibrillator. Should the vicar be the one to say, 'Wait a minute. We all know this lady. Isn't this what she has said she wants? She is old and ill and lonely. She has told many of us she wants to join her husband, who died ten years ago. She should be left to die in peace. Put away your machine, and in the presence of Death, let us pray.'

Pity the vicar who has the guts to say such a thing. It would split the parish down the middle. Half the old ladies would say he is a hero; the other half would call for a public unfrocking. Special meetings of the PCC would be needed; the police, magistrates, the local paper, the bishop – it might even reach the ears of Canterbury or Rome!

The Joint Royal Colleges Ambulance Liaison Committee (JRCALC) issues guidelines to their members on when *not* to start resuscitation. They are in cases of:

1. Decapitation
2. Massive head destruction
3. Massive injuries incompatible with life
4. Decomposition or putrefaction
5. Incineration – full thickness burns greater than 95% of body surface
6. Drowning – known submersion for longer than an hour
7. Rigor mortis
8. Livor mortis (post-mortem lividity)
9. The known existence of a DNAR order.

I suppose it is some small consolation to be told that if I have been decapitated, no one will try to resurrect me!

The ambulance team has an unenviable job. They do their best, but they get a lot of blame from the general public, which is demoralising. In a situation such as the one just described, with Kelly and Beatrice so clearly upset, it must have been profoundly distressing for them. But, legally, no relative can say what medical treatment should or should not be given to another person.

Success for the ambulance team is defined as 'admission to hospital alive', and they are duty bound to strive for as long as necessary – up to one hour – to achieve this objective. They are empowered to declare 'life extinct', but as long as there is the smallest electrical response it can be argued that life is *not* extinct, and they must continue. Even if the ambulance crew get the patient to hospital alive, the side-effects can be severe, especially if the

brain has been starved of oxygen. Some people in long-stay geriatric wards and care homes are there because of brain damage
following a successful resuscitation (see also Appendix I).

Louise Massen is Clinical Team Leader for the South East Coast
Ambulance Service, working in Gravesend, Kent. She was invited
to speak at the National Council for Palliative Care annual conference in March 2009. She called her lecture 'Dying Differently'.
The following is taken from her lecture notes, with her permission:

1. Ambulance clinicians from all services work within the
   Ambulance Service JRCALC Guidelines 2006 (Joint Royal
   Colleges Ambulance Liaison Committee).
2. Ambulance clinicians' role traditionally has been to:
   - Preserve life
   - Prevent deterioration
   - Promote recovery.
3. The role of the modern ambulance service is far more than
   this. Ambulance clinicians have specialist skills in primary
   and critical care, and, increasingly, take healthcare to the
   patient – especially out of hours.
4. The only way that very ill patients are able to get to hospital
   will be when someone asks for an ambulance to attend.
5. The Ambulance Service offers a 24-hour service, seven days
   a week, following the JRCALC Guidelines 2006.

**– the guidelines are specific that in the event of being called
to a cardiac arrest or near-life-threatening event the ambulance
crew is obliged to initiate resuscitation – unless**
1. A formal Do Not Attempt Resuscitation (DNAR) order is
   in place, in writing, and given to the crew.
2. The DNAR order must be seen and corroborated by the
   crew on arrival. If the ambulance crew is *not* satisfied that
   the patient has made a prior and specific request to refuse
   treatment, they *must* continue all critical care in the usual
   way.

3. The condition of the patient must relate to the condition for which the DNAR order is written. Resuscitation should not be withheld for coincidental reasons.

4. Resuscitation may be withheld if a known terminally ill patient is being transferred to a palliative care facility. This can only be valid if Ambulance Control has been given prior and specific information, which has been recorded against the patient's name and address, and the ambulance crew has been informed.

Louise called the second part of her lecture 'The Moral Dilemma'. What happens when an ambulance crew arrives at the house of a patient who has suddenly 'collapsed' and Ambulance Control has received no other information? What will the crew do? Imagine the scene:

1. The ambulance crew will come running into the house laden with response bag, AED (automatic external defibrillator), an airway bag and drug kit.

2. The crew will take the stairs two at a time and rush over to the patient who has collapsed in bed.

3. They will perform a quick primary survey to establish vital signs. If there is no Airway obstruction, Breathing, or Cardiac output (known as ABC), the crew will commence resuscitation.

4. The crew will grab the patient by the arms and legs and lift them on to the floor, and using medical shears slice the nightclothes up the middle to expose the patient's chest and throat.

5. Next, they will place defibrillator pads on the patient's exposed chest and commence cardio-pulmonary resuscitation using JRCALC guidelines.

6. The crew will intubate the patient with an endotracheal tube, or in some circumstances, a laryngeal mask airway.

7. They will gain intravenous access, either using a jugular or peripheral vein; then administer intravenous drugs.

8. The crew will use the AED to deliver defibrillator shocks if necessary.
9. If resuscitation is successful, the crew will lift the patient on to a carry chair, downstairs and out to the ambulance, and race off to the A&E department of the nearest hospital.
10. When resuscitation is not successful, the crew will perform a Recognition of Life Extinct (ROLE), and contact the police, who must inform the coroner's office.
11. The crew will fill out the Patient Clinical Records.

Louise continued her lecture by asking these questions:

Is this right or is it wrong?

Why does it happen?

What can we do to make sure it does not happen?

How can we help?

To which she gave some answers:

1. The Ambulance Service needs to be incorporated into the Integrated Care Approach for all end of life care patients.
2. By having the information recorded in the Ambulance Control Centres, the crew would be forewarned.
3. Having access to a written DNAR/Advance Directive/ Living Will immediately on arrival will prevent inappropriate clinical intervention being performed.
4. Paramedic practitioners and clinical care paramedics have a huge range of medical treatments available. These can include broad-spectrum antibiotics and many drugs for treating minor illnesses, the use of which is controlled by Patient Group Directives (PGDs). All ambulances carry oxygen.

Louise ended her lecture by saying that the ambulance crew is usually first on the scene of a collapse, and that there is still a widespread lack of understanding among the general public about the scope and practice of ambulance clinicians in end-of-life situations. She pointed out that the advanced medical pathways available often put ambulance clinicians in a difficult position, which can be a true moral dilemma for them.

Numerous letters and telephone calls between Louise and myself have impressed on me the truth of these last words. She has told me many sad stories of an old person, obviously at the point of death, or maybe even dead, whom they are obliged to resuscitate and transfer as fast as possible to the nearest A&E department, where more advanced techniques can be administered. She tells me that usually the relatives or friends will say, 'Do all you can,' and insist on transfer to the hospital; and although the crew know that such steps are often pointless and sometimes cruel, they *must* do it.

On the other hand, she told me of a man of forty whom she recently attended after he had suffered a cardiac arrest: the ambulance crew resuscitated him, and took him to hospital. He returned home within four days, and was back at work in a fortnight.

There really is no right or wrong here.

I asked Louise Massen to write a supplement on the training of ambulance crews and the scope of their work, which is reproduced as Appendix II, at the end of this book.

Currently, there is a great deal of anxiety and inter-disciplinary debate about whether or not resuscitation is appropriate in palliative care – this being defined as 'the care of patients with a known terminal disease'. Opinions rage back and forth with extreme views expressed on both sides. A Joint Statement from the British Medical Association, the Resuscitation Council (UK) and the Royal College of Nursing was issued in 2006. It is broadly based and helpful, but very technical. More succinct, and therefore more accessible, is an article published in the *Nursing Times* in April 2009 by Madeline Bass, Senior Nurse and Head of Education at St Nicholas Hospice, Bury St Edmunds, Suffolk. The article shows the insights and instincts that a thoughtful nurse can gain from many years' experience of caring for patients at the end of their lives. This article is reproduced as Appendix III at the end of this book.

Resuscitation in nursing care homes is quite another matter. The people in them generally do not have what is termed 'known terminal illness'. They are old and frail, but with the advent of the National Service Framework for Older People (DOH 2001), age discrimination is illegal. They may have a condition such as Alzheimer's or a neuro-muscular disease, but these are chronic, and a known terminal time span cannot even loosely be ascribed. Some people in nursing care homes have a DNAR order, issued by a doctor. Some people sign living wills that include a DNAR order. For the majority of people, however, no advance decision has been made, in which case whether or not to resuscitate is entirely up to the staff of the care home, and whoever happens to be on duty at the time. There are very few trained, registered and experienced nurses working in nursing care homes these days. These homes are run by managers, who may have no clinical experience, and care assistants, who may have a very skimpy training in basic nursing. But they all know how to use an AED machine.

I have a friend, Sue Theobald, who does a great deal of voluntary work for the elderly and disabled, including running a music therapy group. She tells me that the group was in a small, specialist home that houses about six people with severe advanced Alzheimer's disease. Whilst the group was there, a woman actually died. Within seconds, the staff had her wired up to an AED machine. Sue tells me the speed of their movements was incredible. The electricity was switched on and the woman's heart jerked back into some sort of beat.

Why? The answer is nearly always fear. Fear of litigation haunts the medical world from top to bottom, from the most exalted professor of medicine to the humblest paramedic or care assistant. 'Cover yourself,' is the first rule of practice, 'and if in doubt, resuscitate.'

Today resuscitation in the community is burgeoning, with a
5–8 per cent success rate. However, this figure includes young
patients and success in the resuscitation of older people is not
evaluated separately. The latter is predicted to be 0–2 per cent in
the very short term, and even when resuscitation is successful brain
damage may occur. Automatic External Defibrillators (AEDs) can
now be obtained on the open market, anyone can use one, and
this is causing great excitement. Soon every public place will be
required to have an AED, and once they are available, they will be
used. The force, violence and pain inflicted never seems to be
considered.

I was talking on BBC Radio South on Sunday, 6 February
2011 – it was a phone-in. A lady who said she was sixty rang to
say she had died fifteen years earlier and had been resuscitated. She
told listeners she had experienced an exquisite sense of beauty and
peace and then 'suddenly there was pain. I could never tell you
how dreadful it was, like a great wooden stake being rammed
through my chest.' That must have been the CPR – entirely
justified on an otherwise healthy woman of forty-five, but not
justified on a failing old body for whom there is no chance of
return to a meaningful life.

Five per cent of the population die in an ambulance, but this
statistic can be misleading. Ambulance paramedics are required to
get a patient to hospital alive, so they use every means available to
keep the heart going for the duration of the journey. Something
must be done to protect the elderly who, like me, want to be able
to die quietly without first being subjected to well meant, but
intrusive attempts to resurrect us.

A Commission of Enquiry is needed. I have approached all
members of parliament and many members of the House of Lords.
I have approached DEMOS, the government think tank that acts
as a secretariat for commissions concerning social and medical
issues. In this age of electronic tags and instant access to personal
data surely it should be possible to prevent inappropriate resuscitation attempts.

1980

TIME TO GO

The Appalachian Mountains in 1896, the year Harry Randolph Truman was born, was a wild, rough place and it was hard to scratch a living out of the rocky soil. In a land of rolling valleys of oak and sycamore, beech and birch, it was natural for generations of Trumans to be woodsmen or loggers, and in later years Harry used the skills learned as a boy to construct the lodge, log cabins, boats and boathouse for the visitors' centre he built on the edge of Spirit Lake beneath the brooding presence of Mount St Helens, in Washington State, USA.

Truman possessed a daredevil streak and in 1917, lured into the war in Europe by dreams of adventure, he enlisted in the 100-Aero Squadron of the American Expeditionary Force. He learned to drive and to fly, and trained as an aero-mechanic and electrician – all skills that he would use in later life. Under a veil of secrecy the squadron was sent to Halifax, Nova Scotia, one of the Canadian ports shipping troops to France during the First World War. The boat on which he sailed was hit by a torpedo, and although many died, Truman was one of the survivors. His dreams of adventure were replaced by the cruel reality of war.

In France, he worked first as a mechanic and then as a combat pilot. In later years, at St Helens Lodge, he would tell of flying the French biplanes in an open cockpit, 'a leather cap on my head, a silk scarf round my neck flapping in the wind'. Like many such tales, they improved with each telling.

But war changed Truman, as it did many young men. A friend said, 'He became a kind of loner, I think. He never discussed the war, he wanted to forget it.'

Truman was demobilised in 1919 and he returned to a very different America. He worked as a mechanic for a Ford dealer, but although always polite and courteous, he kept to himself, and seldom confided in or even mixed with his fellow workers. He seldom revealed his deepest feelings to anyone. It was not until later that they learned that he had married a girl called Helen Hughes during this time and that they had had a daughter.

In 1921, Prohibition, forbidding the sale or consumption of alcohol in the United States, became law. Truman was deeply offended. He had fought for his country, and now that same country was telling him he couldn't have a drink! He saw it as a crisis that must be opposed. Besides, the humdrum routine of being a car mechanic, for low pay, was proving irksome; bootlegging offered better prospects. In many ways it was the perfect match of man and occupation. He was adventurous, ambitious, and full of initiative. Taking risks, bending the law, was just a well-paid game for him. He became a rum and whisky runner, picking up supplies smuggled illegally into the port of San Francisco, and running it into Washington State. What his wife had to say about this is not recorded! But bootlegging started by small entrepreneurs like Truman soon came to be controlled by organised and ruthless gangsters. With inevitable disputes over territory and money, Truman escaped just a few steps ahead of a gang who were after him. 'I got in trouble with some big guys. Things got hotter than Hell,' he said later.

He had to leave rum running and tried several low-profile jobs in which he hoped not to be noticed, but the boys were after him and he could not hide. Eventually, he decided that the wilderness was the only place where they would not find him – and that is how he came to Spirit Lake, beneath Mount St Helens, where he remained for fifty-four years until the mountain blew up.

Spirit Lake was over three thousand feet above sea level, and the land belonged to the Northern Pacific Railroad Company. Truman rented fifty acres from them and the rights to boating and fishing. He built his first cabin on the shoreline in 1926, and life was hard, but he had always responded well to a challenge. Few people could live in such isolation, and, inevitably, his marriage suffered. There were no schools for thirty miles, so his daughter had to live with her grandparents. His wife could not stand the separation so she joined her daughter. Divorce followed.

But Truman stayed. Like everyone, he had to earn a living, and he guessed that the beauty of the area would be a draw to visitors. Slowly, he built a holiday centre – cabins for visitors, a boathouse and jetty – offering fishing, riding, and trekking. The dramatic landscape and the solitude drew people from when the snows melted in spring until the cold of autumn. Winters were snowbound, and then he was alone.

Truman was a tall, handsome man and his carefree spirit, combined with rugged independence, made him extremely attractive to women. He tried marriage again, but the loneliness of the winters, being snowed up for months on end with one man – however attractive – proved too much for the poor woman, and she, too, left him.

Somehow, through the 1920s and '30s, Truman managed to continue his bootlegging, and he always kept a supply of illegal spirits for his tough, outdoor friends. He also constructed a still, and made good money from selling moonshine (a home brew, distilled into a spirit of rotgut potential). Truman was hardworking, hard-drinking and hard-swearing. 'That ol' sinner,' said a friend after his death, 'he was just a goddam, hell-bound ol' sinner. Up there in Heaven he'll smuggle whisky in one door and ice and shakers in the other, an' carry on like he always did. Jeez, I really miss that ol' son-of-a-bitch – sure miss him.'

In 1946 Truman married Eddie. She was the woman for him, and they loved each other deeply. Friends said that he worshipped her. Not only did she seem to enjoy the long, cold winters, she could handle his somewhat tempestuous nature, his hard drinking, and his autocratic ways.

When she died, thirty years later, he was devastated. The loss nearly destroyed him. He ceased caring for himself, or his lodge, or the visitors' centre. A friend said, 'If he hadn't been so tough, it would have killed him right away. But the old bugger was tougher than a boiled owl.'

★

Truman would walk to his boathouse as dusk set in, the warm evening wind whispering in his face. Trees, hundreds of years old, surrounded the lodge. 'Bear and cougar, deer and elk grazed in the underbrush, the dense carpet of fir needles silencing any footfall ... He could see the wild orchids and shooting-star wildflowers growing between the low bush huckleberries, the beautiful maid-enhair ferns and delicate violets, yellow, white and blue. Monkey flowers and kingcups bloomed on the banks of the lake.'*Quite often a fisherman would be whipping his line for a cast upstream from the dam. An otter would surface, see the fisherman and dive, splashing the water with its thick tail. As the sun dropped behind the hills, Spirit Lake, the place Truman knew so well, assumed an air of mystery. The light would change, and the snow-capped Mount St Helens would show a different mood before it was swallowed up by purple darkness. The distant snowfields would become incandescent, dimly reflecting a pinkish glow. Then the moon would rise, and the mountain, holding her secrets close, would look as if she belonged to another world.

But in winter the temperature would drop to well below zero for months on end, as snow followed snow and the ice on Spirit Lake froze to five feet deep. Animals and birds would move to warmer grounds, bears would hibernate, and many creatures would die. Storms would come one after another, and the snow would fall six, or eight, sometimes ten feet deep. After every fall, Truman had to climb on to the roof of his lodge to shovel it off, or the weight of snow would have made the roof cave in. The winter months were a constant battle to survive, and Truman turned his talents to trapping and poaching. He had bought in sacks of beans and rice and flour, bacon and salted beef; he had dried fruits and herbs, and stacked wood for the fire.

People who live close to nature have a different take on life from urban dwellers, who think they can control everything. These people recognise the rhythm of life and death in the changing shifts

* From Shirley Rosen, '*Truman of St Helens*', published by Madrona Publishers, Seattle, Washington State, 1981

of the natural world. Truman's years of reflection beside his lake, beneath the shadow of the mountain, had surely formulated his philosophy of life.

In March 1980, Truman was eighty-three years old, fit and strong, but nonetheless old and getting older. Eddie had been dead for five years and he was lonely. He had kept the place going because, if he hadn't, he would not have survived the winter. He had no enthusiasm for the idea of summer visitors, but that was the business upon which he depended for an income.

On Friday, 20th March, at 3.45 p.m., the ground under his feet shook slightly. He was glad, and thought it was a sign that the spring weather had loosened an avalanche down the side of Mount St Helens.

But scientists at the University of Washington, twenty miles to the north, were not so blasé. The seismographs showed an earth tremor measuring 4.1 on the Richter scale, and the location was close to Mount St Helens, which gave cause for real concern. Three days later the earth moved again, measuring 4.4 on the Richter scale, and the quakes were even closer to the mountain. Visitors were urged to stay away, and by the end of March the authorities were considering possible plans for an evacuation. The forest service closed all roads to the area above the timberline. Truman's lodge was *eight miles* above the timberline.

On the last day of March, a state of emergency was declared. Rob Smith, an old friend who lived further down the slopes, was having a drink and a quiet conversation with Truman when 'all of a sudden the whole building seemed like a little cardboard box, rocking backwards and forwards,' he remembered. They went out on to the porch and saw Mount St Helens spit a plume of ash thousands of feet into the air. Quite soon afterwards, the Deputy Sheriff's car came screaming up the approach road, his voice booming from the loudspeaker: 'The mountain's erupting. Everyone out.' Rob quickly made ready to leave, but Truman was not prepared to go. Rob went out and returned with the Sheriff. The two men tried every tactic from threat to guile – 'We're standing on a dynamite keg with the fuse lit. If it goes up, we will die' –

but they couldn't persuade the old man to go with them. They left, and Truman was alone.

Mount St Helens was much changed the following day. A crater had appeared on the summit, two hundred and fifty feet in diameter, surrounded by a dirty black ring of ash, disfiguring the purity of the snow. Large fissures, more than a mile long, were visible, and Truman must have been not just awestruck, but tremblingly afraid. Yet it must have been then that he formulated his unshakeable resolve: 'If that mountain goes, I go with it.' He was eighty-three years old, his beloved wife was dead, he was lonely and he frequently wondered what he had to live for now that she was gone. He had lived beside that mountain since he was a young, virile man of twenty-nine, and it was as much a part of him as his own hands and feet. His soul was in that mountain, and there was no life for him elsewhere. He would stay.

This resolve, spoken by a man in his right mind, started a bureaucratic and legal battle that was to rage for the next eight weeks. It also brought in the press, which exacerbated the sheriff's headaches, and was the cause of many sleepless nights.

The West Coast of America is on a known geological fault line, and tremors and small eruptions are quite common. But a dormant volcano, threatening to erupt, was big news, and all the papers wanted a story. When word got round that an old man was living halfway up the mountain and refusing to leave, editors were ecstatic and ordered their reporters to get the 'human story'.

A 'no entry' zone had been marked out by the authorities. Did the reporters take any notice? Of course not! They swarmed up the roads in droves, panting for a good story. When they met roadblocks, they proceeded on foot, cameramen and all, along the forest paths. If the Sheriff's forest rangers ordered them off, they stuck up two fingers and ignored them. Helicopters came in, and so many flew over the roadblocks that, at times, the highway in front of St Helen's Lodge resembled an air force landing pad.

Truman turned out to be a journalist's dream. He was old and gnarled, he was fast-talking, heavy drinking, and his language was too ripe to put into print. His views were extreme and his contempt for authority was equal to, or indeed exceeded, that of the average reporter. He also proved to be photogenic. At first he was wary of the press boys, and refused to have anything to do with them. But then he began to see the advantages of their attention. They were a lively bunch, mostly young, full of enthusiasm and daring. Their company was stimulating and entertaining, and Truman was lonely. They all had an amusing tale to tell about how they had got in, how they had fooled the Sheriff's men. The situation was heady for an old man who had spent much of the winter alone, and Truman reckoned he could afford to lavish his entire whisky supply on these men. They all drank a toast to the damnation of that goddam Sheriff and his goddam rules and regulations.

But Truman was not doing all this just to be kind or hospitable. He was a wily manipulator with a well-honed talent for getting what he wanted. For one thing, the reporters helped keep his mind off the situation – one big quake prompted him to say, 'You know, I'm scared as hell about earthquakes. I just wish it would all stop' – but, more importantly, he realised the press coverage would be of help to him.

Truman quickly became famous in the Western States, and when the *New York Times* ran a two-page article on him, complete with quotations and pictures, he became a national celebrity.

For the law-enforcement officials charged with keeping people out of the Red Zone, it was a nightmare. The pressure to interview Truman grew as the quakes and avalanches continued, and lightning bolts, some two miles long, flashed above the mountain. A second crater opened up on the summit and blue flames could be seen leaping into the air. But still the press boys continued to dodge the roadblocks.

Truman made his intentions absolutely clear – he was going to stay at the lodge, no matter what. 'You wouldn't pull me out with a mule team,' he said. 'That mountain's part of Truman, and Truman's part of that mountain,' it was reported in one paper. To another, he said 'I tell you; I'm no brave soul. Those goddam

quakes scare the living Hell out of me. But hell, I've lived here
fifty-four years. I might as well stay; I'm not leaving my home
now. You know, the people down town, they don't understand.
They think I'm putting on a false front. Well, Jesus Christ, I'm
going on eighty-four years old. When you've lived fifty-four years
in one place and it's the only home you've got, well, you don't
just walk off and leave it. Well, Christ no. People just don't
understand.'

Another paper reported these words: 'If the mountain does
something, I'd rather go right here with it. If I was out of here and
lost my home, I wouldn't last a week at my age, I'd just die, and
die miserable too. I'd have nothing to live for at all, and I'd just
double up and die. My old heart would stop – if I've got one, an'
a lot of people have said I ain't got no heart.'

The press loved it, and the newspapers lapped it up, printing
rows of dots when the language became too obscene. The public
bought the papers and magazines in their millions. Truman was a
star. The American people like to think of themselves as robustly
independent, like the first settlers, and here was a grand old American backwoodsman, showing them all that the 'spirit of America'
was alive and well.

Meanwhile, in the courts and committee rooms of Washington
State, debate was raging about Truman's status as the only person
remaining inside the Red Zone. Was it lawful? Was he trespassing?
Could the evacuation order be enforced? Should he be forcibly
removed for his own safety?

The land still belonged to the Northern Pacific Railroad
Company, so they enquired if the lease could be revoked in excep-
tional circumstances; the reply was so long in coming that it wasn't
worth waiting for. The Sheriff checked with local prosecutors
about Truman's legal rights. The lawyers conferred and came up
with the conclusion that an independent court would have to
decide, and that, in view of the publicity, it was doubtful they
could find an impartial jury to hear the case. Therefore, they could
not prosecute. Besides, there was no way of avoiding bad publicity,
and the lawyer doubted if there was a law-enforcement official in

the county who would arrest Truman, even if he was breaking the law.

But was he? He was in his own home, doing no harm to anyone, except perhaps himself. Some bright spark came up with the question, was he sane? If not, he could be certified and removed. But the idea of getting in a couple of psychiatrists to examine him, which would undoubtedly reach the ears of the press, leading to a stream of derisive articles, was too much for the poor Sheriff and the idea was abandoned.

The fact is, Truman was saner and a great deal more intelligent than anyone debating his case. He had always been a cute customer when he wanted something. He said once that 'the press is more powerful than the law'. Had he foreseen what was likely to happen to him? It would have been no trouble for two hefty young forest rangers to manhandle an old-timer out of his home, into a car or a helicopter. But with the press reporting every move this would have caused a public outcry. Civil liberties, the rights of man, assault – all would have been evoked. Truman knew what he was doing all along. Not from altruism had he exhausted his stock of whisky and rotgut on the press boys. With public opinion on his side, he was safe.

'Safe' is an odd word to use if you live in the path of an erupting volcano, but his logic was impeccable. We all have to die, and, whatever the circumstances, it is better to die in your own home than in an unfamiliar place surrounded by strangers. He had said, 'If I lost my home I wouldn't last a week at my age. My old heart would stop.' He was probably wrong, there. In modern America old hearts don't just stop, and if they do, life will be forced back into them. For Truman, it would have been a nursing home, confined, confused, drugged and defeated. From that, he was 'safe'.

Truman stayed, and on 18th May, 1980, at 8.45 a.m. Mount St Helens blew and he went with it. A blast of hundreds of millions of tons of rock, ash and magma hurtled into the air at a speed of 900 miles per hour and a temperature of 700 degrees Celsius, then poured down the mountainside. Spirit Lake and the surrounding woodland vanished for ever.

A memorial service was held for Truman a month later at the American Baptist Church in Longview, Washington State. The President of American Baptists took the service. In his commemorative speech he said these words: 'No one lives his life amid the awesome beauty of Spirit Lake and Mount St Helens without a deep theism we could not readily define. Truman was a man of the seasons – he didn't resist nature, he respected it – and he was a creature of the cycles nature brings. Wherever he is now, if he can see what is going on here today, he's saying "don't you dare cry for me! I did just what I wanted. Go have a good time."'

I am indebted to Shirley Rosen's book 'Truman of St Helens', published by Madrona Publishers, Seattle, Washington State, 1981, for the information for this chapter.

'I'm not afraid of dying, not at all, because I know what it's like. I've been there. It was after the birth of my third son, and I had a massive haemorrhage. An artery in or near the vagina had ruptured and fresh arterial blood was literally bursting out of me, like a fountain or a water jet. I felt myself sinking slowly, slowly downward, like a slow spiral. This must have been the blood and the oxygen leaving my body. I couldn't have moved if I had tried. But I didn't want to. I was in a tunnel, a big tunnel and I was walking along it towards a beautiful opening or door or something at the end. It was so beautiful, I could never describe it; not an earthly beauty but peace and quiet and beauty, and I wanted to get to it. I was very near. Another few steps and I would have got to it, which is what I wanted. But then I heard a sound and I felt movement; that must have been when they checked the blood flow and started pumping blood into me. And I looked behind me and saw three little children, and I knew I couldn't go. So I turned around and went back. But, oh, it was so lovely and I so much wanted to get to that beautiful place.'

— *Joanna Bruce, MBE*

(*Jo is my mother's first and favourite granddaughter*)

ACUTE HEART FAILURE

To write about my own mother's death is so painful that I wonder if I can do it at all. I have sat for hours at my desk with a pen and a blank page, and nothing comes but tears and regret. I have shut it out of my mind for twenty-five years, telling no one, unable to dwell on what happened, what might have happened, had I acted differently, what I could have done, should have done, what I did not do, did not know. For twenty-five years I have erased from my mind thoughts of the pain she must have suffered, her fear, her terror, and, worst of all, her anguish at being surrounded by strangers in the hour of her death, because I, her eldest daughter, was not there.

Who can write about their parents objectively? Not me, for sure. The relationship is too personal to be objective. I will say only that my mother loved life and everyone she met. She was full of fun and vitality. It was life-enhancing just to be with her. She was also exceedingly pretty.

In 1986 she was sixty-five and very popular. She had a host of friends, held constant luncheon, tea and dinner parties. She was a brilliant cook and a generous hostess. She swam regularly and enjoyed walking, gardening, and taking her grandchildren on outings. She enjoyed life, and appeared to be in excellent health.

She had arranged to meet some friends for a coffee morning, but did not turn up. They telephoned the house, but there was no reply, so one of them came to the house and knocked on the front door. No reply. The woman looked through the window and saw my mother lying unconscious on the sitting room floor. She immediately called the local hospital, an ambulance came, and my mother was rushed to Accident and Emergency and put straight into intensive care.

My sister and I were informed, and we both arrived as soon as we could. Our mother was attached to a defibrillator, an intra-venous drip and other life-maintaining apparatus, with dials and monitors and flickering graphs and lights. The gentle hum of the machines was reassuring, in a way. My sister and I were both trained and qualified nurses, but no longer practising, and medicine had advanced so rapidly that neither of us had seen such hospital treatment, nor did we know what was going on. We were told that our mother had had an acute heart attack.

'Acute' is the word to understand, and acute heart failure is quite different from congestive heart failure, which is a slow and cumulative process of heart dysfunction, usually occurring in the elderly. Acute heart failure occurs in a second, with no warning, no history of ill health, and it often attacks relatively young people. There are many possible causes, but the most common is a sudden occlusion (obstruction) of one of the coronary arteries. It is usually, though not always, caused by blood clots, developing in an ather-omatous section of a coronary artery. If a clot forms in one of the coronary arteries, the occluded area of heart muscle will die. This is known as an infarction. It is a major catastrophe. Whether the infarction is partial or total will depend on the size of the clot and the size of the artery occluded. Either way, the occurrence is commonly called a heart attack.

Our mother must have had a partial infarction, because she was found on the floor, unconscious, and no one knew how long she had been there. Add to that the time taken for ambulance transfer to the hospital, and several hours must have elapsed. When my sister and I arrived, she was breathing without the aid of a ventilator, but did not appear to be conscious. We stayed with her all night, dozing intermittently in the chairs that the staff had provided for us.

On the second morning she regained consciousness, glanced around her quite brightly, then looked at us in surprise. 'What are you two doing here? What's going on?'

We stayed with her all day. She was very weak, and obviously ill, but she talked rationally and could remember everything up until the moment she had collapsed. She seemed very interested in what must have happened, and in all the medical paraphernalia around her. She remembered her mother, who had suffered a heart attack about thirty-five years previously and died.

'If all this medical treatment had been available for my dear mother, she wouldn't have died. I was there with my Dad. The doctor came, and said there was nothing he could do. I am very grateful to the doctors and nurses here,' she said.

The doctor told us that she was out of danger and that we could go home if we wanted to. As my sister had three children to look after, we agreed that she should go and that I would stay on at the hospital with our mother. I stayed with her all evening and dozed in the chair beside her during the night. The machines hummed and whirred, and nurses came at intervals to check a monitor and offer words of comfort and reassurance. It reminded me of my own years of night duty – the night-time holds a beauty and mystery that we do not know during the daylight hours – but I had to recognise that although I was an experienced nurse, the new machines were quite beyond me.

It was Midsummer Day. Dawn was breaking, and soon brilliant sunshine was streaming in through the hospital window. My mother stirred and looked around her. 'It's going to be a lovely day,' she said.

A nurse came in and removed the drip from her arm. 'You've had a good sleep,' she said.

'Yes, and I feel a lot better. A cup of tea would be nice,' my mother replied. Then she turned to me and said, 'Go and get yourself some breakfast, dear. I'm sure there must be a canteen open somewhere in the hospital. I'm all right. I feel much better.'

The nurse agreed. 'We want to change your mother's bed and give her some breakfast, and we will probably get her up as well. I daresay she will be transferred to the ward when the doctors have seen her.'

I made my way to the hospital canteen with a great sense of relief in my heart. She's going to be all right, I thought. Modern medicine is wonderful. I remembered similar cases of acute heart failure that I had seen thirty years previously, when there was very little that we could do, and when many people died, or survived to be cardiac cripples.

Breakfast was excellent – cornflakes, bacon and eggs, toast and marmalade, coffee – and it increased my sense of well-being. I had intended to go straight back to my mother, but ... but ... All those fatal 'buts' in life; they are as bad as the 'if onlys'. If only I had followed my first intention. If only I had resisted the call of a midsummer morning, the lure of the rising sun casting long shadows over the hospital garden, the sight of small clouds floating in a clear blue sky, the sound of birds singing. If only I had shut my eyes and ears to the beauties of nature. But I didn't. I went for a walk in the morning light.

When I got back to the hospital, the door of the intensive care unit was locked. I could hear sounds from within but could not enter. I knocked on the door several times, my anxiety increasing. Eventually a nurse came out and said that an incident had occurred, and I could not be admitted.

'What incident?' I asked.

'A cardiac incident. We are dealing with it.'

'But I must come in,' I said.

'No, I'm sorry,' was the firm reply.

'But she is my mother. I *must* come in.'

'No. You cannot be admitted. Go to the waiting room and you will be kept informed of progress.'

'What are you doing? What's happening?'

The nurse did not reply, but turned back, shutting the door firmly in my face.

I was trembling and crying. 'Let me in, open the door. You can't keep me out.' That is what I intended to say, but it is more likely that I was inarticulate.

Someone led me to the waiting room and brought me a cup of tea.

I cannot remember my state of mind – confusion, panic, anger, self-reproach were all mixed up and churning around. Time passed.

What were they doing? A 'cardiac incident'? That could mean anything. When had it occurred? Why, oh why did I take that walk? I should never have done it. Never. I should have gone straight back after breakfast, and then I would have been there to protect her. I envisaged her, weak and helpless, wanting me, perhaps calling for me, and I wasn't there. I had abandoned her.

I ran back to intensive care, and banged on the door, calling out, 'Let me in, let me in,' but a man came out and told me: 'No'. I tried to push past him, but he completely blocked my path and held me back. An indistinct picture of white-coated figures, and masses of black machines and wires around a naked body on a bed, was all I saw before the man shut the door. A nurse led me back to the waiting room. She saw my distress and was very sweet. My mother had suffered a second heart attack, she told me, and the resuscitation team were doing all that they could to save her. 'Don't worry,' she said softly, 'your mother is in good hands. They know what they are doing.'

'But why can't I go in?'

'It really would be best if you stay here.'

And so I did, as everyone has to. No one is permitted to see a full-scale hospital resuscitation taking place.

I sat in numb grief for two hours. Self-reproach amounting to self-flagellation haunted me. If I had not taken that damned walk I would have been with her, and protected her from the violence of resuscitation. But would I? Could I? You never know in life, and it is always easy to be wise after the event. Could I have sat there and watched my mother suffer a heart attack, the symptoms of which I was well acquainted with, and done nothing? Could I have calmly observed her sudden pain, my mother clutching her chest with both hands, gasping, throwing her head back, mouth wide open in a frantic attempt to draw air into her lungs, her colour changing rapidly to a pallor that betokens death? Could I have witnessed this and done nothing? Of course not! In any case, my mother was still wired to cardiac monitoring equipment after the first heart attack, and red lights would have been flashing, warning signals screaming way beyond the confines of the intensive care unit in which she was being treated. The resuscitation team would have arrived anyway, and would have taken over. I would have been told to go to the waiting room, which is where I sat for two long, dreadful hours.

Eventually, a doctor came and told me that my mother was dead. They had done all that they could, he told me gently, but she had not responded.

'Since death (take my words literally) is the true goal of our lives, I have made myself so well acquainted during the last few years with this true and best friend of mankind that the idea of it no longer has any terrors for me, but rather much that is tranquil and comforting. And I thank God that he has granted me the good fortune to obtain the opportunity of regarding death as the key to our true happiness. I never lie down in my bed without considering that, young as I am, perhaps I may on the morrow be no more. Yet not one of those who know me could say that I am morose or melancholy, and for this I thank my Creator daily, and wish heartily that the same happiness may be given to my fellow men.'

— *the young Mozart in a letter to his father*

A GOOD DEATH

There are many neuro-muscular degenerative disorders – motor neurone disease, Parkinson's disease, multiple sclerosis, Huntingdon's chorea, among many others. Each follows a similar, though slightly different, pattern. Basically, the nerve endings start to degenerate, and with it, muscular control starts to slip, and the condition is progressive over a number of years. Cognitive function is usually not involved, and there are many examples of a brilliant mind in the wreck of a body – Professor Stephen Hawking springs to mind. However, different areas of the brain can sometimes be affected. If the centres regulating speech are damaged, a misdiagnosis of dementia may be made, with tragic results for the patient. I can think of few conditions more heart-rending than to be trapped, unable to speak, in a degenerating body over which you have no control, yet retaining your full mental faculties, and hearing, on all sides, that you are demented. However, this is not always the fate of a person so afflicted.

Carole and John had been married for ten years. He was a widower of sixty-five and she was a divorcee of fifty when they met. He was the love of her life. Ten years later he started to do strange and unexpected things, and to say things that made no sense. They consulted a doctor, who diagnosed frontal-temporal degeneration with primary progressive aphasia – that is, language mix-up and then loss of speech. John could understand exactly what was being said, and he and Carole listened carefully. They were told that it was not Alzheimer's, but a degenerative disease in which the nervous and muscular system would break down. The ability to make any decisions would go, together with the ability to read and write, but understanding would remain for a long time. They were told that there was no known cure, but that certain drugs could relieve the symptoms and that death could be expected in two to five years. John said, 'At my age, seventy-five, I can expect death in the next two to five years anyway, so what's the big deal?' and they all laughed. Carole was advised to keep a regular domestic routine going, and they were both told to enjoy life as much as possible – stimulation was the thing, physical, mental, emotional, visual, anything that makes you feel good.

They had two years of intense living and loving. They counted each new day as a gift from God to be lived to the full, and every hour was filled with rich experience. He loved music and had been a choral singer all his life, so, with the conductor's permission, he continued weekly rehearsals and could sing in tune, but he did not take part in concerts. They went to new places, saw new things, read new books (Carole reading aloud), met more frequently with their families and grandchildren – it was good for the grandchildren to see John and to know that, in spite of his mental and physical infirmities, he enjoyed life. They went on several holidays together – the Canaries, the Greek Islands, a cruise to the land of the midnight sun – and all of these trips John relished. He loved sitting in the sun.

As time went on, John developed amyotrophic lateral sclerosis, which is a slow creeping paralysis. He was now failing fast, and one by one his muscular controls went, including continence and the ability to chew and swallow. He was at home all this time. The Macmillan and local hospice nurses came daily, and John's son and two daughters (one of whom was a nurse) visited regularly. With their support, Carole managed well, and they were deeply happy. He knew she was always there and, although John had lost the ability to express himself through words and sentences, he spoke with his eyes, which followed her everywhere. Almost until the end – or possibly right up to the end of his life – he retained understanding and responded to those around him. Human interaction is not dependent on speech, and I have even heard it said that language and speech make up only ten per cent of all human communication.

★

One day Carole told me an interesting story. They were both deeply religious people. Carole had found her faith during the trauma of the divorce from her first husband, John when he was eighteen and had been called up for military service during the Second World War. Apparently the sergeant called his unit together and said something like, 'Right, you 'orrible men, tomorrow you go to France, and half of you may not come back. Those of you who feel you might be in need of some horizontal refreshment had better go and see the company doctor and have a talk about sex. Those of you who feel that death might be an uncomfortable experience had better go and have a talk with the padre. Company dismiss.'

John had a talk with the padre.

Both John and Carole were Lay Readers in the Church of England, which is how they had met in the first place. John had now reached the stage of his illness where he could not talk, or if he did try it was unintelligible gibberish. They had, throughout their marriage, said daily prayers together, and Carole continued the practice, although John could not join in. She told me that one morning – and she couldn't say why – she suddenly chanted the Anglican Order for Morning Prayer, 'O Lord, open thou our lips,' on a G.

Immediately, in tune, and with clear enunciation, John responded:

'And our mouth shall show forth thy praise.'

She caught her breath in astonishment, and continued:

'O Lord, make speed to save us.'

He responded:

'O Lord, make haste to help us.'

She continued the centuries-old chant until the conclusion:

'Glory be to the Father, and to the Son, and to the Holy Ghost.'

He completed the ancient response:

'As it was in the beginning, is now, and ever shall be: world without end. Amen.'

All this was accomplished with clear articulation, in a precise rhythm, and in tune.

And although John never spoke again, he sang the morning and evening responses every day until he neared the end.

Carole told the neurologist this story, and he said, 'Well, of course. The back of his mind is still working, but the front's gone wrong.' After that, Carole and other members of the family always talked to John about things from the past, all the events of his life that they remembered, and although he could not speak it was clear that he understood. At a shaggy-dog story his brother had been telling at every family gathering for years, John laughed until tears ran down his face.

About two years after the onset of the disease, Carole took John on holiday, and on the return journey he started to choke. He had not eaten or drunk anything for several hours and he was choking on his own saliva.

Carole took him directly to hospital and his lungs were aspirated. She was told that his glottis had ceased to function. The glottis is the muscle that, by reflex action, covers the windpipe on the instant of swallowing so that food is directed into the stomach. If it does not work, any food or fluid or saliva will pass directly into the lungs. The patient will either choke, or die of starvation or dehydration, or a massive infection will set up in the lungs and overwhelm the body.

Carole stayed with her husband, expecting it to be the end. John's lungs had been aspirated and he had been given morphine and was comfortable. Carole expected to sit with him until he died. However, the staff nurse came to him and started to insert a naso-gastric tube through which he could be fed artificially. Carole was watching. It is not easy to insert a naso-gastric tube, even under the most auspicious circumstances, with a patient who is conscious and fully co-operative. Usually, it is best to give the patient a boiled sweet and tell him to suck and swallow all the time so that the glottis is almost continuously covering the trachea. But

John had no control over his body and therefore did not have the ability to suck.

The tube has to be inserted into the nose and pushed downwards towards the stomach. It is best if the head is arched backwards, which to some extent straightens out the passage. The tube will go through the nose and down fairly easily for about the first third of the passage, but if there is no glottal reflex, a mass of soft tissue will be encountered and the tube may very easily go down the trachea into the lungs. This is very distressing to the patient.

Carole watched the staff nurse try this, with no success. She withdrew the tube and Carole breathed a sigh of relief. But when the nurse attempted it a second time, Carole said, 'This is not going to work, is it?'

'We have to make three attempts to pass a naso-gastric tube before we can say it cannot be done.'

'And what if I say "no"?'

'I would say "Thank God".'

'That is what I do say, now. It is not going to work, and I am not going to see him put through any more. I will take him home to die.'

The nurse breathed a great sigh of relief, and for the first time Carole looked closely at her. She had been so concentrated on her husband that she had not noticed the nurse, but with the long shuddering sigh and the murmured, 'Thank God for that', Carole looked at her face. The woman looked distraught. Carole said softly, 'What's the matter?'

The nurse replied, 'I have three other patients here and none of them can swallow, and I can't get a tube down any of them. I've tried, and I have to try again, and then again a third time, and I have other patients to look after.'

Carole spoke to her about what she had said – three attempts? Why, and what did that mean? Apparently, if a patient cannot swallow, artificial feeding must be started. If three attempts are unsuccessful, then a tube will be inserted under anaesthetic, with scanning equipment, or a feed-peg could be introduced into the stomach through the abdominal wall.

Carole asked, 'Do you mean that for all patients, whatever their condition, three attempts must be made? Is the rule inflexible?'

Apparently, it was.

I was aghast when I heard this. Surely no doctor would be fool enough to issue a blanket rule covering all patients. No experienced nurse would attempt a distressing procedure *three times* on a dying patient without discussing with the doctor the course of action, or inaction, most appropriate. Where did the rule come from? Carole did not know. One can only assume that the rule came from the hospital authorities, or perhaps even some government guideline issued by bureaucrats who are not trained in medicine or nursing. Apparently, the nurse told Carole, the rule had been issued in order to offset any accusations about *not* feeding – in other words, starving patients who could not swallow. This is defensive medicine again – a curse destroying good medical practice.

Carole took John home. It was a very difficult decision, because she knew that at home he would have no food or drink, and would die, whereas if he remained in hospital he could be fed artificially. But he was dying anyway, and had said that he did not want to die in hospital. They had discussed this over the two years they were given in which to contemplate his end. But still she hesitated. It was only with the help and support of John's son and daughters that they jointly decided to take him home.

The Integrated Care Pathway (ICP) for the care of the dying patient at home is based on studies showing that more than half of all terminally ill patients express the wish to die at home. It started as a pilot scheme, set up by the Liverpool Hospitals, to facilitate rapid discharge from hospital and to make available multi-professional care at home. Families looking after the dying need help, and the pilot scheme proved such a success that it is now provided by all NHS trusts.

Carole signed all the necessary papers (of which there were many) and took John home. A team of medical, nursing and domiciliary help was provided by the hospital. Yet such is the lack of understanding in society that someone said to Carole:

'Are you bringing him home to starve him to death?'

Carole was deeply shaken by this ignorant and cruel remark, but she collected herself sufficiently to reply: 'No, I'm taking him home to allow him to go through the process of dying as comfortably and as gracefully as possible.'

John was discharged from hospital on 5th October, 2006, in the care of his family, the Macmillan nurses and the local GP. When they had received him home, the doctor asked the nurses what they wanted to prescribe. Then he turned to Carole and said, 'They know far more about this than I do.' John could not swallow, and so drugs were given to suppress secretions so that he did not choke. The nurses showed Carole how to keep his mouth and throat moist with glycerine swabs, and many other details of palliative nursing.

Carole slept with him every night, which is the closest and sweetest communion two people can have. She said, 'I lay beside him and held his hand. He was so relaxed, and I knew he was happy, and so I went to sleep.'

On the night of 15th October, John Lewis died. Carole told me, 'I woke up at one o'clock, and I knew at once that something had happened. The engine had stopped. He looked the same, but he was not there. He was quite warm and peaceful, and I think he had just slipped away quietly whilst I slept, as though he didn't want to disturb me. It was a beautiful experience. It was a beautiful death.'

She said nothing for quite a while, and then said 'I had twelve perfect years with John, and in some ways the last two were the best of all. Now I can truly say "it is finished".'

2007

THE LIFE FORCE

Leah had been my delightful neighbour for twenty-five years and I had always assumed that she was about ten years older than me. It was not until she broke her leg and went into hospital that I discovered she was thirty years older than me. Leah was a hundred and two.

Leah was a widow and lived alone in her flat, and she fell at about eleven o'clock at night. Somehow, God knows how, she managed to haul herself to the telephone and ring for an ambulance. Steve and Sandy, neighbours who held a key, were awakened by the noise of an ambulance team trying to get in to the building. Steve went with them into her flat and found Leah on the floor, covered in blood, with a trail leading across the carpet from where she had fallen. The break was a compound fracture of the tibia and fibula, about three inches above the ankle, and pieces of bone were sticking out of the flesh. Poor Steve, who is not used to that sort of thing, nearly collapsed, but he controlled himself and helped the men get Leah on to a stretcher. In hospital, the bones were re-aligned, the flesh wound sutured and the leg plastered from thigh to toe. No one expected her to live.

But Leah did live. When I first saw her in hospital, she was virtually immobile because of the weight of the plaster. She was uncomfortable, certainly, but not in pain. She had a corner bed by the window. This was in June 2007. She sighed wistfully. 'I hope this is not the end. Life is so beautiful, so interesting, so exciting. I don't want it to end.' In the year that followed, that was the only time, as far as I know, that she mentioned the possibility of death.

I reflected that, if she had not managed to haul herself across the floor to the telephone, she would undoubtedly have died during the night. Numbness, caused by shock and blood loss, would have

285

engulfed her, and she would have drifted away before the morning light. I wondered what suffering lay ahead for her, what she could have spared herself within a night of fading consciousness. She knew her age; had she not anticipated death? But that is not the way our instincts work. Self-preservation is the first of the primary instincts, so Leah had made a superhuman effort to reach the telephone and seek medical help.

Leah's husband, Alex, had been the artistic director for scores of major films between 1930 and 1975. He had worked all over the world with directors such as David Lean, Alexander Korda, Roman Polanski and Alfred Hitchcock. Leah had frequently accompanied him on location, and met many of the great film personalities of the period.

She told me that her biggest headache had been keeping Alex tidy and presentable, because he never cared a scrap about his appearance, and only wanted to wear old and comfortable clothes. 'I knitted him a cardigan once, and after that he wouldn't wear a jacket. The only things he wanted were these cardigans. I must have knitted dozens of them. They looked quite smart for a few days, but I don't know what he did to them, because after a fortnight they looked dreadful – all out of shape, buttons pulled off, holes in the elbows – I could never understand how he managed it. The worst part was the carbon and charcoal from the sketches and drawings. If he wanted to smear something, or blend shades, he wouldn't use a cloth like anyone else would. No, not him – he would grab the bottom of his cardigan and rub the drawing with that. No wonder his clothes were in such a state!'

She told me that they were asked to meet a new director. 'We were told it was just an informal meeting one evening, so Alex went directly from work. I arrived from home and got there first. I saw at once that it was just about the smartest, most sophisticated cocktail party that film people can put on. Everyone was dressed to the nines, trying to outshine everyone else, the way they do, you know. It was all very pleasant. But when Alex arrived I nearly died of embarrassment. You've never seen such a sight – he looked worse than usual. One side of his cardigan was hanging down to his knees, the other side was up around his waist and it was covered in carbon and charcoal. There was a hole in his trousers. I can't imagine how he had managed to tear his trousers; they weren't like that when he went out in the morning. But he didn't seem to have the slightest idea of how he looked compared to all the other smart people. He went around greeting everyone, charming, affable, friendly. People always liked him. You couldn't help liking him.'

She sighed, and a dreamy look came into her eyes.

'I've been a widow for thirty-two years, but I would never marry again. I've had a couple of offers; but no, not after a man like Alex.'

Another time she said, 'When your husband dies, life changes utterly – everything changes. No one wants to be bothered with a widow. Invitations stop. Friends melt away. It's when you begin to know who your true friends are. I had to start all over again, with a new life and new friends.'

But Leah was not just the wife of a successful artistic director. She was a remarkable woman in her own right and had scores of friends. I was not the only one who enjoyed visiting her in hospital. She sat up in bed, or on a chair, knitting for anyone who wanted anything knitted – indeed, I have a jacket and my husband has two jumpers from this period! I looked around at the other old ladies in the ward and she seemed to be the youngest of them all. She was sitting upright, her back unsupported, her eyes bright, her skin clear, her hair nicely arranged – one would have thought she was a sprightly eighty-year-old. It was a joy to visit her, mainly because she was so interested in everything you were doing, and her memory was phenomenal. Most old people have short-term memory loss. Not Leah. She wanted to know the outcome of something I had told her during the last visit, of which she had remembered every detail. I told her I was going on a cycling holiday with my grandson, and when I next saw her, her first words were, 'How did it go? Did you have fun? You were in the Cotswolds, weren't you?'

Everything interested her, and she remembered things I had

forgotten myself. And as for Scrabble! It was humiliating. I played many games with her and she beat me every time. In fact, she didn't simply win; she wiped the floor with me. My husband played a couple of games with her, but then announced that he wouldn't play any more because he didn't like Scrabble. Men are not very good losers ...

Leah was a Jew, and the rest of her family was in Israel. She was obviously much loved because her daughter, who was seventy-eight, with a husband of eighty, and her grandchildren, in their forties and fifties, came to England regularly with their children, or phoned her every day from Israel. She was not one of those tragic figures, of whom I have seen so many, who are left entirely alone in their old age. Her family was very good to her, right until the end.

Leah spent three or four weeks in the orthopaedic unit of the main hospital. This is much longer than most people stay, but she could not remain indefinitely because the bed was needed for emergencies and she was transferred to what one would call a long-term geriatric hospital. My heart grieved for her when I heard where she was going, because I knew the hospital, and it did not have a good reputation locally. That was, I think, because the buildings had formerly been the old workhouse infirmary, and they had a bleak and forbidding aspect – 'Abandon hope all ye who enter here.' I approached the place with trepidation.

As I found my way to the ward, my attitude changed. A pleasant young nurse directed me to Leah's bed and several others smiled at me as I passed. Leah was just finishing her lunch. I saw that her head was bent over and her shoulders were shaking. I thought she was crying. With great concern I touched her shoulder and said, 'Whatever is the matter, Leah?' She looked up and at once I saw that she was not crying, but laughing!

'I was just thinking about yesterday's lunch. Pass me those tissues, will you dear, and I'll tell you what happened.'

She blew her nose and wiped her eyes.

'The ambulance came to bring me here. Well, I was in the back with a young man and we got talking. He was South African, so I told him that I had been there with my husband when he was working on the film *Gold* with Roger Moore and Susannah York. And would you believe it, it turned out that his father was a stunt man in *Gold*. Well, we had so much to talk about, swapping stories, and he was telling me about his family and how his father came to be in *Gold*, that we didn't notice time passing. This hospital is only about a mile up the hill from the main one, but about half an hour had gone by. We had travelled fifteen or twenty miles, and neither of us noticed.'

She had to have a little cough and wiped her eyes again before continuing.

'Well, we got to the hospital and they lifted me out and carried me up to the ward. A nurse showed them the bed that was ready for me, and they tucked me in. Another couple of nurses made a fuss of me, checking to see I was comfortable, and then the nice young South African boy said goodbye.

'It was nearly lunchtime, so they brought me lunch, which I ate, then they cleared it away, and I was just settling down for a little doze when a young lady doctor came over with a bundle of notes in her hand. She said she wanted to examine me, and pulled the screens around the bed.

'Well, she examined me all over, eyes and throat, and heart and lungs and I don't know what, then she looked at my leg and said, "This is a very long plaster for a fracture in the foot."

'"No, it was the tibia and fibula, a compound fracture."

'"It says here, the fourth metatarsal."

'"Well that's wrong, it was the tibia and fibula."

'"I've got X-rays here, Mrs Wilson, and—"

'"But I'm not Mrs Wilson!"

'And then it all came out. No one knew quite how it had happened, but the ambulance men had been given the wrong instructions. The hospital was expecting a patient, and a bed was ready, so I was put into it, no questions asked.'

She had to cough again, she was laughing so much.

'So I had to be transferred again. I didn't get here until yesterday evening. I've been wondering about Mrs Wilson and what sort of a day *she* had. Mine was highly entertaining.'

In all the weary months that followed, Leah's sense of humour never deserted her, and her interest in life never flagged.

From the beginning, Leah had been on continuous urinary drainage, because it would have been impossible for her to use a bedpan regularly. A catheter into the bladder for weeks on end can cause friction and general discomfort, but she did not complain. I presumed that she was having diuretics to keep the kidneys functioning efficiently, and also some kind of anti-bacterial drug to avoid infection.

I do not know what happened to her bowels. From experience I can say that bowel movements can be one of the biggest problems for geriatric nurses to have to deal with. Constipation usually sets in, and faeces become impacted, leading to nausea, headaches, lethargy, confusion and other nasty conditions for the unfortunate patient. Enemas help, but Leah could not have been turned on her side to receive an enema. Aperients often add to the abdominal pain, or can sometimes cause uncontrollable defecation into the bed, causing a nightmare of shame and humiliation for a sensitive person. How the nurses and carers handle this is one of the greatest challenges of good practice; a bad experience can leave a scar, slow to heal, on the mind of the unfortunate patient.

Weeks passed, and the leg did not heal. I don't know how Leah endured the boredom of those long summer months, trussed up in a massive plaster that was impossible to move. Sometimes she complained of aching and stiffness in other parts of the body, so I massaged her other leg and her back and shoulders, which she said helped. Thank God for those new air beds, I thought, which continuously shift pressure from one part to another. In my nursing days massive pressure sores would have developed.

About six weeks after admission, Leah complained of a slight cough, which she could not shift. The next time I saw her she looked dreadful. It was an embolism in the lungs, I was told. She was on high doses of antibiotics and continuous oxygen and an intravenous drip for fluids. She could scarcely open her eyes or move a hand. Her breathing was laboured, yet she had the courtesy to mouth the words: 'I can't talk. Forgive me.' I sat quietly massaging her upper chest for about an hour. 'This is it,' I thought, 'she won't survive this one.'

From the beginning, when the fracture first occurred, she had been on cardio-vascular drugs and other drugs to maintain circulatory function, as well as diuretics to stimulate the kidneys. When the embolus lodged itself in the lungs, massive doses of clot-busters were added, and all the other drugs were modified or intensified. Daily blood samples were taken for analysis until, she said, she felt like a pincushion.

Leah was on the 'not for resuscitation' list, which meant that, if she actually died, no attempt at resuscitation should be made. In my days of nursing, an embolus on the lungs would almost invariably have been fatal for an old person, and I felt reassured to see that notice at the end of her bed. I was glad to see that she would be left to die in peace.

I was not the only one to expect her death from an embolus. Her granddaughter, who was a practising nurse in Israel, came over to England and stayed in Leah's flat, spending most of each day at the hospital with her grandmother. But the antibiotics, the oxygen, the clot-busters and the drip, combined with the cardio-vascular drugs, did their work. Leah was tougher than anyone had imagined and confounded us all. Two or three weeks later she was as perky as ever, sitting up in bed knitting or sewing, doing the *Times* crossword puzzle, watching *Countdown*, *Mastermind* and *University Challenge* on TV, getting most of the answers right, and beating me at Scrabble.

At some point during the summer months she developed an infection of the lungs. 'It's an MRSA bug,' I thought, 'this will be the end.' But it was not the dreaded MRSA. It was a treatable infection, and another course of antibiotics drove it away. Leah was back on form – on form for her visitors, that is. None of us knew what she really endured as the weeks dragged on into months.

A long-stay geriatric hospital is not a place where any of us would like to end up. Leah was in a smallish ward of fifteen beds that were not too close to each other, but close enough for there to be no privacy. Most of her neighbours were confused in one way or another. Yet Leah never complained, not to me, at any rate. She did not become morose, in-turned or whiny – least of all did she succumb to self-pity. Her thoughts were always focused on those around her. 'Look at that poor old soul over there. She cries all the time, poor soul.' Or, 'That woman over there came in last night. Her son came with her, a man of about fifty. He stayed all night, but he went after breakfast, had to go to work. It was good of him to stay for so long, don't you think?'

The ward was chronically understaffed, and the nurses and care assistants were under great pressure, but they were cheerful and tried to maintain a happy atmosphere. Leah liked them, and knew all about their boyfriends, their children and their holidays. She was obviously popular. The worst thing for her was the boredom – 'There's nothing to do. The day is punctuated only by meal times, nothing else.' Leah continued with her crosswords and books and knitting, which she adored, and I often took her a new commission to be knitted for someone else. Another friend, Suzy, had seen the same need, and also presented her with things to be knitted, until Leah had to draw a line – 'Nothing more till after Christmas. I can't cope.'

Leah's reading would have been impressive for a woman half her age, but for someone of one hundred and two it was formidable. Moreover, she read without the use of spectacles. I saw her reading in hospital a history of Afghanistan in the twentieth century, upon which she commented knowledgeably; a biography of Charlotte Bronte, with a second for comparison; she read novels, biography, social history, poetry and occasionally a newspaper, but never a magazine. 'I can't waste my time on those things,' she said.

She made the best of things with heroic goodwill, but it was not easy. 'Nights are the worst,' she said to me once. 'I hardly sleep. Nights are very long.'

I am sure they were. To be awake, uncomfortable, and scarcely able to move for hours on end must have been a torment. I asked her about getting a nurse to shift her position.

'There aren't any nurses overnight,' she said. 'Well, not what I would call a nurse. There are all these different women who come from an agency. You never see the same one twice, and they are so slow. I don't know what they are supposed to do. They amble around, or sit chatting, but you can't ask them to do anything, because they won't.'

I thought of my own months of night duty as a student nurse, when we were constantly on the move in a ward of thirty beds.

'But what about the night sister?' I said. 'You could ask her to get the nurses to move you.'

'I haven't seen a night sister since I've been here,' she said simply.

The ward was hot and claustrophobic, but the summer wore itself away and autumn brought with it cooler weather, which was a relief. Many times X-rays had been taken, but, to Leah's disappointment, each time they showed that the leg had not healed and the huge plaster could not be removed. She would have to stick it out.

In November, after five months of discomfort and immobility, it was finally taken off and a knee-to-ankle plaster was fitted. She was overjoyed, and when the nurses brought her a Zimmer frame, she practised walking with the zeal of a young athlete training for the Olympics. Finally, she went to a rehabilitation centre where, to her delight, she had a room of her own. There was a high staff/patient ratio there, and she had a lot of physiotherapy. At last, the short plaster was removed, and life skills were introduced, such as walking up and down stairs, taking a bath and shower, using the kitchen, cooking a meal. She was determined to succeed, and within a fortnight, after six weary months in hospital, Leah was ready to go home.

Leah was treated entirely by the National Health Service, and from my observation as a visitor, I would say that she received good treatment throughout. The ambulance emergency treatment on the night of the break was impeccable, and the fact that she survived was little short of a miracle, and due entirely to her hospital care. Having been trained in the old school of nursing, when discipline was rigid, I was a bit shaken by the free-and-easy attitude of the nurses, but I think that is just my age – everything has loosened up in the last fifty years, and no one today would put up with the sort of nonsense that manacled us young nurses. There was, undoubtedly, a relaxed and cheerful atmosphere generated by the nurses. They sat on beds, chatted and laughed with the patients – things we would never have dared to do. I had the uneasy feeling, though, that no one seemed to be in charge, and I discussed this with Leah.

Leah agreed. 'I've been in several different wards, both here and in the main hospital, and I could never have told you who was in charge.'

The main hospital was superior in every way to the long-stay geriatric hospital. But this has always been the situation. There is no point in looking back sentimentally and moaning, 'It was better in my day,' because it was not. The drama and excitement of surgery, acute medicine, emergency care, have always been the aspects of medicine that have attracted staff, and the career structure of the professions reflects this. An ambitious young doctor or nurse will rarely go into geriatrics if he or she wants to get on in the profession.

On the whole, I would say that things are probably better today than they were half a century ago. Staff shortage is no less acute, but at least Leah was in a ward with only fifteen other patients, and there was a reasonable distance between each bed. In my day, wards contained between thirty and forty beds, with about two foot of space between them.

Leah spent about four months in the geriatric hospital. In general, she was treated with kindness, courtesy and pro- fessionalism. The weariness and boredom of her situation she coped with in her own way, through mental activity and engaging with staff, who seemed to go out of their way to keep her spirits up. Quite simply, they were good to her.

HOMECOMING

Leah was discharged in December under the care of her GP, a district nurse and a home help. She occupied a beautiful ground floor flat in a large Victorian house that was divided into twelve. She was the oldest resident and everyone knew and liked her. Something akin to a reception committee was waiting in the hall to greet her when the ambulance brought her home. She was thrilled, and not a little touched, by all the attention.

However, she was basically alone, and had to manage. Indeed, it was what she wanted, as she was fiercely, almost aggressively, independent. Her grandson begged her to come and live with them in Israel, but she refused. It was pointed out that she could afford to pay a carer to live in for a while. 'I should hate it,' she replied. 'I have to learn to manage by myself.' And slowly and surely she did. Every step with the Zimmer frame was tortuous, every turn to get something from a cupboard or the fridge was frightening to watch, but she wouldn't let anyone do it for her – 'I've got to do it myself,' she said. The neighbours, Suzy and Sandy, and her cousin, Carmela, did the shopping for her, and brought in cooked meals.

Predictably, the home help didn't come up to scratch. 'She just flicks a duster around the place, doesn't do anything properly, but I suppose I will have to put up with her until I can do it myself.' And once, 'I was disgusted! I gave her my sheets to iron. I had washed them' – and she had, God only knows how – 'and she only had to iron them, and put them on the bed. When I went to bed that night, would you believe it, I found that she had only ironed the top and bottom of a folded sheet, and not opened it out to iron the middle. I have never been so disgusted in all my life! I had to get up at 11 o'clock, take the sheets off the bed and iron them myself. I will never give her sheets to iron again – never.' The thought of Leah stripping a bed, manipulating an iron and ironing board whilst clinging to a Zimmer frame, then making the bed in the middle of the night, sent a shiver down my spine. But I kept very quiet on that one. I have never ironed a sheet, to my recollection. My attitude is – if you can't give a thing a shake and put it on the bed it's not worth keeping! But I could hardly say that, could I? I didn't want to end up in her 'disgusted' book.

Her social life intensified. She couldn't get out, so people came to her. She revived her former bridge parties, and played with ferocious zeal, I was told. Bridge is a very difficult game, requiring a quick mind and memory skills. I resigned myself to being wiped off the Scrabble board, although she had the kindness to tell me my game was improving. I found, to my surprise, that I was concentrating fiercely, working out all sorts of sly strategies to outmanoeuvre her, but I never did, she was too quick for me. Then I realised, not at all to my credit, that I was getting irritated, and was determined to beat her. But the craftier I became, the more did she, and she was always one step ahead. Incidentally, she also kept the score, adding it up in her head as we went along. I tried score keeping once and got into such a muddle that she took the task from me without a word.

Steve and Sandy were very good to her, coming in each day to see if she was all right and if she needed anything. They had a baby who was between a year and eighteen months old at that time, and they brought him in to visit her every evening when he'd been bathed and was in his pyjamas ready for bed. Some toys were kept in Leah's flat so that he could play. The two seemed to love their time together, and I have seen that little boy in the hallway, crawling towards her flat and lifting his hands up towards the door. Even after she had gone, he continued to do this for several months.

In February, Leah had her 103rd birthday. The whole family, including great-grandchildren, came over from Israel. The flat was so full of flowers you could hardly move.

Leah was determined to do more things for herself. She started by walking one hundred yards down the road and back, unaided. The next thing we knew she had been to Tesco, which was a quarter of a mile away. 'I like to choose my own things. I don't like people shopping for me – they always get it wrong,' she said. In early March she said, 'I've been up to the Town Hall today to get my bus pass. I will need it when the weather gets better.'

Then the ceiling fell in the bathroom. It sounded like an explosion. No one was hurt, but it broke the wash-hand basin into two pieces and cracked the lavatory pan. It would have been a shock to anyone, but Leah took it in her stride, and in the end my sympathies lay with the builders and the insurance men; the stick she gave them about repairs!

Her life force was incredible. She was absolutely determined to cope, and seemed to accept every difficulty as a challenge to be overcome – *nothing* was going to beat her. Nobody knew the mental and physical effort this cost her, no one saw the tears of frustration as muscular weakness took its toll, or the relief as she sank into bed at night. No one saw the effort it cost her to get up in the morning. She once said, 'When I wake up, I can hardly move, my limbs feel so heavy and I ache all over. But I have to make the effort. Sometimes it takes me half an hour to get out of bed. Can you believe it? Half an hour just to get up!' Then she would have a bath, which loosened her up, and, dressed, did her hair, creamed her face, and manoeuvred her Zimmer frame around several awkward corners to go to the kitchen for breakfast. It took her three hours. Many people twenty years younger would simply have stayed in bed and expected someone else to look after them. Not Leah – she would look after herself, thank you. Renewed pleas from her family to go to Israel were all rejected.

It must have been early June when Sandy from next door had cooked a meal for Leah and she said, 'I don't really feel like eating.'

'Try it, dear, it's nice.'

'Yes, of course I will. It looks lovely. You're very kind.' But Leah couldn't eat it.

Quite quickly after that, Leah suffered from nausea and

vomiting, and became constipated. 'If only I could open my bowels I would be all right,' she said. 'What I need is an enema and a good clear out.'

I was sitting beside her. She didn't look herself. I asked her if she would like a game of Scrabble. 'I don't think I could concentrate,' she said. She moved a little and winced. 'I can't seem to get comfortable. This pain jabs at me, here and here.' She pointed to her stomach. I felt the area. It was a mass of hard lumps.

The district nurse came to give her an enema. I met her in the hallway as she was leaving.

'I am going to get her doctor to come and see her as soon as possible,' she said.

'Are you thinking what I'm thinking?'

'I don't know what you are thinking.'

'I think she has cancer of the stomach and abdominal organs.'

'I am sure she has,' replied the nurse.

The doctor came a couple of days later, and arranged for a hospital scan, which showed a massive cancerous growth in the abdomen.

Leah spent a few days in hospital at the time of the scan, then came home, then went back to hospital for more tests, then was sent home again. She was not eating, or at best she was taking only a tiny bit of food, and she lost weight rapidly. She began to look very ill. Her grandson came over from Israel and stayed with her for a week. He put pressure on her to go into a nursing home. 'I will not return to Israel and leave you alone like this,' he said, 'and if I don't go back I will probably lose my job.'

He searched widely, and found a home he thought she would like. She moved in.

I visited her there. It was a lovely day in June, and she was sitting in the garden in the sunshine – Leah always loved the sun. She seemed more relaxed, and therefore a little improved. This is often the way. The hospital or nursing home offers a feeling of security and freedom from the constant tension of struggling to cope with a battle one is going to lose. She was deeply engrossed in a crossword and saw my shadow on the grass before she saw me.

She looked up with a lovely smile. 'You can't stay beyond three o'clock,' she announced. 'It's the finals of *Countdown* on television. I've been following it all through and must see these finalists.' Her passion for word games and mental gymnastics was undiminished. She told me that she liked the new place, though she couldn't eat the food, which she blamed on the cook, not on her digestive system. She felt she ought to stay there, because it was a worry to her family if she was alone at home, though she missed her home terribly.

I suggested again that she could have a live-in carer. Before the sentence was finished she butted in. 'Never. I should hate having someone around me all the time.' Most of us would think like that.

She told me that the previous day she had been taken to the anti-coagulant clinic at the hospital. Whilst I was with her, a carer came and said that the results had come through, and that she must have an increased dose of Warfarin. She handed Leah about six or eight tablets to swallow along with a glass of water. Leah sighed. 'These pills! I'm sure it's all these pills that are making me feel so sick.' But she swallowed them nonetheless.

Suddenly she looked at her watch. 'I've got to go. It's time for *Countdown*.' I tried to assist her indoors, but she resisted help, and in the end I gave up. I left her, paper and pencil in hand, eyes eager, sitting in front of the television, waiting for the first jumble of letters. On my way out I met another of her friends. 'I'm just going to see Leah,' she said brightly. I wondered what sort of dusty reception she would get!

I was bothered by the higher dose of Warfarin, and made a point of seeing the matron to discuss this before leaving. She was very guarded at first, as though I was accusing her or the nursing home of some impropriety.

'It has nothing to do with me. We can only do as we are instructed. You will have to talk to the doctor.'

'I'm not trying to cause trouble, honestly. I am merely puzzled.'

We swapped details on our training and experience. She was a woman in her fifties and was obviously dedicated to the care of the elderly. When I mentioned that I had been sister-in-charge of a cancer ward, she realised we were probably having similar thoughts.

'If you look at her medical record you will see that since January the dosage has been going up after every visit to the Warfarin clinic,' she said.

'On what assessment?'

'On the blood sample analysis.'

'But she's a hundred and three! What do they expect?'

'I'm not sure that age comes into it.'

'Apart from Warfarin, what other drugs does she have?'

'Statins, cardio-vascular drugs and stimulants, anti-coagulants and diuretics, as well as regular analgesics.'

'But that's crazy. She has advanced cancer. It is better to die of heart failure than cancer.'

'I know that. You know that. The doctors know it. But we cannot discontinue the drugs.'

'Why? I don't understand.'

'At the moment she is alive, alert and enjoying life.'

I thought of Leah watching *Countdown*, beating the contestants at their own game.

'You are right,' I said thoughtfully, 'she does enjoy life.'

'If we stop the drugs someone might say that we were deliberately hastening her death.'

'But is that likely? Would anyone say such a thing?'

'It is quite possible.'

'Have you discussed it with the relatives?'

'Yes, and they said they will leave the decision to us.'

'Have you discussed it with Leah?'

'No.'

'Does she know she has cancer?'

'No.'

'No? Why will no one talk about death? That's at the root of the trouble.'

'I know. But I have to safeguard the good name of the nursing home. I can't discuss philosophical issues.'

At that moment a young man in a T-shirt and open-toed sandals breezed into the office.

'Philosophy? Sounds a bit heavy! Is that how you spend your afternoons?' He laughed good-naturedly.

'We were talking about Leah, Doctor,' said the matron.

'Leah? She's fine, going on nicely.'

Encouraged by his obvious good nature I said, 'I was wondering why she is still on cardio-vascular drugs and diuretics.'

His smile vanished. 'What's the trouble? Have you any complaints?' he said abruptly.

'No, not at all. Quite the opposite, in fact.'

'Are you a relative?' he demanded.

'No, a friend.'

'I cannot discuss a patient with friends,' he said curtly, and walked out.

I must have looked really put out, because Matron said, 'You shouldn't have said that. For all he knows you might be a journalist looking for a story about hospitals or care homes. The newspapers could probably do with something like that to boost circulation.'

'I hadn't thought of that,' I said quietly.

The strength of the media, with their seemingly insatiable desire to criticise the National Health Service, came home to me.

'I see what you mean. It would require more courage than the average doctor possesses to say "no more". He would probably have to face an internal enquiry to justify his position.'

'Exactly. And in the meantime, Leah is as well as can be expected.'

'Yes, she is. In fact, she's better than I expected, for which you are to be thanked.'

We shook hands and I left, but before leaving the building I poked my head around Leah's door. She was deeply engrossed in *Countdown*, eagerly writing things down, crossing them out, looking up and thinking, then scribbling again with evident satisfaction. The friend who had arrived at three o'clock was nowhere to be seen. Presumably she had been sent packing by this doughty, irrepressible old lady.

★

Cycling encourages meditation. There is something about the gentle, rhythmic movement, the fresh air, the curve of the road, the passing hedgerows, that promotes thought. As I cycled home from the nursing home, I reflected that I had undoubtedly been in the wrong. Three times in the past twelve months I had thought that Leah would die, and in the back of my mind I had suspected that it would probably be the best thing for her. She would die quickly and peacefully, without suffering. When I had seen her in the hospital after the embolism I had really thought she would not survive the night. But she did survive – triumphantly. She had lived to enjoy six months at home, gaining strength, improving her walking ability, seeing her family and friends ... in short, living life as fully as a lady of her age could expect. None of this would have been possible had it not been for modern medicine. The intervention of cancer was not really surprising. We all have potential cancer cells inside us, and a shock to the body, such as Leah's broken leg, would be enough to trigger a growth. It is quite possible, as medicine advances, and death is pushed further and further into retreat, that many of us may die of some form of cancer. And yet ... and yet ... it nagged in my mind ... isn't it better to die of heart and circulatory failure, before you have to die of cancer? In the end, we are all in the hands of God, and nothing we do will alter our fate.

I had gained a good impression of the nursing home. The matron was the only trained nurse on the staff, but she set a good example and the assistants and carers whom I met *all* seemed pleasant men and women, who looked after the residents with cheerful goodwill. I saw a lot of smiling faces the day I was there. Leah's room was spacious and airy, with two windows facing south and west, both overlooking the gardens, and she had a large bathroom leading off the main room. I felt she would be comfortable and happy there in the last weeks and months of her life.

However, an incident occurred that shattered the calm. Leah was barely digesting food, felt nauseous much of the time, and sometimes she was sick. Both constipation and diarrhoea plagued her. Most of these nasty emissions she could control, but not always. One night, shortly after I had seen her, she tried to get to the bathroom, but what with the struggle to get out of bed and manoeuvre her Zimmer frame, she could not quite make it, and vomited all over the bathroom floor.

Leah called for a member of the night staff, to whom she explained what had happened, apologised, and asked if the woman would clear it up. The woman looked at the mess, looked at Leah, said, 'Clear it up yourself,' and walked out.

Leah told me that she had struggled into the bathroom again, and managed, though she was fearful of falling, to detach the showerhead and spray water all over the vomit. Then she got hold of towels and spread them over the watery mess to soak it up. Finally, she returned to bed and got some sleep.

But that did it for Leah. In the morning she demanded to see the matron, told her what had happened, and said she was leaving that day. Poor matron was profuse in her apologies. She said that the woman came from an agency and would never be employed there again. But nothing would change Leah's mind. 'Because of that woman I am leaving this morning,' she said. A taxi came, and by ten o'clock she had left the nursing home, although she was in no way fit to do so.

Matron was deeply ashamed and embarrassed. None of her staff were trained nurses, and ninety per cent of them came from agencies. Only ten per cent were employed full or part time because of the impossibility of getting rid of anyone who was unsatisfactory. If an agency care assistant did not work properly, the matron could say that she would not have the person back. The care assistants were always being shifted around, and some were trained, some not; some experienced, others not; some were very good, others poor or bad. It was always a lottery who was sent by the agency, and night duty was the hardest to cover satisfactorily.

Poor Leah arrived home, and no one was expecting her. She was seriously ill, and had to climb the front steps to the house, open the front door, which is heavy, cross the hallway, and open the door to her flat, which had been double-locked and is even heavier due to fire regulations. She was cold, and the heating had been switched off. She had to go to the cupboard and pull down the main switch, which is stiff. I just cannot imagine how she managed to do all this in her condition, but she did. Later that day a driver brought a case with her things in it, and left it in the hallway. That was the first clue that anyone in the house had of her return.

Steve went round to her flat and found her in a state of utter exhaustion, collapsed in her armchair. He telephoned the family in Israel to inform them. The doctor and community nurses had been informed by the matron, but visits could not be started straight away and Leah had to wait several days for a district nurse, carer, or home help. Sandy cooked meals for her, but she could not eat.

Once again, though, Leah perked up. Perhaps being at home, which is where she had always wanted to be, stimulated her. Added to this was the knowledge that she *had* to cope, because she adamantly refused to return to the nursing home, and there was no alternative. So each morning she got up, bathed, dressed, and received her friends, with whom she talked intelligently and with humour. She played with Steve and Sandy's baby, did her crossword puzzles and word games, and generally spread around her a love of life that was infectious.

Yet all the time she was growing weaker and losing weight. The weight loss accentuated the growth in her abdomen, and now she looked as if she were seven or eight months pregnant. Her pain was increasing, and the prescribed analgesics no longer relieved it. One night it became so unbearable that she rang her GP, who arranged for hospital admission immediately.

I visited her in hospital towards the end of July. When I walked in, I thought she was unconscious, but no, she smiled and took my hand.

'They've given me something to relieve the pain,' she said. 'It feels easier. I wish they would give me an enema. I feel I need a good clear out.' Her faith in enemas was touching. Had she still not been told, or had she, perhaps, guessed the truth?

Apparently not, because her next remark was, 'I'm wondering if I've got shingles. It can be very painful you know, my cousin had it.'

She drifted off into sleep again and I sat stroking her hand. Then someone came round with a drinks trolley, and she had a little water. A nurse emerged with the evening drugs, but she passed Leah's bed. 'I've told them I'm not having any more pills,' Leah said, 'nothing.' There was a pause, then, 'I'm sure it was the pills that made me so sick. But no more, I've told them. And I don't feel as sick, now. I feel better without them.'

Did she know that it was the pills keeping her heart and circulation going that had sustained life in her through the months since the accident? She was a highly intelligent woman, and it seems unlikely that she did not know. Perhaps she had discussed it with her granddaughter, the Israeli trained nurse.

Yet I had never discussed it with her, or the present fact of progressive cancer, or the inevitability of death. Mutual friends told me that she had never mentioned death to them, either, which is surprising because most old people – well short of one hundred and three – will say things like 'I'll be glad when it's all over,' or 'I've had a good life. I'm tired now, and want it to end.' My grandfather talked of the Angel of Death; others speak of going to meet their loved ones. The only time Leah had mentioned death was fourteen months earlier, when she had looked out of the hospital window at the blue sky and said, so wistfully, 'I hope this is not the end. Life is so beautiful, so exciting, so interesting. I don't want it to end.'

Her passion for life had sustained and driven her through all the months of coping alone. Yet now I felt her life force was waning. She could struggle no more, and she knew it. Was that why she had announced she would have no more pills? Had she known all along that it was the pills that had kept her going and that rejecting them would mean the end? Was this Leah's way of closing the door?

A nurse came up to the bed and gave her an injection.

'Is that morphine?' I whispered. Our eyes met.

'Yes,' she said briefly.

'I'm glad,' I said softly. The nursed smiled and moved away.

It was high summer – long bright evenings with no wind. But the sun sinks eventually, though it seems it never could, and when I left Leah that evening I felt her light was going out, and that I would not see her again.

Leah died on 8th August, 2008. Her family were with her.

Cancer can sometimes lead to a hard and difficult death. It was so for Leah, and her daughter and granddaughters told me of this. They couldn't understand how her body managed to sustain life for so long. I think I can. Her love of life had been her strength and driving force. She had led a privileged life, with a happy childhood and a happy marriage – who could ask for more? She had also enjoyed good health until the age of a hundred and two when she broke her leg. Three times – the break itself, the embolism, the hospital infection – she had nearly died, and each time it would have been a relatively quick and easy death. But three times modern medicine had pulled her through and kept her alive until cancer intervened. I wondered how Leah would have reacted if she had been able to see ahead.

If the Angel of Death had shown Leah the manner in which she would die, I am quite sure she would, like most of us, have said, 'Oh no – not that. Isn't there an easier way? Anything would be preferable.' But if the Angel of Life had stepped in at that moment, and shown her fourteen months of increasing difficulty, but also of friendship and family love, I am quite sure she would have said to Death, 'If yours is the price I must pay, so be it,' and she would have turned and taken Life by the hand.

EUTHANASIA

It is surprising how many people are quite unable to talk about death, yet are happy to talk about euthanasia, and they do so with the assured confidence of one who knows all the answers. Consider the following conversation I had with a neighbour in 2008. He started:

'I've got to go and see my mother in the local care home.'

'I didn't know she was there.'

'Yes. She fell and broke her pelvis last year. She's eighty-six. She'll never walk again.'

'That's very sad, at that age.'

'It was dreadful in the summer. That hospital's a disgrace, you know. It ought to be closed down. She developed MRSA. We nearly lost her.' He sighed. 'They managed to pull her through, but her mind was gone; she doesn't know where she is or who we are.'

'It would have been better if she had died of MRSA, then?'

'Oh no. I'm a great believer in euthanasia.'

'But what's the difference?'

'She was suffering. It shouldn't be allowed. But if they gave her an injection, a little prick, she wouldn't know anything about it.'

'She's probably suffering now, in the care home.'

'Yes, and it shouldn't be allowed. Euthanasia's the answer. I'm a firm believer in it. You want to read up about it on the web.'

I wrote this conversation down verbatim immediately, so that I would not forget it. He was obviously shocked when I suggested that she could have died of MRSA, but then immediately said that she should be 'euthanised'.

In May of this year, I asked my neighbour's permission for this story to be published, and I asked him about his mother's present condition.

He said: 'She is in a dementia care home. It costs us £500 a week. She is doubly incontinent, she can't really walk, she has no real mental understanding. Does she have any quality of life? No.'

I asked him, 'Is your opinion about euthanasia the same?'

He was very clear in his reply. 'Oh yes, definitely. And my father had the same belief.'

'And would you still say that she should have died three years ago when she broke her hip, which was the beginning of the end?'

He was thoughtful for a very long time, and then said, 'Yes. Euthanasia is the best, but as it's not legally possible, I think she should have been allowed to die of the MRSA infection.'

Later in the conversation he repeated his opinion about the hospital being a disgrace because of MRSA. This attitude is heard all too often. When I was a young nurse, old people in hospital frequently developed pneumonia and died. In the 1950s massive doses of antibiotics started to be given to kill pneumococcal organisms and every other infection. But micro-organisms are the basic life form, and, when attacked, they adapt and mutate in order to survive. This is the Darwinian law of life. So these simple cells have developed a resistance to antibiotics, and no hospital can be blamed. There have always been infections in hospitals, and always will be. These 'super-bugs' are no more than a variant of 'the old man's friend'.

The remark that suffering shouldn't be allowed is widely held, and many would agree with him. Yet suffering is a part of life, just as happiness is, and it is certainly not a justification for ending life. Suffering stalks the wards of all hospitals, but it is not senseless; if it was, all life would be senseless, and it is not. Indeed, suffering is a mystery that we cannot fathom, and never will be able to. The mystics embrace suffering, as one of the steps towards perfection.

I remember a lady whom I nursed when I was at the Elizabeth Garrett Anderson Hospital. I will never forget her, or what she said. She was a nun from a prestigious Roman Catholic teaching order, with schools in France, Belgium and England. She was a Latin and Greek scholar, and was deeply respected not only for her intellect but also for her teaching skills and her administrative abilities.

She was only forty years old, but her body was inflamed and distorted by rheumatoid arthritis. Her joints were virtually locked, like those of a wooden doll, and any movement was agony for her. We made matters worse by administering quite the wrong treatment. At the time it was thought that aspirin helped arthritis. Perhaps it did, sometimes, but this lady was allergic to aspirin, and she developed a duodenal ulcer. Nothing was known about allergies in those days, and it was thought that milk was the best treatment for a duodenal ulcer, so she was put on a milk diet, which meant about six pints of milk a day. This caused an irritable bowel and constant diarrhoea, but still we persisted with milk and aspirin, not knowing that both were causing the violent reaction. At no time of the day or night was this poor lady without pain. She could not move because of the arthritis, and her inflamed gut allowed her no rest. She could barely sleep. We had to turn her hourly, sometimes more frequently, to clear the frothy faecal fluid and blood that poured from her. Moving her was agony for the arthritic-locked joints, but she never complained, nor even let out a moan of pain – yet we could see the suffering in her eyes.

One day she said to me, 'I used to think that I was doing God's will in my religious vocation. I used to think that by teaching the girls, and instilling a love of classical learning, and the knowledge of Holy Scripture, that I was serving God. But now I know that I was wrong. God does not need my intellect, my learning, or my teaching. All that God requires of me is that I should lie here and suffer.'

This lady had entered the hell of physical suffering and, in its depth, found spiritual peace.

The prospect of state-sanctioned euthanasia sends a chill of despair down the spine of most medical people. Medicine is a vocation, not a job. It is a calling, comparatively rare, to care for and, if possible, to heal the sick. To promote death is contrary to the Hippocratic oath and inimical to the heart of medicine. If euthanasia became law, medicine, as we understand it, would come to an end.

The vast majority of people are simple, trusting souls who lead decent lives, go to work, raise their families, meet their friends, and, when they get sick, they go to their doctor in the hope that he or she will be able to make them better. If there was the smallest chink of suspicion, especially in the minds of the helpless or the chronically sick, that they could be 'put down', the trust would be destroyed. 'Put down' is emotive language, usually best avoided, but it is the language of ordinary people, it is the way most of us think and feel about these things.

I am a Christian; with every breath of my body, every beat of my heart, I trust and love God. Christian teaching guides my thoughts and my life. But when it comes to euthanasia, I flounder in a sea of uncertainty. It is horrifying, and contrary to the ten commandments, to think of killing the weak and helpless. Yet I also believe in evolution, and it may be that the necessity to decide the time of death for ourselves and others is part of God's purpose for the evolutionary development of mankind towards responsible maturity, to which we will have to adapt mentally, spiritually and emotionally. Yet still it shivers me, and I don't know the answer.

State-sanctioned euthanasia would open the floodgates for the entry of unimaginable wickedness. Not everyone is well motivated, not all families are loving, not all people wish their neighbours well. Doctors are not all wise and good, and it is quite possible to become addicted to killing, as the career of Dr Harold Shipman has shown us. The Devil is alive and well in the twenty-first century, and will no doubt exploit the opportunities for evil.

Yet a paradigm shift in the evolution of man has occurred in the last seventy years, which has altered birth, life and death, totally and irreversibly. Scientists can now confidently say that human life could be extended to two hundred or three hundred years, and some even say a thousand! Having seen, in my own lifetime, the miracles (that is not too strong a word) that medicine can achieve in saving and extending lives, I do not doubt that this will be possible. But given the difficulties this could imply – questions of quality of life, overpopulation, human and natural resources – a cut-off point will have to come somewhere. If it does not come from natural death, or individual decision to die, it will have to be imposed. This is euthanasia.

The personal decision to die at the right time, and in the right way, is the ideal promoted by those who would legislate for voluntary euthanasia. But will it really end there? If medicated life can be extended, decade after decade, with no end in sight, surely someone will have to make the decision to end it?

To 'turn off the machine' is the expression most people use to mean ending life by turning off life-support equipment, such as a ventilator or a kidney machine. But, although the ethics are exhaustively debated, and a legal decision is required before it can be done, it involves relatively few people and occurs only in special circumstances. Yet the issue is more complex. As with everything in life, it is the little things that shape our destiny. Millions of people daily take drugs that keep death at arms' length for a few more weeks, or months, or years. Should that switch be turned off? In other words should we, who are dependent on drugs, cease to take them and allow death to come? And if so, when? This does not require the decision of a judge or magistrate. It is a personal choice.

I have heard several ageing people, who enjoy robust good health thanks to cardio-vascular drugs and other life-maintainers, tell me quite cheerfully that when the time comes they will want to 'take something to end it all'. When I point out that it would be far easier to stop taking life-maintaining drugs, or have the pacemaker disconnected, their smile vanishes. The muttered response is usually something like, 'But I couldn't do *that*,' and the person looks profoundly unhappy, and sometimes even shudders. The reaction is muddled thinking, certainly, but understandable. Which of us does not cling to life? When dying seems years away, we can be objective, even blasé, about it; but when it is to be next year, next month, next week – oh no! – and we reach for the pills that will prolong our time on earth.

Yet I am convinced that within a short time – a generation, perhaps, or two at the most – we will all have to take responsibility for our own deaths, and we will have to get used to it.

But what of those who cannot take the responsibility, or cannot articulate it? Most people would say that the doctors must decide. Under common law today, and perhaps more subtly, social pressure, doctors have to be very careful of withdrawing life-maintaining drugs. It is not strictly speaking euthanasia, but it is close.

The people who run Dignity in Dying (formerly the Voluntary Euthanasia Society) fear being kept alive unwillingly more than they fear death, which is understandable. However, to me at any rate, their mantra of dying with dignity is less easy to understand. Dying is a biological process, and there is no dignity to it, as anyone who is familiar with death will tell you. But the departure of the soul from the body is spiritual, which is altogether different. Even people who do not believe in God, or the human soul, will tell you that at the moment of death something mysterious, even awe-inspiring, occurs which they cannot explain or understand.

'To die in peace' is the biblical expression, which I prefer. To be allowed the space, the time, and the silence in which to know that I am going to die, to contemplate death and to come to terms with the inevitable, and above all to become friends with and welcome the Angel of Death, is what I pray for. All dignity will go as control of bodily functions goes, and I will become totally dependent on others, but if peace remains, that, for me, would be the perfect end.

Yet I am realist enough to know that such an idyll is unlikely. A hospitalised death amongst a crowd of other old ladies is what I can expect, and must accept. There will be no peace, and this, too, must be accepted. I anticipate rejection, because the old and ill are not a pretty sight, and few people want to enter these places. Few people want to draw close to death, so I must accept that I will probably die alone. It is widely assumed that the dying will be in pain, and the kindest thing is to drug them, so I accept that I may be drugged stupid, and my role will be simply to submit.

This is not an inspiring end, but it is already the norm, and few of us will escape it. We can cry aloud: 'Do not go gentle into that good night ... Rage, rage against the dying of the light.'* We can huff and puff about our dignity and our rights, but it will avail nothing. Death, the great leveller, makes fools of us all. The Grace of Humility, and her sister Acceptance, will be a better and surer guide on the hard and stony path that lies ahead.

But what have we to complain about? Practically everyone of my generation leads a life enhanced by, or even dependent upon, medicine. We have grabbed greedily the extra years and called them our 'right'. So perhaps we should simply accept that a hospitalised death is the price that must be paid.

Euthanasia is not the same as suicide, which is no longer a criminal offence. On 9 July, 2009, Sir Edward and Lady Downes died in the Swiss clinic, Dignitas. Lady Downes was seventy-four, riddled with cancer, and had been told she had only a few weeks to live. Sir Edward was eighty-five. He was comparatively healthy, but his hearing and eyesight were going, and he was finding it increasingly difficult to cope with the infirmities of old age.

Sir Edward had been a very distinguished opera conductor. I knew his name fifty years ago when I was a young girl haunting Covent Garden Opera House, queuing for hours for a cheap ticket. Edward Downes was a repetiteur in those days, occasionally taking the baton when someone fell sick. Later, he earned international acclaim. I was stunned to read of his death, and of the way it had occurred.

This clinic, Dignitas, gives me the creeps. What sorts of people administer it? I shut my mind to such thoughts. But when it came to contemplating the death of Sir Edward, it seemed to me entirely logical. He had married the ballerina Joan Weston in 1955 and theirs was a true love match, lasting for fifty-four years. The thought of life without her must have been intolerable to him.

* Dylan Thomas, 1951.

313

Had her illness come ten years earlier, when he was still conducting, he might have seen things differently. But at eighty-five, with his life's work over, due to failing sight and hearing, and beset with the usual problems of old age, and above all, the loss of his wife, he wanted to go with her.

In the olden days – as my grandchildren would say – a man like Sir Edward would probably not have survived for long after the death of his wife. Grief-laden, lost and disorientated, unable to cope, perhaps not eating, not taking care of himself, he would have wandered aimlessly around and ultimately 'taken to his bed', from which he would neither have had the strength nor the will to rise. No one would have been surprised. It would have been a welcome and merciful end to a long, happy, and fulfilled life.

But we are not living in the olden days. We are living in the twenty-first century, when it is not lawful for an old man to die of old age. A team of doctors and nurses and social workers would have been on to him, assessing and monitoring every function of his mind and body. Dozens of things would have been found to be 'wrong' with him, for which drugs could be prescribed. Had he attempted to refuse treatment, psychiatrists would have been called in to assess his mental capacity. It could have gone on for years. Sir Edward was having none of it. He wanted to go with his wife, and he chose to do so in the only way that he felt he could.

Less than a month after the deaths of Sir Edward and Lady Downes the Law Lords required the Director of Public Prosecutions (DPP) to clarify the law on assisted dying. Hitherto, to aid, abet or assist anyone to commit suicide had been a criminal offence with a maximum penalty of fourteen years in prison. However, no one in the UK has ever been prosecuted for doing so.

In February 2010 the DPP confirmed that someone who was 'wholly motivated by compassion' should not be charged with a crime. This is one of six factors for prosecutors to consider as they decide on the merits of each case. Assisting suicide is still a criminal offence, but the new guidance means that it may not be regarded as being in the public interest to prosecute.

We are on the cusp of a seismic legal change concerning the condition of human life at its close. Events are moving so fast that, at the time of publication, this section of my writing may already be out of date.

A Commission on Assisted Dying was set up in 2010 and is expected to continue until the end of 2011. After that it may well be that new legislation comes into place.

HELGA

Is there anything more enduring than an old friendship? Beautiful, elegant ... Helga will always be associated in my mind with Paris in the mid-1950s, where we both worked as *au pairs*. She was about twenty-eight, and I seven years younger. She was German, from Munich, where her father was an opera singer at the State Opera. The Nazi Party, the war, and the virtual destruction of Germany had overshadowed all her early life; she had known nothing else. Her mother had died, and, after the war, Helga and her sister were homeless – I never knew exactly why, because her father was still alive. She hinted that her father was a very difficult man, a musician and singer, wrapped up in his art, expecting and revelling in the adulation of his fans (mostly women), and quite incapable of looking after two teenage girls. The two sisters walked hundreds of miles to an aunt who lived in or near Hamburg. They ate whatever they could find, and slept where they could. She told me that the American soldiers stationed in Germany were always very good to them, and it was through contact with them that she learned to speak English, which she spoke all her life with a delightful touch of an American accent.

When the girls got to Hamburg, they found it to be in complete ruin. They had heard that the city had been badly damaged, but their imagination had not prepared them for the reality. Chaos reigned, and of the suburb in which their aunt's home had been, nothing was left. Their aunt was presumed dead. How the sisters lived, I just do not know, because she said nothing of the years between 1946 and '56. At some stage she must have learned shorthand and typing, and worked as an English/German secretary, and then decided to come to Paris to learn French and become a trilingual secretary, which was better paid. This was where we met.

Helga was so beautiful, that particular type of German beauty, rather like that of Marlene Dietrich, with lovely blond hair, finely chiselled features, and a slightly superior look that irritated some people but intrigued others. She was tall and slender with such stunning looks she attracted many men. She had had very little formal education because of the war, but she was so intelligent, and so artistic, that it did not matter. She had received no musical education, but seemed to know all about music. She had no training in the fine arts, yet knowledge of painting and sculpture seemed to come naturally to her. She had had no guidance in the appreciation of architecture, but nothing missed her eye. She had something informed and insightful to say about everything and taught me, her younger friend, so much, not just about the arts in the abstract, but about the humanity behind the creation.

We lived in central Paris, I with the family I worked for, and she, independently, in a tiny attic room at the top of an apartment block that was always hot in summer and cold in winter. Could I ever forget it? The concierge who opened the door, grumbling at having been disturbed, the lift to the fourth floor, which looked as though it had been constructed in the days of Napoleon Bonaparte – perhaps it had! Then two or three flights of stairs, each one steeper and narrower than the last, to the ill-fitting door of Helga's fortress where she slept, lived, studied and entertained her friends. Everything was always in perfect order, in a space about nine feet square. With a camper burner on a tiny cabinet, and one saucepan, she produced delicious meals and delicacies.

We both studied at *L'Alliance Française* and met a lot of international language students, but in the evenings we went out with her artist friends, earnest, excitable young men trying to put the world to rights after the war. They brought their canvases to her, seeking her opinion and advice, which she always gave after a careful study of the painting. Obviously, they respected her opinions, because they came back with more. Although not much older than they were, she could always be relied upon to comfort and console and, though she had very little money, to provide food, paint, a canvas, a book or a record. Throughout her life she had a wonderful kindness, which drew people towards her.

Helga probably had short-term affairs with some of these artists; she was young and vibrant. I would never have enquired – it was entirely her business – but I doubt if she was ever wantonly promiscuous, she was just not the type. Admirers surrounded her all her life, but she never married.

The Paris days came to an end. I returned to England to do midwifery, and she returned to her homeland to work in Baden-Baden as a trilingual secretary and interpreter. She remained there for the rest of her life. It was there, when she was about thirty-five, that she met a man whom she truly loved. He was a German pilot named Hans, who had been severely wounded in the abdomen during the fighting. She nursed him for two years and gave him the love he needed. They could not marry, because he already had a wife who did not want the trouble of nursing a sick man. After his death, she said she cried for two years, and for thirty years she took flowers each Sunday to his grave. I was with her on one occasion (she was probably around seventy at the time) and I remember a very beautiful graveyard on a hillside, quiet in the sunshine, with vineyards spreading to the south. She said, 'It makes me happy that he is here, in this beautiful place.'

Helga was getting on for fifty when she and Eugen met. He was only thirty, so there was a big age gap. They were lovers, but she would not marry him. 'I do not want him to be burdened with an old woman,' she said. They did not even live together. 'I do not want him to become too dependent on me. He is too young. It would not be fair. He must be absolutely free.' I met Eugen several times and although, sadly, we did not share the same language, I could see that he adored Helga, and was a constant support and companion to her. Throughout her long life, Helga retained that feminine beauty and fascination that is more than sex appeal.

Helga was around seventy when she developed cancer of the breast. A mastectomy and chemotherapy were effective, but she was very much weaker and during the next ten years suffered many falls, both in the street and in her home. She told me about these, saying, 'I am afraid to go out in case I fall again. I have no confidence.' I last saw her in 2005 in Baden-Baden, and she fell and broke her shoulder. She was in great pain, but her concern was for my husband and me, that she had spoiled our holiday! I remarked with wonder at her stoicism; she smiled. 'That is my way; I do not want to burden others with my pain. I just put up with it.'

A break of the shoulder can be very serious, because healing of such a complex joint is difficult. It is also very painful. She told me that, after this accident, Eugen left his own apartment and stayed with her, day and night, looking after her. The shoulder took seven months to heal, and she told me that the experience really deepened the love between them. She also said that she hoped that Eugen would find a younger woman with whom he could share a more meaningful life than 'looking after a broken old woman like me'.

Helga had read my books, and one day asked me on the telephone if I was writing anything new. I told her I was writing about death. She chuckled. 'Ah yes, death, we think more about it as we grow older, don't we?' Then she told me she hoped for death all the time, because life had become so burdensome.

A little while later I received a letter dated 14th March, 2009, which contained the following sentences:

Two years ago I tried to contact death-help organisations in Holland and Switzerland. But of course, I am uncertain if I will choose this way because of Eugen. I do not want to shock him.

The letter speaks of other things, then goes on:

My last remaining energy is now searching for the way for eternal release. In my opinion it is inhuman to extend lives in hospital that are not serviceable any more. I hope you understand me, in spite of religious doubts. Did I tell you about my black-out in my bathroom at the beginning of December, when I lay almost six hours helpless on the cold marble floor? The next day Eugen found me and drove me to hospital. They started to X-ray me all over and, surprisingly, nothing was broken, in spite of my osteoporosis, but they discovered metastases in my body (I had had two cancer operations in earlier years). I told them that I would not agree to any more operations, and therefore do not care for more details. The chief doctor touched me on both shoulders, and then said kindly, 'According to your wish you are herewith released from hospital.'

A friend in Baden-Baden now explained to me the way to get into contact with the Swiss organisation, where she is already admitted in her wish to die. It seems very complicated, but makeable.

A funny point: she has postponed two times her final 'ceremony' which she payed for beforehand and now moves into a first-class clinic in Baden-Baden. Who knows if Helga will not end up with a similar solution? I don't think so, but I find the story quite amusing.

I wrote to her, but do not have a copy of my letter. A reply came on 18th June:

My dear Jennifer

I can hardly believe that your letter dates from May 11th, but time seems to pass more and more quickly to a very tired old woman. Probably because she needs so much time for each daily task or good intentions (telephoning old friends etc.) So I spent several hours on the outline of this letter, my English having diminished like my mind!

Many many thanks for your letter, so beautifully hand-written. It has touched me because of your understanding reaction upon my intentions, And of course I was especially impressed by your announcement that you are preparing a new book with respect to peaceful and human release. In fact there are too many artificial prolongations, which I observed not only during my own stays in hospitals but also during long lasting cares of old friends. Not to forget my fiancé, who suffered a lot due to the consequences of his war-injuries (belly shoots). We had just installed our small appartment in Baden-Baden, when he started to spend most of the time in hospitals. During the last weeks of his life I remained every night with him in a Karlsruhe-hospital, taking an early train to my office in Baden-Baden. During these nights I observed how much he suffered. One morning I decided not to drive to my office but wait for the doctor in chief. I prayed to release him and glanced into understanding eyes – he became [gave] an injection I suppose of morphium. I stayed next to him all day long. At about noon-time my dear Hans took my hands reposed on his pillow and kissed them. 'Es ist alles so schön mit dir' (everything is so good with you) were his last words. Then he fell asleep, still breathing for several hours, before his final release.

Where are such physicians nowadays? In earlier times, where many people died at home, the 'house-doctor' released his patients from more suffering in due time.

Right you are, dear Jennifer, at the moment my 'Suisse-endeavour' seems unachievable. This organisation is confronted with different sorts of troubles parts of the due to plotting actions. So I have to look out for another way of release, at least what my house-wife obligations are concerned, also to release Eugen, who is still sacrificing so much time and money for me. He is 18 years jounger than me and must prepare his new life with his new girl-friend, 20 years jounger than I am. This is the better solution for his future. I have the impression that they will become an ideal couple, as soon as she achieves her pension-time in summer of next year. So I have started to visit old-people's homes in Baden-B., but the achievable ones are still too expensive for me, and once again Eugen offered his financial help. But then I wood soon end up in hospitals again, because of the condition of my body. Recently they have discovered new metastasis, but after two cancer-operations I certainly would not agree to support a third one in my age of 82. Eugen repeats toujour that I should stay in his appartment, and that he would always take care of me as much as possible in his new situatian of life. But I realise more and more that my mind is in permanent reduction as far as the sense of registration is concerned, I am still quite good in reaction and even in organising the necessities of household etc. But I am more and more troubled by my permanent trouble: Whom did I meet or talk to on the telephone to-day or yesterday, what did we talk about, what did I see on the TV last night? I never swith arround, as many of my friends do. I choose beforehand out of the programm and then listen to these broadcasts with interest. But nevertheless!

The biggest trouble became my frightful emotions when I am allone. I remember now that it was the same with my father when he had about my age. My much jounger step-mother took attentively care of him, in spite of a younger friend and lover. When she married our father she was not so thoughtful and patient. She did not support any longer the step-daughters, only 6 and 8 years younger than herself. My sister and I left the house and so began the adventure of our life and professional possibilities.

Sorry for the length of my biography. To my excuse: The title of your book inspired me, and also your remark 'Life is sweet – and death always fearful'. I cannot agree to this formulation. On my opinion life in age becomes more and more fearful and painful, and death is – at least for me – a hopeful aspect. One could endlessly discuss about different opinions, but you, my dear old friend, have the courage to resume them in book-form. Congratulations to your human engagement!

Finally many many thanks for the new CD's of your last book-success. I have not yet found the calme hours to listen to them, because of many tiresome household happenings and visits from good old friends. The next ones – comming from Bruxelles – will arrive at the end of the month, staying for one week. I have found a rather cheep lodging place for them, which is not so unreliable as yours turned out to be. But as soon as I will find the time for quiet listening, I'll send you my 'echo' by telephone or by letter. I admire your numerous physical and spiritual engagements, dear Jennifer. As to myself, the burn-out condition dominates, nevertheless I have succeeded in writing this much too long letter!

    Much love to both of you

    Helga

P.S. The main trouble is probably that I have no self-confidence anymore.

During the summer months we had telephone conversations. On 14th December, 2009, she wrote the following letter:

My dear old friends

    I take leave of you with just a few words: I finally succeeded in becoming [getting] the 'green light' from Switzerland. It was probably the last moment, as they only accept people still being decisive, which means self-responsible, and my mind has been drifting away rapidly during the last months. I can still react and organise, but the sense of registration has collapsed. In addition I became more and more frightful – just as my father did in my age – so I cannot plan any own ways on the street any more.

    I am so glad that Eugen has meanwhile found a friend, younger than he is (he approaches to the seventies) with whom a positive future seems possible. She has a house in the same village where he neglected his very attractive apartment since 2004 because of all my accidents etc. I found several younger friends interested in my house-wares and book collections (of course I did not want to irritate them by my true intentions, so I pretended to move to old Swiss friends of mine) hoping that my wonderful friend Eugen will not be overcharged with the evacuation of my apartment.

    'Take my warm-heartiest wishes, my dear, unforgettable

friends Jennifer and Philip, for a long continuance of your wonderful partnership, and all your spiritual impulses!

Helga

I received the letter on 17th December and at once rang her telephone number. It was unobtainable, and has remained so ever since.

It is impossible to exaggerate the state of shock I was in after receipt of this letter. Uncertainty about what had happened tormented me and in any mental or emotional crisis I need spiritual help and guidance, so I rang the Reverend Mother of the convent with which I am connected, and told her the terrible story. The vocation of the Sisters is prayer and meditation, and, without such contemplatives I believe the affairs of man would long ago have sunk into chaos. The Reverend Mother told me that the Sisters would pray for Helga and the medical dilemmas that we have to face. Nuns are not just about prayer; they are usually very practical. She said, 'You must find out what happened to Helga in her last days and hours. Can't you get hold of the address, or better still the telephone number, of this place in Switzerland and find out?'

Thankful that Helga would be safe in their prayers, I immediately obtained the telephone number of Dignitas in Zürich. Fortunately, there were no electronic voices to contend with. A man who spoke very good English answered. I gave him the name Helga Wieter, and mentioned her intentions and her last letter. I said, 'That letter was written on the 14th; today is the 17th. Is she expected to come to you? Is she with you? Please tell me. Is she alive or dead?'

The man would tell me nothing. He said, 'It is confidential; I cannot tell you; it is against the law.' He repeated this phrase, 'against the law', several times. I persisted, saying, 'She would have come alone; I know she would. Her friends must know what has happened to her.' He said, 'I cannot tell you. We have people ringing us to enquire about a husband or wife, but we cannot tell them anything; it is against the law. We even have the police contact us in their enquiries trying to find a missing person, but we cannot disclose information. It would be illegal to do so.'

Still I persisted, saying, 'Why illegal? That makes no sense. Illegal to whom?'

He told me, 'We are an association of forty thousand members worldwide. Our members expect and receive confidentiality from us. Any association with a private membership is the same. I cannot help you; it would be illegal.'

I could get nowhere with him. I was left in a burning rage – so it is perfectly legal to give someone a dose of barbiturate knowing that it will kill them, but not lawful to reveal who it has been given to? What sort of law operates in Switzerland? Registration of births and deaths is surely a statutory obligation in any civilised country, and these are public records. At the very least, a funeral cannot be conducted in secrecy, and no one informed.

I have long had severe reservations about Dignitas though I could never clearly say why; its philosophy seems so logical and, in a way, humane. And yet my experience regarding Helga's death leaves me very uneasy.

All over Christmas I grieved for Helga, and wondered what had happened. Not knowing is probably the hardest thing to cope with. The winter was extreme – a sheet of ice gripped the whole of Northern Europe – and I thought of a frail old lady leaving her home and travelling by train, alone, to Zürich. Did she ever get there? Did she slip on the ice and break another bone, and if so who picked her up? Perhaps she arrived in Zürich and simply got lost in bewilderment in a strange city. I imagined her misery, not knowing where she was, in freezing weather, wandering helplessly around. But perhaps she *did* arrive at the Dignitas premises, and two doctors examined her and assessed that she was not mentally competent to make a decision for herself. What then? Would she have been sent away, and who would have taken the responsibility of bringing her home? It doesn't bear thinking about, does it?

Christmas is not a good time to have your mind burdened with such thoughts, nor is it a good time for communication. I tried several times to contact Helga by telephone, but the line was always unobtainable. I resolved to do my best to contact Eugen.

We have a friend, Carole, who speaks German. She agreed to write to Eugen on my behalf, telling him all that I knew, and sending him a copy of her last letter to me. I am sure he had no idea of her intentions. We agreed not to post the letter in the middle of Christmas and New Year festivities, but to send it in early January, three weeks after Helga's letter of 14 December. I did not know Eugen's surname, nor his address, so the letter had to be sent to Helga's apartment, with no more than his Christian name on the envelope in the hope that he would find it. I also wrote to the director of the company for which she had worked for twenty-eight years. Though Helga had retired long since, I felt there might be *someone* who still knew her. Then I waited.

I waited, but no reply came.

After our Paris days, Helga and I seldom met, but our friendship continued through our letters. We both enjoyed sharing news and views, ideas and reflections. Grieving usually involves going back over the past. I could not visit the place where Helga had died, so I found pleasure and relief in writing several letters to her, as we had done over the years, although I knew there could be no reply. Here are some of the thoughts contained in these letters:

Dearest Helga,

In your earlier letter you say, 'I hope you understand, in spite of religious doubts.' Of course I understand, dear brave Helga, struggling with burdens you no longer have the strength to bear, knowing that things can only get worse. But: 'in spite of religious doubts'? There I am not so sure. I have doubts aplenty, but they are not based on religion, because there is no religious teaching on the subject. As far as I am aware, none of the world religions – Christian, Muslim, Hindu, Jewish – or any philosophical teachers of any era can help us. What did Socrates or Aristotle have to say? Or Jesus Christ or Mohammed? Nothing. They had plenty to say about death, but not about man's ability to *prevent* death. We are entering a new phase of history and we cannot look to the past for guidance. Religious teaching has to adapt and find a new way. No, Helga, I do not have doubts because I am a Christian. And if anyone starts telling me they 'know the mind of God', I think I will scream!

You also said, 'In my opinion life in age becomes more and more fearful and painful and death is, for me at least, a hopeful aspect.' These are beautiful and inspiring words, especially as you have always said you do not consider yourself to be a true believer like Eugen (a Catholic) or me (an Anglican). I am sure that your attitude that death is a hopeful prospect is echoed by millions of people worldwide.

Of course, ten or twelve years ago, when you were around seventy, you could have died of cancer. When we were young girls, no one would have been surprised; after all, threescore years and ten was the span of life for mankind. But medicine saved you and you had ten more years of active and happy life. But now you say, 'Life in age becomes more and more fearful and painful,' and this leads to suicide. I hope and pray that all went smoothly for you on your last journey, and that none of my worst imaginings came to pass. I wish you had had someone to accompany you, just to make your journey easier . . . but . . .

Dear, lovely Helga, you have always been an inspiration to me, and I lament your passing and grieve for your suffering, and hold you in my prayers with love and memories of youthful happiness.

Rest now in peace eternal. Jennifer

Helga was a very considerate and thoughtful person. She wanted to die and she was determined not to trouble anyone. These desires are entirely understandable, and I have heard many people say something similar. Yet, in acting as she did, she has probably caused more turmoil than she could ever have anticipated. For those left behind, the knowledge of suicide is harder than any other death to get over. Shock, grief, guilt and bewilderment are all mixed up in the mind. An endless cycle of self-reproach is common – 'What could I have done? Where did I fail?' Even I, hundreds of miles away, feel this. What must it be like for Eugen? Helga told me that she wanted him to have a new life with a new partner, but, in fact, she may have inflicted a wound that could trouble him for the rest of his days.

Helga's fault was secrecy, but even that is understandable. No one talks about death, and she felt unable to discuss her fears and intentions with Eugen who, she had convinced herself, would be shocked and try to stop her. It is easy to imagine that she could not bring herself to raise the subject, even though, dozens of times, she may have wanted to. She was trapped in the taboo, which is as strong in Germany as it is in England. So she took her last steps alone.

IN THE MIDST OF LIFE WE ARE IN DEATH

Much of this book is dark and dreadful, and the reader could be forgiven for thinking I must be a miserable old stick, best avoided. Hotly, I refute the allegation!

It is true that I have contemplated death throughout my life, but not negatively. In fact, it has been the spur and stimulus of all my many activities and interests – life is short, enjoy it while you may. If you cannot envisage your own death, how can you enjoy life? Or, to put it another way, it is impossible to live life to its very fullest if you fear death, which is our certain end.

'It is finished,' were Christ's last words from the cross. His life's work was done and he could say 'Into Thy hands I commend my spirit'.

Old age has been kind to me, so far. The years are short and getting shorter.

I look at those I love so much and ask nothing more than to enjoy their company and do all the things I enjoy doing whilst I am still able. The very fact that I know that I will soon (how soon? Too soon!) *not* be able to do so much, gives these activities an added zing.

2007

Clonakilty, Ballygarven, Skibbereen, the music of the language sings of ancient Celtic peoples. Ballybunnion, Maudawadra, Cappoquin, Skull. Only in southern Ireland could such names be found, tiny hamlets existing for centuries amidst the hills, valleys, rocks and endless waterways. How much more beauty can the soul sustain, I mused as I cycled alone, every turn in the road revealing a new vista of sea and sky and estuaries and little islands, home only to seabirds. I sang to myself as I cycled amid the silence and awesome beauty of the Kerry coastline.

It had been a long day, and some of the hills had been daunting. By five o'clock I was getting tired and looking forward to the hotel, a shower, and a good meal. The hotel was beautiful, perched on a cliff overlooking the Atlantic, about as far west as you can go, and it had every facility, including a gym, saunas, a massage room and an open-air swimming pool. I enquired about a massage and was told I would have to wait half an hour. Never mind, thought I in my folly, I will have a lovely cool swim first. The pool gleamed blue in the evening sunlight. I was hot and tired after a long day cycling, and jumped straight in.

I was dead when they pulled me out.

Apparently, I had been spotted lying at the bottom of the pool, not moving, and two men had dived in and got me out. They held me upside down by the legs, and shook me vigorously to get the water out of my lungs. Someone rushed into the massage room to alert the therapist, who came immediately. Whilst I was upside down, she thumped my back hard repeatedly. Then they laid me down, and the therapist started manual compression of the rib cage, forcing the heart to beat again. At the same time, someone else started mouth-to-mouth resuscitation, forcing the lungs to function. They continued in this way until a weak pulse could be felt.

Half the residents and staff of the hotel were now crowded round. I was breathing and coughing, but still unconscious, so someone suggested carrying me into the hot sauna, to raise my blood temperature. This was no doubt a good idea, because the evening air was chilly, and I was wearing only a swimsuit. It was in the sauna that I came to. I remember finding myself lying on a wooden bench, surrounded by steam, and the hazy faces of people around me. A doctor was leaning over me, listening to my chest with a stethoscope.

'Where am I? What happened?' I enquired.

'You had a lucky escape,' the doctor said.

330

*

I was indeed lucky, and millions of people can say the same – their lives have been saved by modern medicine, for which we can be deeply grateful.

Yet life remains finite, and we go through agonies of indecision about whether or not to prolong it. Should drugs and treatments be continued or withheld? Is it futile? To resuscitate, or not? Finally, should euthanasia be legalised? These matters are so complex and so dreadful that they blow the mind. It is like being out at sea in a thick fog, and the compass fails. We don't know in which direction to steer the boat.

The great and good of the professions debate these issues end-lessly. But that is not enough. *Everyone* must enter the debate, because we are all involved; and this is where most people fall lamentably short. It is well nigh impossible to talk to anyone about death, I find. Most people seem deeply embarrassed. It is like when I was a girl and nobody could talk about sex. We all did it, but nobody talked about it! We have now grown out of *that* silly taboo, and we must grow out of our inhibitions surrounding death. They have arisen largely because so few people see death any more, even though it is quite obviously in our midst. A cultural change must come, a new atmosphere of freedom, which will only happen if we open our closed minds.

I have the impression that things are already changing. Around 1975 I spoke at a sixth form college. The subject was, 'Should drugs and advanced medical treatment be given to an old person who is dying?' When it came to questions and debate, there was an ominous silence. Twenty boys and girls gave me some very suspicious looks, making me feel uncomfortable. When it came to a response, every one of those young people said that, of course, all available treatment should be given, no question about it, there was nothing to debate. I remembered my matron's words: 'This is a dangerous subject,' and her caution not to be too free in what I said and to whom, because I would be misunderstood.

Last year, 2009, my granddaughter, who is doing A-level phil-osophy, religion and ethics at school, asked her course teacher if

I could address the class on the same subject. Afterwards, about twenty-five young people couldn't stop talking. Debate, opinions, examples were thrown back and forth. The bell went, it was the last lesson on Friday, and still they couldn't stop. I seem to remember we overran by about twenty minutes, until the caretaker came in to say he was locking up. This is the healthy attitude, and our hope is in the young. My thanks to staff and pupils of Townsend C of E School, St Albans.

However, the dilemma remains. Life used to be so much simpler, as it still is in many parts of the world. Birth, life and death were seen as part of a great whole, ordained by God. This has largely been eroded by the steady decline in faith. But it seems that Man is a believing animal; we absolutely must believe in something outside ourselves, and preferably something beyond our under-standing. Having lost faith in God, we place it uncritically else-where. Huge numbers of people now cling to faith in science, which, it is thought, can be controlled.

This is the root cause of all our problems. The dilemma has not come upon us through science or medicine, *per se*, nor even from social attitudes to death. It has crept up on us through lack of faith, and hidden between the lines of this book is a plea for a return to the simple understanding that life and death are in God's hands, not ours.

Reverence at the time of death used to be accepted without question. All religions require it. 'A peace beyond understanding', the Christian church calls for; Buddhists see death as the gateway to Enlightenment, and demand calmness in death; reincarnation is central to Hinduism, and the laws of Karma teach death as a step towards Nirvana; ancient Jewish law has described death as 'God's kiss'; Moslems see death as part of Allah's plan for mankind, against which it is wrong to struggle. Death and religion are closely linked.

In the secular, and increasingly atheistic age, in which we now live, this ancient teaching has, to a large extent, been denied and discarded, and we find ourselves with a medical dilemma beyond parallel.

I find it hard to understand the mind of the true atheist, who believes that life is nothing more than a series of electrical impulses and biochemical reactions to chemical stimuli. Presumably, such thinkers see death as the worst thing that can occur, because it means the end of everything. Therefore (logically), maintaining the continuance of physical existence, under any circumstances, is entirely justifiable.

But I do not see things that way. Death may be the end of what we presently call 'life', but it is not the end. There is another dimension, a spiritual life that we are all caught up in and cannot escape, which is eternal. I believe that we come from God, and return to God. The awesome mystery of birth and death, both of which I have handled, convinces me of this truth. As the physical body grows weaker and draws near to death, the soul yearns, with unspeakable longing, to return to God, the source of life.

I have seen this many times, and one cannot say that it is consciously 'longing for God'. It is yearning for the peace and contentment that enfolds the dying body and calms the dying mind, and, in my view, this comes from, and is part of, God. It is 'a peace beyond all understanding', to which we, as human beings, are all entitled.

LAST THOUGHTS

Only six months after this book was first published, I was diagnosed with cancer of the oesophagus and with secondaries in the bones. I want anyone reading the book to know that I am completely at ease with the diagnosis. I have no fears, no worries, no regrets. I do not try to struggle against this – I accept it as part of life. I shall be sorry to leave my dear husband and this beautiful world, but I do not fear what is to come. In fact, I am grateful, very grateful, because we all have to die, and it could be so very much worse. As it is, my family will see probably only a brief period as the cancer takes over. At the moment, I feel only weakness. I can see death coming, but if it is to be no more than weakness increasing day by day, then it is no bad thing.

I feel that everything is slipping away from the periphery, which is rather nice. There are, I am sure, hundreds of things I could, or should, or must be doing, but they become less relevant as the days go by. They just slide away. As everything slides away, what I am left with is faith and love. Faith, which has been the cornerstone of my life, and love, which has been always with me. Love of my husband; our love for each other; love of my daughters and my grandchildren, and their surpassing care of me. And overall, and around all, the love of God. Thanks be to God.

Jennifer Worth, April 2011

'Lord, grant us a quiet night and a perfect end,
so that we who are wearied by the changes and chances
of this fleeting world
may rest upon Thy eternal changelessness'

— *The Anglican office of Compline from the Book of Common Worship*

APPENDICES

Appendix I: Medical aspects of cardio-pulmonary resuscitation, *David Hackett*

Appendix II: The Paramedic's Tale, *Louise Massen*

Appendix III: Should patients at the end of life be given the option of receiving CPR?, *Madeline Bass*

Appendix IV: Principles of Palliative Care, *Madeline Bass*

APPENDIX I

Medical aspects of cardio-pulmonary resuscitation
David Hackett, MD, FRCP, FESC.

Consultant Cardiologist, West Hertfordshire Hospitals
NHS Trust, and Imperial College Healthcare NHS Trust;
former Chairman of the Resuscitation Committee, West
Hertfordshire Hospitals NHS Trust; and former Vice-
President of the British Cardiovascular Society.

During the Second World War and in the Korean War the severe
injuries inflicted led to surgeons having to extract bullets and
shrapnel from many locations in the body including the heart.
Previous medical teaching had assumed that any cardiac surgery
would be fatal, but many foreign bodies were successfully extracted
from the heart without mishap. This led to the dawn of modern
heart surgery, and the recognition that many serious heart conditions could be treated. Doctors observed that ventricular fibrillation, a fatal abnormality in cardiac rhythm, could occur in certain
circumstances such as during induction of anaesthesia or in the
early stages of heart attacks in hearts that were otherwise healthy,
'hearts that were too good to die'. It was also known that accidental
electrocution could induce ventricular fibrillation, and that powerful electric shocks could reverse it. In 1947, the first successful
internal defibrillation was performed during an open chest surgical
procedure. The first successful external defibrillation was performed in 1955, and in the early 1960s portable defibrillators were
developed. In 1967 mobile coronary care units were introduced in
Belfast, with successful out-of-hospital defibrillation in patients
with acute heart attacks. These developments led to the concept
of Emergency Medical Services, to bring medical care to resuscitate
the victim at the scene, rather than 'scoop and run' to the hospital.

It has been known since the late 19th century that open chest cardiac massage could maintain an effective circulation. Closed chest cardiac massage by compressing the front of the chest against the vertebral spine resulting in compression of the heart and ejection of blood into the arteries was rediscovered in 1960. Mouth-to-mouth ventilation, often used to initiate breathing in a newborn, was shown to maintain oxygenation, and resulted in a switch from more cumbersome manual ventilation techniques. The combination of chest compression and mouth-to-mouth ventilation, or cardio-pulmonary resuscitation, became known as basic life support; this could maintain life for a short time until defibrillation or another definitive procedure was performed.

Recent developments in cardio-pulmonary resuscitation
It has long been recognised that the key elements of survival from cardio-respiratory arrest are early recognition and prompt call for help, early cardio-pulmonary resuscitation, early defibrillation and early advanced medical care. Recent developments to aid out-of-hospital resuscitation include Automated External Defibrillators (AED), which use electrode pads attached to the chest to diagnose the heart rhythm. If ventricular fibrillation is confirmed then both screen display and verbal advice is given to press a button and deliver a defibrillating electric shock. These devices have led to first responder defibrillation, public access defibrillation and home defibrillation. If an ambulance has been called, the dispatcher can provide telephone instructions to direct bystanders to initiate resuscitation while awaiting the arrival of the emergency medical services.

Modern cardio-pulmonary resuscitation – A B C
The Resuscitation Council (UK)* publishes various guidelines for cardio-pulmonary resuscitation, which are internationally accepted. If someone collapses or is found to be unresponsive, the

* The Resuscitation Council. http://www.resus.org.uk/SiteIndx.htm

standard approach follows the pattern Airway, Breathing, Circulation or A B C. Detailed guidance and flow-chart posters can be found in various publications available from the Resuscitation Council website.* On discovering a collapsed or unresponsive person, the bystander or professional should call for immediate professional help if in hospital, or telephone the national emergency number if out of hospital. Resuscitation is a team effort, and cannot be performed effectively by an individual.

The first action is to ensure the airway is clear of obstruction from the tongue, mucus or a foreign body. If the circulation is working adequately, the subject is placed in the lateral recumbent or recovery position on their side, which prevents the tongue from obstructing the airway. If there is cardiac arrest, and the patient should remain lying on their back to allow resuscitation, a short plastic tube known as a Laryngeal Mask Airway (LMA) or other oral airway such as an oro-pharyngeal or Guedel airway is inserted into the throat to keep the upper airway open. In unconscious patients with ongoing cardio-pulmonary resuscitation, a longer tube called an endo-tracheal tube can be inserted from the mouth directly into the windpipe to allow direct ventilation with a manual bag or ventilator; insertion of an endo-tracheal tube is a highly specialised skill usually undertaken by trained paramedical staff or anaesthesiologists.

The second action is to ensure that the subject is breathing. If there is no spontaneous breathing, then mouth-to-mouth ventilation should be commenced, although with this technique there is a risk of infections being transmitted.

The third action is to ensure there is a circulation. If there is no effective circulation, then chest compressions should begin. The most effective circulation is achieved with chest compressions at a rate of about 100 times a minute, or just less than two per second. Ventilation can interfere with chest compressions as the lungs expand, so it has been found that the most effective

---

* The Resuscitation Council. http://www.resus.org.uk/pages/mediMain.htm

combination is two ventilations for every thirty chest compressions.

Advanced life support

Advanced life support relates to the underlying causes of a cardio-respiratory arrest. If there is no circulation because the heart is in ventricular fibrillation, then only prompt defibrillation with an appropriate electric shock can restore the normal rhythm. If the heart is in an abnormal rhythm and going very fast, such as in ventricular tachycardia, then a defibrillating electric shock can also restore a normal rhythm. Various other treatments can help or restore normal circulation. For example, if during basic life support the circulation is inadequate because of a very slow pulse from heart block (when the electrical impulses that control the beating of the heart are disrupted), medications such as atropine or adrenaline can be given by intravenous injection to speed up the heart rate, and many modern defibrillators can perform external electrical stimulation, which can also increase and pace the heart rate. If blood pressure is inadequate because of a weakened heart, then medications such as adrenaline can be injected to stimulate the force of contraction of the heart thereby raising the blood pressure. Abnormally fast heart rhythm disorders can be treated with anti-arrhythmic drugs, such as amiodarone.

Results of cardio-pulmonary resuscitation

The results of resuscitation depend crucially on where the cardio-pulmonary arrest has occurred, and the previous medical history. Resuscitation in hospital should be, and usually is, prompt and more likely to be effective, whereas outside hospital there may be a delay and therefore the outcome is less likely to be as good. Secondly, if there is no previous medical history of cardio-pulmonary disorder, and there is good cardiac and lung function, then the outcome can be good; in this circumstance, successful resuscitation can usually result in the patient returning to normal activities and having a normal life expectancy. On the other hand, if there is a history of advanced heart failure or end-stage lung disease, then the outcome is often poor; in this scenario, resuscitation can be technically successful in the very short term, but is unlikely to result in the patient surviving to discharge from hospital.

The success rates reported as regards resuscitation from cardio-respiratory arrest will also depend crucially on the selection of patients. If every patient who is dying is resuscitated, then the success rate to survival at discharge from hospital will be low. Conversely, if resuscitation is not attempted on all those patients who are near death from an untreatable condition, and in all others who are considered medically inappropriate to be resuscitated, then the success rate will be much higher.

Results of cardio-pulmonary resuscitation in hospital

An audit of 1,368 cardiac arrests occurring in forty-nine hospitals in the United Kingdom in 1997 showed that eighteen per cent of patients were discharged alive, and of these eighty-two per cent were still alive six months later.* In thirty-one per cent of these patients there was a treatable cardiac rhythm disorder such as ventricular fibrillation or ventricular tachycardia, and within this group forty-two per cent were discharged alive. If the cause of the cardiac arrest was not an easily treatable cardiac rhythm abnormality, then only six per cent were discharged alive. In this audit, factors associated with an improved chance of survival included an easily treatable cardiac arrhythmia as the cause of the arrest, a prompt return of the circulation in response to cardio-pulmonary resuscitation, and the age of the patient, with those under seventy being more likely to survive. The Resuscitation Council (UK) and The Intensive Care National Audit & Research Centre (ICNARC) are collaborating to develop a national database regarding cardio-pulmonary arrests that take place in hospital† to enable analysis of the frequency of, and outcome from, resuscitation

* Gwinnutt C, Columb M, Harris R. Outcome after cardiac arrest in adults in UK hospitals: effect of the 1997 guidelines. Resuscitation 2000; 47: 125–135. http://www.resuscitationjournal.com/article/S0300-9572(00)00212-4/abstract
† National Cardiac Arrest Audit (NCAA). https://www.icnarc.org/

in the United Kingdom. This should result in more consistent reporting and a better understanding of what might result in improved success rates.

The statistical likelihood of success in cardio-pulmonary resuscitation is not reflected in popular television dramas! A study of ninety-seven episodes of television medical dramas in the United States of America in 1994–1995 analysed sixty occurrences of cardio-pulmonary arrest; sixty-five per cent of these arrests occurred in children, teenagers, or young adults and sixty-seven per cent appear to have survived to hospital discharge.* Such rates are significantly higher than even the most optimistic survival rates in the medical literature and the portrayal of cardio-pulmonary resuscitation on television may lead the viewing public to have an unrealistic impression of the procedure, and its chances of success.

Results of resuscitation for out-of-hospital arrest

In 2004 the Ontario Pre-hospital Advanced Life Support Study of 5,638 patients who had had an out-of-hospital cardiac arrest reported that only five per cent survived to discharge from hospital.† There did not seem to be any trend towards improved survival over time with the introduction of community-based initiatives. The registry of cardiac arrests in the community of Göteborg in Sweden reported that of 5,505 patients who had suffered an out-of-hospital cardiac arrest between 1980 and 2000, between eight and nine per cent of these survived to hospital discharge.‡ Again there was no trend towards improvement in

---

* Diem SJ, Lantos JD, Tulsky JA. Cardiopulmonary Resuscitation on Television – Miracles and Misinformation. *New Engl J Med* 1996; 334: 1578–152. http://content.nejm.org/cgi/content/short/334/24/1578

† Stiell IG, Wells GA, Field B et al, for the Ontario Prehospital Advanced Life Support Study Group. Advanced Cardiac Life Support in Out-of-Hospital Cardiac Arrest. *New Engl J Med* 2004; 351: 647–656. http://content.nejm.org/cgi/content/short/351/7/647

‡ Herlitz J, Bång A, Gunnarsson J, Engdahl J, Karlson BW, Lindqvist J, Waagstein L. Factors associated with survival to hospital discharge among patients hospitalised alive after out-of-hospital cardiac arrest: change in outcome over 20 years in the community of Göteborg, Sweden. *Heart* 2003; 89: 25–30. http://heart.bmj.com/content/89/1/25.abstract

survival rates over the time period of the study. A systematic review and meta-analysis published in 2010 detailing seventy-nine studies of out-of-hospital cardiac arrests involving 142,740 patients reported that twenty-four per cent reached hospital alive, but the rate of survival to hospital discharge was 7.6 per cent overall and this survival rate has remained unchanged over the last thirty years.* Again survival ratio depended on many of the same factors as in-hospital cases i.e. the speed of response, whether the patient received cardio-pulmonary resuscitation from a bystander, if the cardiac rhythm abnormality was easily treatable, or if there was an early return of spontaneous circulation.

In 2004, a study of nearly 1,000 communities in twenty-four North American Regions reported that survival to hospital discharge was twenty-three per cent in those areas equipped with staff trained in using Automated External Defibrillators (AEDs), whereas survival was fourteen per cent in those areas without.† Increasingly, cardiac arrests which occur out-of-hospital are also being automatically treated by a special type of implanted pacemaker known as an Internal Cardiac Defibrillator (ICD). These have been available for more than ten years, and have been implanted in those people at the highest risk of developing lethal cardiac rhythm disorders. When implanted, the devices promptly diagnose and treat almost all lethal cardiac rhythm disorders within a few seconds, using an internal electric defibrillator shock. The widespread use of these devices might paradoxically skew the statistics regarding survival rates, as those not fitted with the device are likely to have less easily treatable conditions and are therefore less likely to be successfully resuscitated following a cardiac arrest.

---

* Sasson C, Rogers MAM, Dahl J, Kellermann AL. Predictors of Survival From Out-of-Hospital Cardiac Arrest. A Systematic Review and Meta-Analysis. *Circulation: Cardiovascular Quality and Outcomes*. 2010; 3: 63–81. http://circoutcomes. ahajournals.org/cgi/content/short/3/1/63

† The Public Access Defibrillation Trial Investigators. Public-Access Defibrillation and Survival after Out-of-Hospital Cardiac Arrest. *New Engl J Med* 2004; 351: 637–646. http://content.nejm.org/cgi/content/short/351/7/637

In 2006 the Termination of Resuscitation Study investigators in Ontario reported on the development of a theoretical rule which would predict a low chance of survival from out-of-hospital cardiac arrest to hospital discharge.★ Where there was no return of spontaneous circulation, no defibrillation shocks had been administered, and the arrest was not witnessed by the emergency services, the rule recommended termination of resuscitation. Of 776 patients with cardiac arrest for whom the rule recommended termination of resuscitation, only four survived (0.5 per cent) to hospital discharge. If the additional criteria of an emergency services response interval of more than eight minutes, were included, together with the arrest not being witnessed by a bystander, then this rule would have proved 100 per cent accurate. These factors should not be used to avoid resuscitation in all such cases, and they should not be applied automatically or be allowed to over-ride clinical assessments. However, they can be very helpful in judging the value or futility of attempting resuscitation or continuing resuscitation of victims of an out-of-hospital cardiac arrest.

Many resuscitations on out-of-hospital cardiac arrest victims are inevitably delayed, and the consequence can be brain injury or damage from lack of circulation and oxygen. It is very difficult to predict the likelihood of recovery from acute brain injury at the time of the arrest, and some patients do make a full recovery.

There are specific circumstances when a full recovery can occur after a long delay, such as cases of electrocution, drowning, hypothermia, poisoning, or anaphylactic (allergic) shock. According to the Resuscitation Council, by three days after the onset of coma related to cardiac arrest, fifty per cent of patients have died.† The International Liaison Committee on Resuscitation consensus statement on 'post cardiac arrest syndrome' states that the most

★ Morrison LJ, Visentin LM, Kiss A, Theriault R, Eby D, Vermeulen M, Sherbino J, Verbeek PR, for the TOR Investigators. Validation of a Rule for Termination of Resuscitation in Out-of-Hospital Cardiac Arrest. *New Engl J Med* 2006; 355: 478–487. http://content.nejm.org/cgi/content/short/355/5/478
† The Resuscitation Council. http://www.resus.org.uk/pages/als.pdf

reliable predictor of a poor outcome (vegetative state or brain death) is the absence of a pupillary light response, corneal reflex, or motor response to painful stimuli at seventy-two hours.* On the basis of a systematic review of the literature, absent brain-stem reflexes or a low Glasgow Coma Scale motor score at seventy-two hours is reliable in predicting a poor outcome.

The frequency of prolonged coma or permanent brain disability after resuscitation will depend on the underlying cause of the cardio-pulmonary arrest, and the speed with which resuscitation was undertaken. A study published in 1997 of 464 out-of-hospital cardiac arrests in Bonn over three years reported that seventy-four patients (sixteen per cent) were discharged from hospital.† Thirty-four (7.3 per cent) were discharged alive without neurological deficit, twenty-two patients (4.7 per cent) were discharged with mild cerebral disability, nine (1.9 per cent) were discharged with severe residual cerebral disability, and a further nine (1.9 per cent) were in a persistent coma.

Should resuscitation always be attempted?

Traditionally it has been taught that resuscitation should always be attempted in people who have collapsed or in patients whose condition has suddenly deteriorated. The case of Karen Ann Quinlan in the United States of America changed medical practice and provided a focus to moral teaching about death and resuscitation.‡ In 1975, aged twenty-one years old, Karen Ann Quinlan was found unconscious and not breathing in bed shortly after consuming alcohol and drugs at a party. Resuscitation was performed, but she did not regain consciousness and remained in

---

* Neumar RW, Nolan JP, Adrie C et al. Post–Cardiac Arrest Syndrome. Epidemiology, Pathophysiology, Treatment, and Prognostication. A Consensus Statement From the International Liaison Committee on Resuscitation. *Circulation* 2008; 118: 2452–2483. http://circ.ahajournals.org/

† Fischer M, Fischera NJ, Schüttlerb J. One-year survival after out-of-hospital cardiac arrest in Bonn city: outcome report according to the 'Utstein style'. *Resuscitation* 1997; 33: 233–243. http://www.resuscitationjournal.com/

‡ http://www.karenannquinlan.org/

a persistent vegetative state for several months. Her family felt that she would never recover, and wanted to withdraw medical treatment including mechanical ventilation. Medical and hospital staff refused, on the basis that this would result in her intended and hastened death; the New Jersey Supreme Court ruled that the patient or their guardian had the right to determine their treatment, that medical staff had no rights independent of the patient, and that there was no obligation for medical staff to use extraordinary means to preserve life. This ruling confirmed the principle that medical treatment could be withdrawn, and resuscitation did not necessarily have to be attempted. Karen Ann Quinlan became known as the 'right to die' case.

The case also resulted in clarification of the legal status of 'Do Not Attempt Resuscitation' orders, and the concept of advanced directives with regard to possible future scenarios or treatments. It reaffirmed the idea that a patient always has the right to refuse extraordinary means of treatment, even if it will hasten their death. Furthermore, the Karen Ann Quinlan case resulted in the establishment of Ethics Committees in many hospitals to provide guidance to clinical staff in situations where patients do not consent to recommended treatments, or where unreasonable treatment is demanded.

Do Not Attempt Resuscitation

If a heart attack is treated promptly with defibrillation, and if other emergency treatment prevents damage to the heart, the patient can often return to a normal life and have a normal life expectancy. Clearly resuscitation in this circumstance would be worthwhile. On the other hand, if a patient with an advanced disease, such as terminal cancer or terminal lung failure, develops a sudden lethal cardiac rhythm disorder, successful resuscitation might result in limited benefit, such as survival for a few more days or weeks, potentially in the context of receiving intensive medical care. Many people would regard this second example of resuscitation as futile, or of limited value. Between these two examples are many shades of grey, and it is good medical practice to try to establish the likely value or futility of emergency resuscitation in each patient during acute illness or admission to hospital. It is also good medical practice to try to think about the likely value of undertaking emergency resuscitation if someone has a chronic progressive and untreatable condition.

A discussion about the benefits or futility of resuscitation can be difficult for someone if they have not considered the matter beforehand, particularly in the case of a newly diagnosed acute illness with limited treatment or with a grave prognosis. On the other hand, most people will want to talk, learn about and discuss their illness, especially when they are anxious or frightened. Talking about the prognosis should be a natural part of the discussion, although doctors often do not raise the subject of death if patients do not ask, and patients can be too uncertain or too frightened to ask. In my experience most people prefer quality of life to longevity but occasionally people will want to keep going for a specific reason even if they are very unwell, such as a family event like the wedding of a son or daughter, the birth of a grandchild, or the completion of an important project.

Questions about resuscitation are not usually a simple yes or no decision. For example, most people who are not in an advanced terminal illness would want to be resuscitated from a simple cardiac rhythm disturbance or from transient difficulty in breathing due to infection, but often would not want prolonged intensive care with supportive treatment on an artificial ventilator or on kidney dialysis. Thus, any clinical discussion of resuscitation should include what types of resuscitation might be undertaken, and how far-reaching these directives might be. If the conclusion is that the person does not want to be resuscitated from their current illness, then this wish must be respected, and a note or statement made in their medical records to this effect. This statement should be as precise as possible, for example: 'this person does not wish to be resuscitated from a cardio-respiratory arrest'. When patients have decided that they do not wish to be resuscitated, almost all hospitals have specific 'Do Not Attempt Resuscitation' (DNAR) forms for completion by an experienced doctor. There is a model DNAR form, as well as a model patient information leaflet, available on the Resuscitation Council website.* Most hospitals also have a resuscitation committee, which will agree local policies on the application of Do Not Attempt Resuscitation decisions, and audit the appropriateness of these orders.

It can take a considerable amount of time for doctors to explain resuscitation issues to patients, and for clinicians to understand the wishes of the patient – such discussions are usually sensitive, exploratory and wide-ranging, and often require several conversations. Modern hospital practice usually involves shift work, and often there are several different doctors looking after each patient. It is essential that the clinical team makes time to discuss resuscitation decisions with each patient, and that there is a consistent response from each clinician.

Almost every hospital has introduced Do Not Attempt Resuscitation policies, procedures and forms, and clinical staff have become better at discussing death and resuscitation with patients. For those involved in hospice care and palliative care teams, however, the management of death goes well beyond the issue of whether to resuscitate or not. An alternative, more positive way of thinking about death in people with advanced disease is labelled 'Allow a Natural Death' (AND).† Allowing a natural death simply means not interfering with the dying process whilst providing care that will keep the patient as comfortable as possible. Allow a Natural Death orders are intended for terminally ill patients who are being cared for in hospices, care homes or at home, but there is no reason why these should not be applied to patients in acute hospital wards as well. The NHS Gold Standards Framework enables generic care providers, such as primary care, care homes, and palliative care settings to deliver a gold standard of care for all people nearing the end of their life,‡ and there is an 'Allow a Natural Death' form

---

* The Resuscitation Council. http://www.resus.org.uk/pages/DNARrstd.htm
† Allowing a Natural Death: http://allowingnaturaldeath.org/
‡ The NHS National Gold Standards Framework Centre. http://www.goldstandards framework.nhs.uk/

on their website.* The Avon, Somerset and Wiltshire Cancer Services also have an 'Allow a Natural Death' form on their website.† Dignity in Dying is an organisation dedicated to ensuring choice about where to die, who is present during death and treatment options, and provides access to expert information, good quality end-of-life care, support for loved ones and carers, together with advice on symptoms, and pain relief.‡ A decision to 'Allow a Natural Death' should be communicated in writing by professional clinicians to the local Ambulance or Emergency Services dispatch control centre to avoid resuscitation if that person should unexpectedly collapse. However, at present there are no national arrangements or systematic ways of communicating DNAR orders across *all* potential healthcare settings. We already use national NHS consent and DNAR forms in our hospitals, so it should not be difficult to extend this and register such forms with the emergency services; Advanced Directives or "Living Wills" could also be included. Of course, a DNAR form or Advanced Directive would need to satisfy the various legal requirements of a written document: it must be signed by the patient and a witness, the patient must have demonstrated adequate mental capacity to make the decision at the time, and the order or directive would have to be applicable to their current illness or condition. Safeguards against fraudulent entries and the influence of overzealous relatives would be necessary – for example, the witness and co-signatory might be a person who knows the patient in a professional capacity, such as their GP, solicitor, priest or minister. Arrangements could be made for patients to reregister or renew these documents annually. Obviously, legal and confidentiality safeguards would also be required with regard to the sharing of the information contained in these forms across different emergency services and healthcare

* The NHS Gold Standards Framework. http://www.goldstandardsframework. nhs.uk/
† Avon, Somerset and Wiltshire Cancer Services Allow a Natural Death (do not attempt resuscitation) Order. http://www.aswcs.nhs.uk/
‡ Dignity in Dying. http://www.dignityindying.org.uk/

organisations. Such forms could be stored electronically and shared online so that when an emergency call is received about a patient with a DNAR order or Advanced Directive, this would immediately be flagged up and the contents notified to the emergency controller.

Clinical staff are not obliged to offer resuscitation to every patient; doctors do not have to offer or provide treatments that are futile. If a patient has an advanced terminal illness with no realistic chance of improvement, doctors do not have to undertake resuscitation in the event of a cardio-respiratory arrest; it would be considered unethical. However, sometimes a patient or their family cannot accept that unavoidable death may be close, and insist that 'everything must be done'. Where there is a persistent discrepancy between the views of the patient or their family and the clinical staff, it is good medical practice to seek additional opinions and advice from experienced doctors not directly involved in the case.

The General Medical Council in The United Kingdom has published guidance on 'Treatment and care towards the end of life: Good practice in decision making'.* This guidance is based on long-established ethical principles, which include a doctor's obligation to show respect for human life; to protect the health of patients; to treat patients with respect; and to make the care of their patient their first concern. Patients who are approaching the end of their life need high-quality treatment and care to help them to live as well as possible until they die, and to die with dignity. The guidance identifies a number of challenges in ensuring that patients receive such care, and provides a framework to support doctors in addressing the issues in a way that will meet the needs of individual patients. It emphasises the importance of communication between clinicians and healthcare teams when patients move between different care settings (hospital, ambulance, care home), and during any out-of-hours period. Failure to com-

---

* Treatment and care towards the end of life: Good practice in decision making. http://www.gmc-uk.org/End_of_life.pdf_32486688.pdf

municate relevant information can lead to inappropriate treatment
being given or failure to meet the patient's needs.

Mental capacity to decide on resuscitation

Decisions relating to resuscitation cannot be made by patients who
are not mentally capable of understanding their condition, the
obvious example being when the patient is unconscious. A patient
must be able to understand, retain, and weigh information about
themselves, and be able to communicate in some form, in order
to make a rational decision about their medical care.

There are variations in different jurisdictions regarding the legal
tests and requirements to determine whether a patient has the
mental capacity to make such decisions, but the general medical
principles are common to most circumstances. In order to dem-
onstrate effective mental capacity, a person should be able to
understand what the medical treatment is, its purpose and nature,
and why it is being proposed; as well as comprehending its benefits,
risks and the alternatives; they must understand, in broad terms,
what will be the consequences of not receiving the proposed
treatment; be able to weigh the information in the balance to
arrive at a choice; retain the information for long enough to make
an effective decision; and make a free choice without external
pressure. Different medical treatments may require different levels
of mental capacity; for example, the consent process for having a
blood sample taken requires a lower degree of weighing and retaining information, compared with the consent process for major,
life-threatening cardiac or abdominal surgery. If a patient lacks the
mental capacity to make a decision about their care, this should be
noted in their medical records, and the clinical reasons for it.

If a patient lacks adequate mental capacity, then the decision
must be made for them in their best interests and urgent medical
interventions can be performed, particularly in the case of emergency or life-saving treatments. In the case of serious procedures
to be done without consent, it is good medical practice to consider
alternative, less invasive treatments; to discuss treatment with all
members of the healthcare team; to discussing treatment with

the patient as far as possible; to consult with other healthcare professionals involved with the patient's care (for example, their general practitioner); to consult relatives, partners and carers; to obtain further opinions from experienced doctors if the patient or their family do not agree with the proposed treatment; and to ensure a record is made of the discussions and any decision taken.

Again, there are variations on the legal requirements in different jurisdictions. Good medical practice would include consultation with relatives, partners and carers to ascertain what the expected wishes of the patient might be. In England and Wales, the Mental Capacity Act of 2005 has brought a legal obligation for clinicians to take into account the views of anyone named or appointed with power of attorney by the patient for this purpose, their carers, or any deputy appointed by a court.★

Initial decision to resuscitate

In an unexpected or out-of-hospital cardiac arrest, when the patient cannot consent to treatment, the assumption has to be that resuscitation should be performed. Death can be verified by any appropriately qualified person, but this is usually done by a doctor, and in the United Kingdom only a doctor who has provided care during the last illness and who has seen the deceased within fourteen days of death or after death can sign a death certificate. If someone is found to have collapsed and died, the emergency services are still obliged to attempt resuscitation as they cannot in general immediately ascertain the underlying condition of the victim. Of course if a person has been dead for some time, for several hours or longer, death will be obvious and resuscitation attempts will not be appropriate.

Age itself should not be a deciding factor when discussing whether to resuscitate someone who has collapsed, when discussing whether to continue resuscitation attempts, or when discussing whether a patient would wish to be resuscitated or not

★ Mental Capacity Act 2005. http://www.opsi.gov.uk/acts/

from a cardio-pulmonary arrest. In general, the success of any medical treatment decreases with age, but there is no specific cut-off point concerning the success of resuscitation from cardio-pulmonary arrest. Furthermore, clinical policies should not be ageist in terms of specifying treatments that are not provided to people over a certain age, unless there is very good medical evidence to suggest a lack of benefit. In the medical literature about resuscitation, there is no evidence that the outcome is dependent on being under a certain chronological age, or that failure occurs over a certain age. The benefits of most medical treatments depend on the general condition of the patient, therefore discussions about the value or futility of resuscitation should be based on that rather than the patient's chronological age.

This is a reason why the most useful information when deciding whether to undertake or continue cardio-pulmonary resuscitation is the medical history. If, for example, a patient has presented with an exacerbation of breathlessness from chronic, extensive and end-stage respiratory failure, uses home oxygen and is house-bound as a consequence of their condition, then resuscitation from a cardio-respiratory arrest is less likely to be successful, and the prospect of a full recovery is unlikely. If such a patient is placed on a mechanical ventilator to take over their breathing and oxygenation, it could be very difficult to wean them off. If, on the other hand, a patient has been healthy and active until recently, and presents with respiratory failure due to extensive pneumonia, then resuscitation is more likely to be successful, and the chances of a full recovery are good. It is often the current or future quality of life that is the influential factor when assessments about resuscitation are being made by clinicians and families or carers on behalf of a patient.

A successful resuscitation can be evident within minutes, but it may not be evident for perhaps thirty minutes or more that resuscitation has been unsuccessful; basic and advanced life-support measures can maintain the breathing and circulation for this length of time and longer. Decisions about when to stop resuscitation attempts are usually made by an experienced doctor when there has been no response, and there is no treatable or reversible cause of the initial collapse. As previously observed, resuscitation should be continued for longer than usual in specific circumstances, such as in the case of children or where the collapse has been caused by electrocution, drowning, hypothermia, poisoning, or anaphylactic shock.

Advanced Decisions

Advanced Decisions, advanced directives, or 'living wills' can be made to specify treatment that a person might or might not want in the future. There are three legal requirements for Advanced Decisions to be honoured – existence, validity and applicability – and these have been set out for England and Wales in the Mental Capacity Act (2005).

For an Advanced Decision to be considered existent, it must be put down in writing, and be signed by the patient and a witness. For it to be valid, the Advanced Decision must not have been withdrawn or overridden by a subsequent Lasting Power of Attorney, and the patient must not have acted in a way that is clearly inconsistent with the Advanced Decision. To be applicable, the person must have had the mental capacity to make the decision about the proposed treatment at the time of writing. The Advanced Decision will not be applicable to treatments or circumstances that are not specified in the document. If there is any doubt or dispute about whether a particular advanced decision meets all the requirements, action may be taken to prevent the death or serious deterioration of the patient, whilst the dispute is referred to legal authorities. It is always very difficult to anticipate every possible scenario with regard to your health and healthcare, and therefore advanced decisions can be very limited in scope, especially when a patient presents with a new illness or condition.

Should relatives witness resuscitation?

Parents will almost always ask to be present when their child is being resuscitated. Historically, as with most medical procedures, relatives have been kept outside when cardio-pulmonary resuscitation is being performed. However, there are differing views between the public and healthcare professionals and the Resuscitation Council has published a useful document on their website about this issue.*

From the relatives' and partners' point of view, being present may help them come to terms with the serious illness or death of a loved one, especially when they can see that everything medically appropriate has been done. The disadvantage is that the reality of resuscitation may prove distressing, particularly if it is traumatic or if they are uninformed. Furthermore, they may physically or emotionally hinder the staff involved in the resuscitation attempt. However, it seems likely that for many relatives it is more distressing to be separated from their family member during these critical moments than to witness them. From the patient's point of view, most would probably want to have their family present but it would be unusual for the patient to have expressed an advanced directive stipulating the inclusion of specific relatives, partners, carers or friends. For the clinical staff undertaking resuscitation, the presence of relatives could increase stress, affect decision-making, and affect the performance of the staff involved. On the other hand, verbal or physical interference by a relative could be prevented by close supervision and restriction of numbers.

Progressives believe that relatives or partners should be given the opportunity to be with their loved ones at this time, and proper provision must be made for those who indicate that they wish to stay. If resuscitation is to be witnessed by relatives, partners or carers, it is essential that they be supported throughout by appropriately trained clinical staff, and that the resuscitation team leader is prepared for and aware of their presence. Every hospital should have a written policy about the procedure to be followed when relatives, partners or carers request to be present during cardiopulmonary resuscitation and this would normally be the responsibility of the local Resuscitation Committee.

* The Resuscitation Council. http://www.resus.org.uk/pages/witness.htm

★

Summary and conclusions

Modern resuscitation methods and techniques date from the many major advances in research and development of medical practice in the 1950s and 1960s. Changes since then have mainly resulted in improvements in existing procedures, rather than in the development of new medical treatments; consequently, improvements in the outcome of cardio-pulmonary resuscitation have been relatively small. The introduction of cardio-pulmonary resuscitation in the 1960s, as with many new drugs or medical procedures, resulted in initial scepticism, followed by enthusiasm, leading to over-enthusiasm and over-use, until a more precisely defined usage becomes established. With the development of procedures, medical practice has run ahead of many of the moral and ethical issues involved in resuscitation decisions. Most of these issues, such as the applicability of Do Not Attempt Resuscitation orders and Advanced Decisions, are now being reassessed so that they come into line with current medical practice.

In general, the success rates of cardio-pulmonary resuscitation remain disappointingly low, especially in out-of-hospital resuscitation, and it does not seem likely that developments in the near future will substantially help to improve the situation. In my view, the most helpful development would be for clinicians to be able to define in advance which people and which conditions are most likely to have a successful outcome, and which will not; there is an obvious need to be more selective about for whom, when and where we undertake cardio-pulmonary resuscitation although this is clearly much easier to do for patients in hospital.

Sudden collapse and death are in fact very rare in healthy people, and are probably becoming even rarer in countries that have falling mortality rates from heart disease. The greatest challenge is to understand when there is likely to be little or no benefit from cardio-pulmonary resuscitation, and to identify more systematically those people in advance. By doing this, death could be managed in a better and more humane way – which is the whole point of this book.

In the end, doctors cannot cheat death; we can only delay it.

APPENDIX II
THE PARAMEDIC'S TALE

By Louise Massen, Clinical Team Leader, Thameside Ambulance Station, South East Coast Ambulance Service (SECAMB)

I joined Kent Ambulance Service on the 1 April 1993. I am second-generation ambulance service and absolutely love my job with a passion! There is nothing else I ever want to do.

We received a three-month residential training course, which was run by a specialist ambulance training college. The course encompassed emergency driving, manual handling, and the specialist ambulance aid skills required to use the equipment we need to treat a whole host of medical, traumatic and obstetric calls.

I graduated in July 1993 and was posted to Dartford Ambulance Station of North Kent. I was proud to work at the station where my father had worked for twenty years. In his day, the ambulance equipment consisted of a basic stretcher, some oxygen, a few bandages and wooden splints, and lots of blankets. I was trained in manual cardiac defibrillation, could take a blood pressure, and use a whole host of splinting and moving equipment to handle the high-speed trauma that we were increasingly being called to deal with.

By 1995 I had completed the extended training by the National Health Service Training Directorate (NHSTD), and was deemed a 'qualified ambulance paramedic'. My new skills included intravenous cannulation and infusion (this meant I could insert a needle over a catheter into a patient's vein to administer IV drugs or fluids), endotracheal intubation (a plastic tube which sits in the patient's trachea or windpipe to facilitate a patent airway whilst unconscious), intraosseous cannulation (screwing a needle into a bone to allow drug access), and a more detailed approach to cardiac ECG interpretation.

Surely and slowly, medical progress has been made and many new protocols, policies and procedures have found their way into the ambulance service. Paramedics these days are proficient in 12-lead ECG interpretation, can diagnose and provide definitive treatment for myocardial infarction by administering thrombolytic clot-busting drugs – every minute a coronary artery is occluded depletes life by about eleven days – so our early intervention and treatment in the pre-hospital setting is improving the quality of many patients' lives, as well as the quantity who survive.

New paramedics, these days, are trained by universities with the emphasis more on education and less on the sort of vocational training that I completed. The new cohorts of paramedics are selected from those who successfully complete a three-year degree course, with the opportunity for all paramedics to extend their training to become paramedic practitioners (PPs) and critical care paramedics (CCPs).

The paramedical degree courses are separated into academic modules covering a range of subjects such as introduction to medical care, trauma care, public health immunology, and foundations of paramedic practice, which covers use of ambulance equipment and clinical skills, and the different sections of anatomy and physiology which are broken down into the various systems of the body – cardiology, neurology etc.

In the first year, the student paramedics cover all the basic education, and by year two they train alongside established paramedics and work as part of an ambulance crew (although they are not allowed to practise autonomously). As the course continues, they learn new practical skills, and complete various hospital and clinical placements to complete their education. Clinical skills are practised under the supervision of experienced paramedics, who have also completed a practice placement educators' (PPEDs) course.

At the end of three years, all the education, clinical skills and experience from working on the front line allows the students to join the ranks of the rest of us registered as paramedics by the Health Professions Council. Every paramedic has to re-register every two years and maintain evidence of clinical professional development to remain on the register – failure to do so could result in a paramedic losing their registration and being unable to practise, in the same way as doctors and nurses must show development.

Our PPs and CCPs undergo degree-level education for an additional eighteen months, and, once qualified, have even more developed examination skills, and can provide more comprehensive roadside care to the patients in the community and at home – our PP clinicians can provide catheter care, perform suturing and wound closure, prescribe broad-spectrum antibiotics and, in some areas, are working alongside general practitioners in facilitating diabetic or asthma clinics.

Our CCPs are working alongside doctors and anaesthetists in providing cutting edge front-line care to those patients most critically ill, working on helicopters and specialist ambulances equipped to transfer patients in drug-induced comas safely between hospitals. This reduces the need to use doctors to look after anaesthetised patients.

Our area now encompasses Kent, Surrey and Sussex in the South East Coast Ambulance Service or SECAMB. The newest advances include a FASTrack Stroke Pathway – we work very closely with all our hospitals so that, when we are dispatched to a patient showing a positive test for a stroke, we can deliver them directly to the nearest hospital able to deliver thrombolytic therapy to dissolve the clot. Stroke patients are now being discharged home and are back at work in weeks – a long way from the treatment a few years ago, when a stroke victim was likely to be paralysed for months, years, or worse.

SECAMB is also the first ambulance trust in the UK fully to follow a new cardiac arrest protocol for out-of-hospital cardiac arrest where the first rhythm is ventricular fibrillation.

SECAMB is now delivering resuscitation based on emphasis for effective cardiac compression, which has been championed by our honorary life medical director, the world-renowned cardiologist Professor Douglas Chamberlain, CBE, who has, for many years, been our greatest advocate, and has worked tirelessly training paramedics.

Our Protocol C resuscitation procedure for patients presenting in ventricular fibrillation is leading the way in pre-hospital resuscitation in the UK. Some of the latest clinical audits published in 2009 for survival following cardiac arrest rate SECAMB as the highest performing ambulance service in the country.

Dying differently

So what exactly does happen when a member of the public dials 999 to a collapsed patient who is terminally ill? Our role is to preserve life, prevent deterioration and promote recovery – but can we always achieve this? What is the dilemma that we, as ambulance paramedics, face when we are called to a patient at the end stage of their illness?

All ambulance service clinicians – technicians, paramedics and advanced paramedics – work within the guidelines of the Joint Royal Colleges Ambulance Liaison Committee (JRCALC). These guidelines are very specific, and state that in the event of being called to a cardiac arrest or near life-threatening event we are obliged to initiate resuscitation unless we have sight of a formal Do Not Attempt Resuscitation (DNAR) order or an Advance Directive to Refuse Treatment.

A patient who is deemed to have mental capacity has the right to refuse treatment, even if not having that treatment leads to deterioration in health and ultimately death. A patient who is unconscious cannot make that decision; it has to be made for them – and in those circumstances, in the absence of any lasting power of attorney by a relative, all steps of active resuscitation would be undertaken unless a DNAR is shown to the ambulance crew.

This formal DNAR must be in writing and given to the crew on arrival at the call. The condition must relate to the condition for which the DNAR is written, so resuscitation should not be withheld for coincidental conditions.

In the case of a known terminally ill patient being transferred to a palliative care facility, the DNAR can be verbally received and recorded by ambulance control.

In an out-of-hospital emergency environment, there may be situations where there is doubt about the validity of an advance refusal or DNAR order. If the ambulance crew are not satisfied that the patient has made a prior and specific request to refuse treatment, they are obliged to continue all clinical care in the normal way.

I am constantly reminded of how my decisions to provide clinical care for patients I attend can have a lasting effect on quite often distressed and highly emotional relatives, who have witnessed the sudden collapse of a cherished one and act on impulse by calling an ambulance ... I have the equipment, the knowledge and the clinical skills to initiate and continue advanced life support and resuscitation, and in the absence of any written order I have to do so ... Or is this always the case?

I may be 'just' a paramedic, but I have empathy with the suffering of the sick. That's why I am a paramedic and do the job that I do, surely?

Dealing compassionately with end-of-life patients

Whilst I am very aware that many members of the public urge us to do 'everything we can' to save a life, my seventeen years of ambulance service experience have shown me that a good many elderly or terminally ill patients do not require the services of a paramedic; in their time of need, they want peace, or a priest, or, in some cases, both. That is the area that I will now go on to discuss.

About ten years ago I was working on the night shift. It was a little after midnight when the crew received a call to attend a 'ninety-six-year-old female, breathing difficulty'. We arrived shortly after the call was made and knocked on the door at the address we were given. An elderly man opened the door, and gestured for us to follow him. We traipsed into the house with our equipment and were led into the front room where a very elderly lady lay on a single bed in front of a fireplace.

The lights were dimmed, but I could see that the lady was dying. Her breathing was bubbly, laboured and intermittent. She was unconscious and her eyes were shut, but she was twitching a little bit. My eye caught an empty ampoule of diamorphine discarded on the mantelpiece.

The man began to tell us his story. The lady in the bed was his ninety-six-year-old sister. He was ninety-four, and had lived with her all of his life. My crewmate and I exchanged nervous glances, and the distress visible in her face was most probably echoed in mine. He continued that she had been diagnosed with cancer a couple of years ago and had fought it bravely, but was now nearing the end and had expressed her wish to die at home – in the comfort of her own bed, in the house where she was born, with her brother for company. He realised that the time was near and was scared. He was terrified of her dying, and wanted to make sure she wasn't suffering.

The family doctor had visited in the afternoon and given her a pain-killing injection. She had been sleeping peacefully ever since, but in the last hour her breathing had become increasingly worrying to him and she had begun twitching.

He couldn't get hold of his doctor, and the GP surgery had redirected his enquiry to the out-of-hours doctors; they had simply instructed him to dial 999. That is how we ended up there.

We sat down and reassured the man. 'We'll phone the out-of-hours doctor back, ask for the palliative care nurses to come and be with you and get her some more pain relief so she isn't in any pain.' He was so grateful; you could see the tension lift from his face.

I made the phone call and explained the situation to the out-of-hours doctor, and said that we required a palliative visit. He refused point blank to attend and ordered me to take that poor dying lady from her nice warm bed to the accident and emergency department. I was nearly speechless, but attempted to reason with him that it was inhumane to suggest such a thing, the lady was dying and nothing we could do could halt the fact. He adamantly refused to consider it. He was the doctor, I was only the ambulance 'driver' and was not in a position to disobey his request. 'Compassionless' was my thought, or maybe something stronger, I regret to admit.

How do you explain this to a distressed relative? That you have to drag his dying sister unceremoniously out of her deathbed and cart her off to the local accident and emergency centre, to be poked and prodded, and then breathe her last on a hospital trolley surrounded by the drunks and assaults that frequent A&E during the night shift? But he was understanding; we had no alternative but to obey medical orders.

We went and fetched our carrying chair, two big warmed blankets and a pillow to prop her up. I knelt on the bed behind her, and, as we lifted her into a semi-sitting position before settling her into the chair, she died.

I looked at my teammate and she nodded. We laid the woman straight back down in the bed, still warm from where we had lifted her up, smoothed her eyes over and covered her with the quilt.

I went to fetch her brother from the kitchen, and we all cried. How unprofessional, I hear you say! I knew in my heart it was the best thing for her. I phoned the out-of-hours doctor again, informing him that now the lady had died, he would *have* to visit and confirm death (in those days we did not perform recognition of life extinct).

Having personal experience as a relative also puts a whole new perspective on the whole end-of-life-care issue. This is something that I experienced for myself in 2008 when my own mother died from a chronic lung condition. It was the spiritual epiphany of this event that spurred me on to help our ambulance service develop a better insight into end-of-life care and how we can be of benefit to patients who are dying.

The death of my dear mother was, without a doubt, the most life-altering event of my existence.

She had a condition known as chronic obstructive pulmonary disease (COPD). She had lived with this for many years, but had been particularly unwell for the year preceding her death, and was being looked after mainly by the respiratory team at home where she had her own oxygen and nebulisers. She had suddenly been admitted to hospital with an exacerbation of the condition. The consultant told my elderly stepfather, Bernard, that there was nothing more they could do for her except 'keep her comfortable'.

Mum was only sixty, and it was not until I went to visit her in hospital and saw her so ill that the terrible truth dawned on me that she was dying. I gathered the family round.

It was the most numbing and distressing thirty-six hours of my entire forty years. My brother Matthew (also a paramedic) rushed down from his home in East Anglia. We sat beside her all night and had some deeply intriguing conversations during those dark hours.

'It's quite ironic, isn't it?' mused Matt. 'If either one of us received an emergency call to a patient of Mum's age, who was unconscious and breathing like this, we would be intubating her, nebulising drugs, giving intravenous diuretics and rushing her into A&E as fast as we could.'

He had a point, and yet we sat there, helpless, while Mum's breathing continued to bubble and struggle, the relentless dull sound of the oxygen hissing away, a constant background noise making my head spin. In the small hours of the night she grew distressed and started moaning and twitching. I went to find a nurse for some help. The doctor wrote her up for some morphine which the staff nurse administered. I asked her how long it would be; Mum's vital signs were all over the place, her breathing and pulse rate were hugely elevated and her oxygen saturations very low. She had a raging temperature of 40.1. I wasn't used to watching people die – I was meant to stop that sort of thing from happening. I was shivering on the little chair next to her, my hand tightly grasping hers, its heat keeping me warm in the depth of the night. Another doctor popped in to see Mum. I was beginning to panic.

'I want to take her home to die,' I stuttered.

'It's not an option now,' replied the doctor. 'I cannot discharge her like this, so close to death.'

It was a truly desperate feeling watching my mother dying,

aching to swing into action and 'do my paramedic stuff', when, deep inside, I knew there was absolutely nothing I could do to prevent the inevitable slide into death. Mum's was as dignified as it could be in the little side room. Both Matthew and I held her hands and watched as her breathing slowly began to fail – when we were finally able to rid her of the oxygen mask – and saw the peaceful look come over her face when her exhausted heart eventually stopped beating.

It gave us both a whole new perspective on death and how it affects those it leaves behind.

We both returned to work, vowing to look into the end-of-life care policies our respective ambulance trusts had in place.

As a coincidence, in June 2008, the Darzi Report was issued by the Department of Health, with the title *High Quality Care for All*. Some of the concerns raised by Lord Darzi included those surrounding end-of-life care. I happened to glimpse some information on this review and begged my Chief Executive Paul Sutton to consider the possibility of championing end-of-life care for SECAMB NHS Trust. He was enthusiastic about my interest, and, with his encouragement, I attended a conference on the subject in November, and found it extremely engaging.

On the back of that conference – and by talking and writing to some of the speakers and delegates – I was invited to speak at the National Council for Palliative Care conference at Guy's Hospital in March 2009 on the subject of 'Dying Differently'. My intention was to speak to the delegates and impress on them the fact that ambulance crews are not just there to perform CPR and dash the patient to hospital, but we can also have a place with palliative care patients, even if it is just to administer pain relief or oxygen.

In the past year our Trust has implemented a general policy surrounding Do Not Attempt Resuscitation and Advance Directive to Refuse Treatment. Any palliative care team can email our Trust with a copy of these orders, and we have the facility to add a history marker linked to an address where a palliative care patient lives, so if an emergency call is generated for that person, the information is passed to the crew that the patient is not to be resuscitated.

Indeed, this facility also extends to GPs and hospital consultants who have patients who have requested DNAR for a·variety of conditions – COPD (like my mother), advanced Alzheimer's, Parkinson's, or any other illness or condition where CPR is deemed inappropriate. The only thing we require to enable us to safeguard ourselves is the sight of the original unaltered document that is signed by the doctor on arrival at the call.

These DNAR documents have no expiry date and, once signed, are valid until the patient dies or the order is changed for whatever reason.

DNAR in most cases would refer to CPR only, but also has the flexibility to allow withholding other treatment such as artificial nutrition and hydration – although these treatments tend to apply to patients already in hospital. Other ambulance services are working around the Allow a Natural Death (AND) procedure.

What is encouraging, of course, is that the ambulance service is now very much part of the integrated multi-disciplined team, and is consulted by the various primary care trusts in end-of-life care issues; and our concerns and wishes are being registered and used, helping us all with the treatment and services we can offer to patients as they reach the end of their natural lives.

What the future holds

Advancement in training, education, and the ever-increasing policies and protocols we follow now, will no doubt lead to an older, and healthier, nation. It is an amazing fact that treatments that we currently use already lead to heart attack and stroke patients recovering fully and going back to 'tax paying' status in a few short weeks. Twenty years ago, these patients would have died, or become paralysed for the rest of their lives.

I often chat with my work colleagues and ask them the searching question, 'Have you thought about how and where you would prefer to die?'

I am surprised that most of them haven't even thought about

their own death, or what their personal preference is. This alarms me, considering the amount of death we actually deal with in our line of work!

For my own part, should I be suffering from an incurable illness, I will be instructing my GP and get my own DNAR written out, and I will leave it in a big white envelope just by the front door – in the hope that the young, keen ambulance crew who come rushing in will take note, and leave me to die in the peace I hopefully have earned!

APPENDIX III

Should patients at the end of life be given the option of receiving CPR?

by Madeline Bass, BSc, RGN, Head of Education,
St Nicholas Hospice, Bury St Edmunds, Suffolk

First published in *Nursing Times*; 105 4, 26–02–2009.

Cardio-pulmonary resuscitation (CPR) is often unsuccessful and may not always be appropriate at the end of life. This article debates whether the use of cardio-pulmonary resuscitation by healthcare professionals in situations when it is unlikely to be successful feeds an unhealthy appetite to intervene just because it is possible. It explores the problem of offering patients and relatives the choice about CPR at the end of life when it is likely to be unsuccessful.

End-of-life and palliative care has become an increasingly important area of healthcare professionals' work following publication of the End of Life Care Strategy (Department of Health, 2008).

Good communication between patients and staff is essential for those who are making choices and decisions about care at the end of life. This may include discussions about cardio-pulmonary resuscitation.

We can now treat disease and disability in ways that would not have been thought possible sixty years ago. These achievements have also created bioethical dilemmas. The advent of new treatment interventions has brought its own unhealthy appetite – the more treatments healthcare workers have to offer, the more they intervene. To them, this equates with doing the best for patients and knowing that everything has been tried.

However, in some cases, interventions can mean poor outcomes for the patient and result in low staff morale. One area of particular concern is the decision about when it is appropriate to perform CPR.

Misconceptions about CPR

The media's interpretation of CPR, primarily through TV drama, has led to a misunderstanding that it is a quick intervention that guarantees success without any side-effects (Bass, 2003; Diem *et al*, 1996).

CPR was first used in its present advanced life-support format of chest compressions, ventilation and defibrillation in 1960 (Kouwenhoven *et al*, 1960). The main problem associated with CPR is identifying when it is appropriate to instigate it as a life-saving measure. The concern is that the decision to proceed is often viewed as the default if a decision about resuscitation has not been made.

CPR was devised as an emergency intervention for unexpected cardiac or respiratory arrest (Kouwenhoven *et al*, 1960) and the majority of healthcare professionals are not aware that the success rates for CPR are very low (Wagg *et al*, 1995; Miller *et al*, 1993) (see Table 1). Only a small percentage of people will survive to leave hospital following a cardiac or respiratory arrest.

Ewer *et al* (2001) looked at the success rates of CPR undertaken on patients with cancer. They asked whether patients were expected to have an irreversible cardiac or respiratory arrest. The results showed that, of patients having an unexpected, reversible arrest, there was a 22.2% success rate. However, for those who were expected to have an irreversible arrest and were at the end of life, there was 0% success.

The effects of inappropriate CPR are often not considered. These include post-resuscitation disease (complications caused by resuscitation itself) (Negovsky and Gurvitch, 1995), an undignified death for the patient, and distress to relatives. Paramedics and resuscitation teams may also become demoralised by repeated failures (Jevon, 1999).

Table 1. Success rates for CPR

Author	Success of CPR, enabling patient to be discharged from hospital	Initial success
Karetzky et al (1995)	3–29%	Not stated
McGrath (1987)	15%	53%
Vitelli et al (1991)	10.5%	65.7%
Varon et al (1998)	9.6%	Not stated
Wallace et al (2002)	2%	Not stated
Sandroni et al (2007)	15–20% for in-hospital arrest	Not stated
Nolan et al (2007)	Not stated	5–10% for in-community arrest

Factors influencing success of CPR

The success of CPR is often measured in terms of initial success – the return of heartbeat and breathing, controlled independently by the patient. It is also measured in terms of survival to discharge (see Table 1). The chances of successful CPR are improved if:

- There is early access to a cardiac arrest team
- Basic life support is commenced immediately
- Defibrillation is carried out as quickly as possible in cases of ventricular tachycardia or pulseless ventricular fibrillation (Jevon, 2002).

Other positive factors associated with a successful CPR attempt include:

- A non-cancer diagnosis
- Cancer without metastases
- The patient is not housebound
- Good renal function
- No known infection

- Blood pressure within normal range
- The patient has robust health (Newman, 2002).

The Gold Standard Framework (GSF) suggests that cancer, organ failure, general frailty and dementia are not associated with success (NHS End of Life Programme, 2007).

The BMA *et al* (2007) recommended that CPR should not be attempted when patients have indicated before the cardiac arrest that they would refuse it or if the attempt is likely to be futile because of their medical condition.

Resuscitation decisions

Discussions about resuscitation at the end of life raise a number of questions.

- Are public expectations of healthcare and technology unrealistic?
- Do healthcare professionals pursue the possibility of an immediate positive outcome from CPR without considering the long-term consequences of the intervention?
- Does inappropriate CPR raise false hope in patients, relatives and staff? (Jevon, 1999)

Awareness and knowledge of CPR guidance among healthcare professionals is poor (Bass, 2003), with knowledge focusing on local policy rather than research evidence and national guidance.

In addition, healthcare professionals often fail to recognise when a patient is dying, which can result in difficulty making an appropriate decision about whether to resuscitate in the event of a cardiac or respiratory arrest. The Liverpool Care Pathway (LCP) is a recommended national tool that can assist professionals to make an accurate diagnosis of dying (Ellershaw and Ward, 2003). This diagnosis can help to inform discussion about when to initiate CPR.

Reducing the inappropriate use of CPR

The inappropriate use of CPR can be reduced by improving

communication between all members of the multidisciplinary team. The End of Life Care Strategy (DH, 2008) gives guidance and outcomes for care at the end of life, including dignity, appropriate care and comfort – appropriate care should include refraining from undertaking inappropriate CPR.

The Mental Capacity Act 2005 allows patients to make advance care plans and allows them to have choices at the end of life. If they are to support patients in making such plans, healthcare professionals need to discuss appropriate choices with them.

It is good practice to have a local Do Not Attempt Resuscitation (DNAR) policy, and use the documentation from the GSF for patients in their own home. The framework prompts healthcare professionals to initiate discussions around advance care planning, such as about what patients want at the end of their life and whether they have choices.

The GSF also encourages healthcare professionals to ask the question: 'Would I be surprised if this person died in one year/one month/one week/one day?' The patient is coded and specific guidance for this coding is given. The coding is:

A: prognosis of years

B: prognosis of months

C: prognosis of weeks

D: prognosis of days.

Guidance relating to the coding provides information about what professionals should discuss with patients and care that should be planned and provided.

For example, if a patient is in the last few weeks of life, then drugs such as analgesics should be available in the person's home in case they are needed. This can prevent a crisis if these drugs are required at short notice. Depending on the patient's condition, the coding is reviewed regularly to take into account any changes.

The majority of GP practices in England have now adopted the GSF in some format, but how it is adopted and adapted depends on individual GP practices.

Choice and misconceptions about CPR

Patient choice is high on the health and social care agenda (Department of Health 2008; 1991; Mental Capacity Act 2005) but this can lead to patients being offered unrealistic choices that are not supported by expert professional opinion. The wrong choice can result in a negative outcome for the patient.

In my experience, there is a misconception among some nurses, doctors and patients that all patients/carers should be given a choice about resuscitation.

Many nurses will have experience of doctors entering a patient's room when they are in the last few days of life and asking the family carers: 'If your relative's heart and lungs stop working, do you want us to resuscitate them?' In some situations, the family carers are adamant that they do not want this. However, where death is approaching much more quickly than expected, or when it has been difficult for family carers to accept their relative's approaching death, they may decide that they want CPR.

This can leave healthcare professionals with an ethical dilemma – the family carers want everything to be done, but CPR itself is not an appropriate intervention, so what should they do when the patient dies? The choice is to initiate CPR or to risk a complaint and possible litigation if they do not.

CPR guidance from the BMA *et al* (2007) does not help healthcare professionals with this dilemma. It states that if patients insist they want CPR, even if it is deemed to be futile, it should be carried out but, when an arrest occurs, the situation should be reviewed. In reality, this means that the patient is offered an intervention that will not be given. This does not support a trusting relationship between healthcare professionals and the patient (Bass, 2008).

Patients or family carers cannot demand CPR and healthcare professionals are not required by law to give a futile treatment. So why is CPR offered at the end of their life when other interventions, such as surgery, would not be considered?

The National Council for Palliative Care (2002a) states that: 'There is no ethical obligation to discuss CPR with the majority of patients receiving palliative care for whom such treatment, following assessment, is judged futile.'

Written guidance on how to decide if someone is appropriate for CPR has been developed by Randall and Regnard (2005). They produced a flow chart that asks whether the person is expected to have a cardiac or respiratory arrest from a reversible or irreversible cause. If the cause is reversible and there is a chance that CPR would be successful, the patient should be asked whether they would or would not like it, should they go into cardiac or respiratory arrest. If the cause is irreversible and there is no chance of success from CPR, then it should not be offered.

Practice points

- End–of–life care does not have to be complex.
- Patients and family carers need to be kept informed about care plans.
- Keep the treatment plan simple by only offering interventions that are appropriate for that individual as this is less confusing.
- CPR should not be offered when it is deemed to be futile.
- Involve the multidisciplinary team in discussions about end of life.
- If your place of work does not have a Do Not Attempt Resuscitation (DNAR) policy, it is important to highlight this. All staff should also be aware of the BMA *et al* (2007) resuscitation guidelines. The National Council for Palliative Care (2002b) has published a document that offers guidance on how to write a local DNAR policy. If you work for an NHS trust, always consult your local policy and guidelines group.
- If there is a chance of successful CPR, then the intervention should be discussed with the patient. If the patient does not have capacity, then evidence of advance care planning, either written or verbal, should be sought. If there is no evidence of either, the patient's representatives should be asked what they think the patient would want. Alternatively, an independent mental capacity adviser (IMCA) or a court of protection decision may be required.

- If CPR is not going to be successful, it should not be offered. The aims of care should be discussed with the patient.

Implications for practice

I would argue that nurses are not equipped through basic training to deal with the stress and psychological trauma that patients and family carers are dealing with at the end of life. Nurses develop these skills through experience, reflection and self-awareness. Nurses can support those who are at the end of life by:

- Refining their communications skills
- Offering appropriate interventions
- Checking the patient understands what is happening
- Using appropriate terminology.

Good communication skills

Good communication includes active listening – this is hearing what is said as well as paying attention to what is communicated in non-verbal ways such as body language.

It is not possible to guess how someone will feel about CPR as there are huge discrepancies between what we think patients want and what they actually want (Jevon, 1999).

We need to make sure that patients and families understand that saying no to CPR does not mean they are saying no to all interventions.

Offering appropriate interventions

Treatment interventions that are unlikely to be successful should not be offered.

The CPR guidelines state that each resuscitation decision should be discussed, where appropriate, with the individual or their representative (BMA *et al*, 2007). However, 'discussion' does not necessarily mean asking the patient or family to make a decision. Discussion may involve talking things over, finding out what the person's understanding of the current situation is, and outlining the treatment aims (Bass, 2006). This can be achieved by asking the question, 'What is your understanding of what has been happening to you/your relative up to now?' Alternative questions such as 'Are you the sort of person who likes to know what is going on?' can be helpful.

These questions may show that the patient understands much more than first thought, or that they would rather you discussed interventions with someone else, for example their family or carers.

Check the patient's understanding

Patients may have heard what has been said but have not retained the information. They may have difficulty taking in what has been said either because they cannot believe it, or they do not understand the terminology used. It is important to check a patient's under-standing and provide written information if appropriate to reinforce what has been said.

Using appropriate terminology

It may not be appropriate to use the term 'resuscitation' when discussing end-of-life care with patients. Simple phrases stating that at the time of death you will not attempt 'anything heroic', but will 'do all we can to make sure you are comfortable', are extremely useful.

Conclusion

By making sure we communicate well, and by using tools such as the GSF, LCPI, DNAR policies and advance care planning documentation, nurses can ensure that they are supporting their patients at the end of life.

Awareness of when CPR is appropriate and careful assessment and care planning by the multidisciplinary team will ensure that patients are only offered interventions that are beneficial.

References

Bass, M. (2008) Resuscitation: knowing whether it is right or wrong. *European Journal of Palliative Care*; 15:4, *175–178*.

Bass, M. (2006) *Palliative Care Resuscitation*. Chichester: John Wiley and Sons.

Bass, M. (2003) Oncology nurses' perceptions of their role in resuscitation decisions. *Professional Nurse*; 18:12, 710–713.

British Medical Association, Resuscitation Council (UK), RCN (2007) *Decisions relating to Cardiopulmonary Resuscitation. A joint statement from the British Medical Association, the Resuscitation Council UK and the Royal College of Nursing.* London: BMA, RCUK, RCN.

Department of Health (2008) *End of Life Care Strategy*. London: DH.

Department of Health (1991) *The Patient's Charter.* London: DH.

Diem, S J *et al.* (1996) Cardiopulmonary resuscitation on television. *New England Journal of Medicine*; 334: 24, 1758–1582.

Ellershaw, J, Ward, C. (2003) Care of the dying patient; the last hours or days of life. *British Medical Journal*; 326: 7374, 30–34.

Ewer, M S *et al.* (2001) Characteristics of cardiac arrest in cancer patients as a predictor of survival after CPR. *Cancer*; 92: 7, 1905–1912.

NHS End of Life Programme (2007) *Prognostic Indicator Guidance.*

Jevon, P. (2002) *Advanced Cardiac Life Support: A Practical Guide.* Oxford: Butterworth Heinemann.

Jevon, P. (1999) Do not resuscitate orders: the issues. *Nursing Standard*; 13: 40, 45–46.

Karetzky, P E *et al.* (1995) Cardiopulmonary resuscitation in intensive care unit and non-intensive care patients. *Archives of Internal Medicine*; 155: 12, 1277–1280.

Kouwenhoven, W B *et al.* (1960) Closed chest cardiac compressions. *Journal of the American Medical Association*; 173: 1064–1067.

McGrath, R B. (1987) In-house cardiopulmonary resuscitation after a quarter of a century. *Annals of American Medicine*; 16: 12, 1365–1368.

Miller, D L *et al.* (1993) Factors influencing physicians in recommending in-hospital cardiopulmonary resuscitation. *Archives of Internal Medicine*; 153: 17, 1999–2003.

National Council for Palliative Care (2002a) *Ethical Decision-making in Palliative Care.* London: NCPC.

National Council for Palliative Care (2002b) *CPR Policies in Action.* London: NCPC.

Negovsky, V A, Gurvitch, A M. (1995) Post-resuscitation disease: a new nosological entity. Its reality and significance. *Resuscitation*; 30: 1, 23–27.

Newman, R. (2002) Developing guidelines for resuscitation in palliative care. *European Journal of Palliative Care*; 9: 2, 60–63.

Nolan, J P *et al.* (2007) Outcome following admission to UK intensive care units after cardiac arrest: a secondary analysis of the ICNARC Case Mix Programme Database. *Anaesthesia*; 62: 12, 1207–1216.

Randall, F, Regnard, C. (2005) A framework for making advance decisions on resuscitation. *Clinical Medicine*; 5: 4, 354–360.

Sandroni, C *et al.* (2007) In-hospital cardiac arrest: incidence, prognosis and possible measures to improve survival. *Intensive Care Medicine*; 33: 2, 237–245.

Varon, J *et al.* (1998) Should a cancer patient be resuscitated following an in-hospital cardiac arrest? *Resuscitation*; 36: 3, 165–168.

Vitelli, C *et al.* (1991) Cardiopulmonary resuscitation and the patient with cancer. *Journal of Clinical Oncology*; 9: 1, 111–115.

Wagg, A *et al.* (1995) Cardiopulmonary resuscitation: doctors and nurses expect too much. *Journal of the Royal College of Physicians*; 29: 1, 20–24.

Wallace, K *et al.* (2002) Outcome and cost implications of cardiopulmonary resuscitation in the medical intensive care unit of a comprehensive cancer centre. *Supportive Care in Cancer;* 10: 5, 425–429.

Related articles in Nursing Times

Acute respiratory failure 2 – nursing management. 16 September 2008

An audit of nursing observations on ward patients. 24 July 2008

Guidelines focus on improving patient safety in mental health. 28 November 2008

National Patient Safety Agency issue an alert on mental health resus. 2 December 2008

Should patients who are at the end of life be offered resuscitation? 23 January 2009

APPENDIX IV

The Principles of Palliative Care

Palliative care is governed by certain principles, which guide the care given. It:

- Provides relief from pain and other distressing symptoms
- Affirms life and regards death as a normal process
- Intends neither to hasten or postpone death
- Integrates the psychological and spiritual aspects of patient care
- Offers a support system to help the family cope during the patient's illness and in bereavement
- Uses a team approach to address the needs of patients and their families, including counselling, if indicated
- Will enhance quality of life and may positively influence the course of the illness
- Is applicable early in the course of the illness, in conjunction with other therapies that may prolong life, such as chemotherapy or radiation therapy, and includes investigations needed to better understand and manage distressing clinical complications. (World Health Organization, 2004)

Other principles of palliative care promote:

- Quality of life: palliative care tries to enhance this as much as is realistically possible
- Patient choices: patient autonomy is respected and encouraged as much as possible
- Open communication
- Looking after the whole person which includes physical,

emotional, psychological, spiritual and intellectual issues
- Looking after the whole family because the patient is not an isolated unit but part of a whole social unit. Their disease, and its effects may have catastrophic influences on this social unit and its dynamics.
- Involving support from the whole multi-disciplinary team (MDT): this includes professionals in the hospital and community such doctors, nurses, palliative care specialists, hospice services, dieticians, physiotherapists, occupational therapists, and chaplaincy. (Regnard and Kindlen, 2002)

Hydration, nutrition, sedation and pain relief in end-of-life care
Adapted from *Palliative Care Resuscitation* by Madeline Bass, published in 2006 by John Wiley and Sons: pp. 8, 13–14 and 113–115.

The subject of whether to use artificial hydration and nutrition in terminally ill patients, which could be included under the cloak of 'active treatment', has brought about different points of views. Rousseau (2000) states that many doctors and nurses feel food and fluid is always a basic need for human existence. However, although this is true, tube-feeding terminally ill patients (either via nasogastric, nasojejunostomy, gastrostomy or via parenteral routes, such as total parenteral nutrition – TPN) has not been found to enhance or prolong life. Remember, tube-feeding in no way resembles normal eating since it is a passive process that totally bypasses the sensory part gained from oral feeding: there is no smell, taste or texture of feeling food in the mouth. Tube-feeding can also have serious complications such as aspiration, nasal cartilage erosion, and tube displacement, which may require an uncomfortable, perhaps even painful, replacement.

It is important for healthcare professionals, patients and their family carers, to realise that weight loss and anorexia are part of the dying process and that the absence of tube-feeding does not lead to death caused by starvation or dehydration; tube-feeding does not lengthen life. In fact it may encourage tumour growth (Rousseau, 2000).

It may be felt by some that artificial hydration is not required for various reasons, a feeling echoed by the National Council for Palliative Care (NCPC, 2002). Their reasons include that, towards death, the person's need for nutrition and fluid is lessened, and evidence suggests that artificial hydration in terminal illness neither prolongs life nor helps symptom control (see list of references for more details). Artificial hydration is not usually needed if good mouth care is given – think how quickly thirst is quenched when a few mouthfuls of drink are taken: it is some time before the fluid is actually absorbed by the body's system, yet almost immediately there is some relief from the thirst. Hence, it is felt that good mouth care can achieve the same results.

The NCPC (2002) continue that certain medications the terminally ill patient may be receiving can cause a dry mouth, such as morphine. Simply adding artificial hydration will not lessen this. They state that artificial hydration being used to correct the correctable is appropriate, such as in hypercalcemia, diarrhoea and delirium caused by electrolyte imbalance. Rousseau (2000) also argues that artificial hydration may cause a complication known as 'third spacing', which can cause peripheral and pulmonary oedema from low oncotic pressures, secondary to low blood albumen [protein] levels and poor nutritional status. It can also increase gastro-intestinal and pulmonary secretions, increase urinary output, and in the end probably cause more patient discomfort then less (Printz, 1992; Kinzbrunner, 1995). It helps, if needing to stop fluids for these reasons, that the family carers are supported during this decision. If they feel they would prefer artificial fluids or nutrition to continue, sensitive explanation why they need to be stopped (because they are causing more side effects than benefits) would need to be given. However, if there are no noticeable side effects from the fluids or nutrition already being given, then there is no reason to stop them.

A blanket policy on artificial hydration is not an individual approach to patient care. Each terminally ill patient should be assessed according to their personal need, present symptoms, and family carers' concerns. Although caring for the patient and their symptoms is important, the patient needs to be cared for as part of a social unit, and it must be recognised how this will affect those close to them. The patient is not a solitary unit: they are part of a family unit, which needs care as a whole.

Other thoughts concerning artificial hydration are that it is necessary, particularly when sedation is being used (Craig, 2002). This will help flush out the toxins from the medication used, and prevent over-sedation. If the aim of sedation is to cause the patient to become unconscious, hydration must be used to prevent death through dehydration (unless of course there are counter-indications for the use of fluids). Hydration may also be useful in patients experiencing delirium caused by abnormal electrolyte levels as it can increase the elimination of opioid metabolites. If a patient is experiencing terminal agitation and requiring sedation, it may be appropriate to continue the fluids unless the patient develops terminal secretions, at which point their body would not have been able to cope with the extra fluids. If fluids are not started, the nurses and doctors need to observe the patient to prevent too much sedation being given: enough to hold the symptoms at bay but not enough to sedate unnecessarily. This is done by starting with a low dose of sedative in a syringe driver and giving extra doses as required, and thus increasing the doses in the syringe driver accord-ing to requirements. If there are concerns about the patient needing hydration, as long as there are no terminal secretions present some fluids could be commenced subcutaneously. However, good mouth care can also help prevent [the patient] experiencing thirst. Remember, the assessment of the need for fluids is an individual one, based on many issues.

Beauchamp and Childress (2001) describe the Doctrine of Double Effect as, 'a single act having two foreseen effects, one good and one harmful'. In palliative care an example of this is the giving of an analgesic to a dying patient who is in pain. If a doctor or nurse gives something to intentionally kill them, this act is actually murder. However, if they give something for pain relief at an acceptable dose, but the patient quickly deteriorates and dies, then this is acceptable because the intention of giving the analgesic was good. There are four elements to the double effects doctrine described by Beauchamp and Childress (2001):

1. The nature of the act: the act must be good in itself.
2. Intention: this must be for good effect. The bad effect may be noted but must not be intended.
3. Distinction between means and effects: the bad effect must be means to the good effect. If the good effect was the result of the bad effect the person doing the act would intend the bad effect in pursuit of the good.
4. The good effect must outweigh the bad: the bad effect is permissible only if a proportionate reason compensates for permitting the foreseen bad effect.

The important thing about any patient care, whatever the disease, illness or situation, is that it must be appropriate. In end-of-life care there are now many drugs that can manage particular symptoms, such as pain, in the majority of patients. However, it is important not to reach for the drugs first, before ruling out other more simple interventions. For instance, if a dying patient seems agitated or in pain, they will be twitching, perhaps frowning, or groaning. Many healthcare professionals would assume the person is agitated either because of pain or simply because of terminal agitation (agitation which occurs when a patient is dying). This certainly may be the case. However, there are many causes of pain and agitation, not simply disease and the dying process. These must be ruled out first. For instance, simply changing a patient's position can make a big difference and settle them immediately. Imagine lying in a bed in exactly the same position for several hours, and not being able to move yourself at all: you can begin to imagine why some patients do indeed become agitated. And dying patients still may need to empty their bowel or bladder, and because they cannot verbalise this, it needs to be checked by those caring for the person. These issues can be settled relatively simply with the insertion of a catheter into the bladder, or by a professional assessing whether they have a full rectum and therefore administering an enema to relieve the symptoms. Other causes may be a dry or sore mouth, stiff limbs, which can be settled with some gentle passive movements, and painful wounds, or the developing of pressure sores. The latter may indeed require medications to manage symptoms of pain: however, simply changing a soiled dressing and repositioning the patient may often be enough to assist.

The golden rule is always to firstly treat anything which can be reversed without drugs. Some of these may take time to work, such as administering an enema: in this case it may be appropriate to give a small amount of medication to settle the patient in the meantime, as it is very hard for relatives and family to watch them in this way.

To illustrate, here are two examples of when simple measures are more appropriate than medications. The first one concerns a gentleman who was dying. He was not expected to live for more than a few days and he appeared agitated. The professionals caring for him administered opiates, which appeared to settle him, but only for very short periods. On visiting him, a nurse specialist giving mouth care noticed his mouth was very sore, full of ulcers and thrush. She suggested regular mouth care with thrush medication and oral gels to hydrate the mouth. Within a few minutes he became very settled, and with a routine of good mouth care he did not require any further medication, and died peacefully the next day.

The other example concerns a lady who had had a massive stroke and was deteriorating in a care home. She, also, appeared very agitated, and was also given strong pain relievers, which did settle her. However, she was becoming more and more drowsy, less responsive, and was requiring quite large amounts of medication to keep her comfortable. One very attentive care assistant noticed that one of her hands was curled tightly into a fist caused by the stroke. She carefully uncurled the hand to find that the lady's nails had grown considerably and were digging into the palm, had broken the skin and the wounds had become infected. With some careful and much needed dressings and cushioned protection to the hand, as well as by cutting this lady's nails, she became much more comfortable and again did not require the massive amounts of medication she had appeared to need before.

When someone is dying, those caring for them must act as their advocates: they must be the eyes and ears for that patient, and careful assessment and interventions can make sure they are comfortable, and that their family and friends recognise how respected and cared for they are.

References: artificial hydration and nutrition:

Andrews, M, Bell, E R, Smith, S A, Tischler, J F, Veglia, J M (1993). Dehydration in terminally ill patients: is it appropriate in palliative care? *Postgraduate Medicine*: 93: 201–208.

Burge, F (1993). Dehydration symptoms of palliative care patients. *Journal of Pain and Symptom Management*. 8: 454–64.

Dunphy, K *et al* (1995). Rehydration in palliative and terminal care: if not, why not? *Palliative Medicine* 9: 221–228.

Ellershaw, J E, Sutcliffe, J M, Saunders, C M (1995). Dehydration and the dying patient. *Journal of Pain and Symptom Management* 10(3) 192–197.

Fainsinger, R L, MacEarchen, T, Miller, M J *et al* (1994). The use of hypodermoclysis for rehydration in terminally ill cancer patients. *Journal of Pain and Symptom Management* 9: 298–302.

National Council for Palliative Care (2002). Ethical decision-making in palliative care: artificial hydration for people who are terminally ill. *NCPC*, London.

Oliver, D (1984). Terminal dehydration (letter) *Lancet*, 11: 631.

Regnard, C; Mannix, K (1991). Reduced hydration or feeding in advanced disease – a flow diagram. *Palliative Medicine*, 5: 161–164.

Rosner, F (1987). Withdrawing fluids and nutrition: an alternative view. *NY State Journal of Medicine*. 87: 591–593. In: Rousseau, P (2001). Ethical and legal issues in palliative care. *Palliative Care*, 28 (2) 391–399.

Sommerville, A (1993). Cessation of treatment, non-resuscitation, aiding suicide and euthanasia. In: Fisher, F, Mcdonald, N J,

Weston, R (1993). *Medical Ethics Today: its Practice and its Philosophy.* BMJ Publishing Group, London.

Tattersall, M H (1993). Hypercalaemia: historical perspectives and present management. *Supportive Cancer Care*: 1: 19–25.

Twycross, R G, Lichter, I (1993). The terminal phase. In: Doyle, D, Hanks, G, MacDonald, N (Eds) *Oxford Textbook of Palliative Medicine.* Oxford University Press.

Other references:

Beauchamp, T L, Childress, J F (2001). *Principles of Biomedical Ethics* (5th Edition). Oxford University Press.

Craig, G (2002). Terminal sedation. *Catholic Medical Quarterly*, February.

Kinzbrunner, B M (1995). Ethical dilemmas in hospice and palliative care. *Support Care Cancer* 3: 28–36. In: Rousseau, P (2001). Ethical and legal issues in palliative care. *Palliative Care*, 28 (2) 391–399.

National Council for Palliative Care (2002). Ethical decision-making in palliative care: artificial hydration for people who are terminally ill. *NCPC*, London.

Printz, L A (1992). Terminal dehydration: a compassionate treatment. *Archives of Internal Medicine*: 152: 697–700.

Regnard, C, Kindlen, M (2002). Supportive and Palliative Care: An Introduction. Oxford: Radcliffe Medical Press. Cited in Bass, M (2006). *Palliative Care Resuscitation.* John Wiley and Sons: Chichester.

Rousseau, P (2000). The ethical validity and clinical experience of palliative medicine. *Mayo Clinical Proctology* 75: 1064–1069. In: Rousseau, P (2001). Ethical and legal issues in palliative care. *Palliative Care*, 28 (2) 391–399.

FURTHER READING AND INFORMATION

Books

Palliative Care Resuscitation by Madeline Bass (2006) Published by John Wiley and Sons. *A guide for professionals, patients and families alike on the ethical and legal issues relating to resuscitation when someone has an incurable illness.*

Person to Person: Guide to the Care of Those with Failing Mental Powers by Tom Kitwood and Kathleen Bredin (1992): *very good guide but not up to date, as it was written before the Mental Capacity Act came into force in 2007.* Published by Gale Centre Publications.

Dementia Care Training Manual for Staff Working in Nursing and Residential Settings by Danny Walsh (2006). Published by Jessica Kingsley Publishers.

How We Die by Sherwin B Nuland (1993). Published by Chatto & Windus/Vintage Books.

Staring at the Sun: Overcoming the Terror of Death by Irvin Yalom (2008). Published by Piatkus Books.

How to Have a Good Death by J Ellershaw, *et al*, ed D Beckerman (based on the BBC documentary by Esther Rantzen). Published by Dorling Kindersley.

Caring for Someone With a Long-Term Illness by J Costello (2009). Published by Manchester University Press.

Caring for Dying People of Different Faiths by Julia Neuberger. Published by Radcliffe Publishing Ltd.

Dying Well: A Guide to Enabling a Good Death by Julia Neuberger (2004). Published by Radcliffe Publishing Ltd.

On Grief and Grieving: Finding the Meaning of Grief Through the Five Stages of Loss by Elisabeth Kübler-Ross & David Kessler (2005). Published by Simon & Schuster.

On Death and Dying: What the Dying Have to Teach Doctors, Nurses, Clergy and Their Own Families by Elisabeth Kübler-Ross (introduction by Allan Kellehear) (2009). Published by Rout-ledge.

Oral Feeding Difficulties and Dilemmas: a guide to practical care, particularly towards the end of life. A report of the working party under the chairmanship of Dr Rodney Burnham (2010). Published by the Royal College of Physicians, together with the British Society of Gastroenterology.

Other books and journal articles: although a long list, this will be particularly useful for health and social care professionals.

Ballinger, D. Is it ever acceptable to deceive a patient? *Nursing Times* (1997); 93 (35) 44–45.

Bass, M. Oncology nurses' perceptions of their goals in the resuscitation status of oncology patients. *Professional Nurse* (2003); 18 (12), 710–713.

Bass, M. Resuscitation: knowing whether it is right or wrong. *European Journal of Palliative Care* (2008); 15 (4) 175–178.

Bass, M. Should patients who are at the end of life be offered resuscitation? *Nursing Times* (2009); 105 (3) 19.

Bass, M. CPR decisions in palliative care should allow for a good death. *Nursing Times* (2009); 105 (15) 11.

Bass, M. Advance Care Planning for the end of life. *Oncology and Palliative Care* (2009); 3 (2) 42–43.

Billings, J A. Comfort measures for the terminally ill: is dehydration painful? *Journal of the American Geriatric Society (1985); 33: 808–810.*

Birtwhistle, J, Nielson, A. Do not resuscitate: an ethical dilemma for the decision-maker. *British Journal of Nursing* (1998); 7 (9) 543–549.

British Medical Association. Withholding and Withdrawing Life-prolonging Treatments: Good Practice in Decision-making (2002); *BMA*, London. Available to download from: *www.gmc-uk.org*.

British Medical Association, Royal College of Nursing, and Resuscitation Council (UK) Decisions relating to cardio-pulmonary resuscitation. *A joint statement from the BMA, RCN and RC* (2001). *www.resus.org.uk.*

Burge, F. Dehydration symptoms of palliative care patients. *Journal of Pain and Symptom Management (1993); 8: 454–64.*

Clark, D. Between hope and acceptance: the medicalisation of dying. *British Medical Journal* (2002); 324, 905–907.

Conroy, S P., Luxton, T., Dingwall, R., Harwood, R H., Gladman, J R F., Cardiopulmonary resuscitation in continuing care settings: time for a rethink? *British Medical Journal* (February 2006); 332: 47–482.

Cooley, C. Communication skills in palliative care. *Professional Nurse* (2000); 15 (9) 603–605.

Craig, G M. On withholding nutrition and hydration in the terminally ill: has palliative medicine gone too far? *Journal of Medical Ethics* (1994): 20: 1339–143.

Dallain, L. Cardiopulmonary resuscitation in the hospice setting. *Cancer Nursing Practice* (2004); 3 (9) 35–39.

Dean, J A. The resuscitation status of a patient: a constant dilemma. *British Journal of Nursing* (2001); 10 (8) 537–543.

Diem, SJ *et al.* Cardiopulmonary resuscitation on television. *New England Journal of Medicine* (1996); 334 (24) 1758–1582.

Dimond, B. Not for resuscitation instructions: the law for adult patients in the UK. *British Journal of Nursing* (2004); 13 (16) 984–986.

Ebrahim, S. DNR decisions: flogging dead horses or a dignified death? *British Medical Journal* (2000); 320 (7243) 1155–6.

Ellershaw, J E, Sutcliffe, J M, Saunders, C M. Dehydration and the dying patient. *Journal of Pain and Symptom Management* (1995); 10 (3) 192–197.

Ewer, M S, Kish, S K, Martin, C G, Price, K J, Feeley, T W. Characteristics of cardiac arrest in cancer patients as a predictor after CPR. *Cancer* (2001); 92: 1905–12.

Field, D. Palliative medicine and the medicalisation of death. *European Journal of Cancer Care* (1994); 3, 58–62.

Firth, S. Wider horizons: care of the dying in a multicultural society. (2001) *National Council for Palliative Care*, London.

Fleming, K. The meaning of hope to palliative care cancer patients. *International Journal of Palliative Nursing* (1997); 3 (1) 14–18.

George, A L, Folk, B P, Crecilius, P L, Campbell, P L. Pre-arrest morbidity and other correlates of survival after in-hospital CPR. *American Journal of Medicine* (1989); 87: 28–34.

Goss, R. *(Letters)* Do not resuscitate orders: without discussion these orders are unethical at any age. *British Medical Journal* (2001); 322 (7278), 105.

Hayward, M. Cardiopulmonary resuscitation: are practitioners being realistic? *British Journal of Nursing* (1999); 8 (12) 810–814.

Herth, K. Fostering hope in terminally ill people. *Journal of Advanced Nursing* (1990); 15: 1250–1259.

Jevon, P. Do not resuscitate orders: the issues. *Nursing Standard* (1999); 13 (40) 45–6.

Kouwenhoven, W B, Knickerbocker, G G, Jude, M D, James, R. Closed chest cardiac massage. *Journal of the American Medical Association* (1960); 173 (10) 1064–1067.

Low, J S; Payne, S. The good and bad death perceptions of health professionals working in palliative care. *European Journal of Cancer Care* (1996); 5, 237–241.

McNeil, C. A good death (editorial). *Journal of Palliative Care* (1998); 14: 1; 5–6.

Mayo, T W. Forgoing artificial nutrition and hydration: legal and ethical considerations. *Nutrition in Clinical Practice* (1996); 11: 254–264.

National Council for Palliative Care. *Ethical decision-making in palliative care*: artificial hydration for people who are terminally ill. (2002) *NCPC*, London.

National Council for Palliative Care. *CPR: Policies in action*: proceedings of a seminar to inform best practice with CPR policies within palliative care. (2003) NCPC, London.

Regnard, C, Mannix, K. Reduced hydration and feeding in advanced disease – a flow diagram. *Palliative Medicine* (1991); 5: 161–164.

Rousseau, P. Ethical and legal issues in palliative care. *Palliative Care* (2001); 28 (2) 391–399.

Safar, P. On the history of modern resuscitation. *Critical Care Medicine* (1996); Feb, 24 (2 supplement) s3–11.

Sweet, S J, Norman, I J. The nurse–doctor relationship: a selective literature review. *Journal of Advanced Nursing* (1995); 22: 240–1.

Thomas, A. Patient autonomy and cancer treatment decisions. *International Journal of Palliative Medicine* (1997); 3 (6) 317–323.

Tschudin, V. *Ethics in Nursing* (2nd Edition) (1992). Oxford: Butterworth-Heinemann.

Vitelli, C; Cooper, K; Rogatko, A; Brennan, M (1991) Cardiopulmonary resuscitation and the patient with cancer. *Journal of Clinical Oncology 9(1) 111–115*.

Willard, C. The nurse's role as patient advocate: obligation or imposition? *Journal of Advanced Nursing* (1996); 24, 60–66.

Willard, C. Cardiopulmonary resuscitation for palliative care patients: a discussion of ethical issues. *Palliative Medicine* (2000); 14: 308–312.

Woodrow, P. Nurse advocacy: is it in the patient's best interests? *British Journal of Nursing* (1997); 6 (4) 225–229.

Younger, S J. Who defines futility? *Journal of the American Medical Association* (1988); 260: 2094–5.

Websites

Dementia

- Dementia, from NHS Choices website. Information about the disease and a short video about living with dementia.
  http://www.nhs.uk/conditions/dementia/Pages/Introduction.aspx
- Alzheimer's Society website: information about the different types of dementia and where to access help.
  http://alzheimers.org.uk/site/scripts/home_info.php?homepageID= 29

- Also information available from BBC Health website: *http://www.bbc.co.uk/health/conditions/mental_health/disorders_dementia.shtml*
- British Society of Psychiatrists has a useful leaflet online: *http://www.rcpsych.ac.uk/default.aspx?page=1427*

Cancer

- Cancer Research UK website: information about different types of cancer and about present research projects: *http://www.cancerresearchuk.org/*
- Macmillan Cancer Support website has a multitude of information about cancer, treatments, and cancer survivorship. *http://www.macmillan.org.uk/Home.aspx*
- For professionals: Macmillan has a very informative 'learn zone' website which can be accessed following this link. It's free, but you need to register to use it. *http://learnzone.macmillan.org.uk/*

Hospice care

- To find your local hospice visit: *http://www.helpthehospices.org.uk/about-hospice-care/find-a-hospice/uk-hospice-and-palliative-care-services/* By typing in your postcode you can access the contact details for your closest hospice.

Palliative care

- Health talk online: Set up by the DIPEx charity, this is a very useful website both for the public and professionals, using real-life people to talk about their own stories. Some of these are to do with having a terminal illness, personal experiences of chronic illness and also mental health: *http://www.healthtalkonline.org/*
- MND Association: helpful website for anyone living with motor neurone disease: *http://www.mndassociation.org/*

- Heart failure: NHS Choices website:
  http://www.nhs.uk/conditions/heart-failure/Pages/Introduction.aspx
- Chronic kidney Failure: UK National Kidney Federation
  http://www.kidney.org.uk/Medical-Info/ckd-info/
- The National Council for Palliative Care is a national organisation which supports people with terminal illness and professionals: *http://www.ncpc.org.uk*
- NHS Choices: information for anyone with a palliative illness. Includes a link to the Carers Direct helpline, and information on some possible grants to help with the financial costs of caring
  http://www.nhs.uk/CarersDirect/guide/bereavement/Pages/Grants
- Marie Curie offer free support to people who want to die in their own home: *http://www.mariecurie.org.uk/*

Advance decisions to refuse treatment

- Useful in finding out more information about recording your own, or your patients', wishes. *http://www.adrtnhs.co.uk/*

The Mental Capacity Act

- Direct.gov is a useful website for lots of different things, the mental Capacity Act being one of them:
  http://www.direct.gov.uk/en/DisabledPeople/HealthAndSupport/YourRightsInHealth/DG_10016888
- The Department of Justice now governs this, but information can be found from the Department of Constitutional affairs, an archive website. This link will take you to the list of booklets available for professionals and the public:
  http://www.dca.gov.uk/legal-policy/mental-capacity/publications.htm#booklets

Enteral/artificial feeding
- Information about patient selection, and complications:
  http://www.patient.co.uk/doctor/Enteral-Feeding.htm
- For people with cancer, this site gives information on what enteral feeding is all about:
  http://www.cancerhelp.org.uk/coping-with-cancer/coping-physically/diet/managing/drip-or-tube-feeding

Do Not Attempt Resuscitation
- The Resuscitation Council (UK) guidance, which has been written with the British Medical Association and the Royal College of Nursing:
  http://www.resus.org.uk/pages/dnarrstd.htm

For anyone living with, or caring for someone with, a long-term illness, or terminal illness
- Financial support if caring for someone with a terminal illness, available at Direct.gov:
  http://www.direct.gov.uk/en/CaringForSomeone/CaringAndSupportServices/DG_10035718
- If I should Die: a very informative website covering lots of different subjects, such as funeral plans, benefits and how to comfort those who are grieving:
  http://www.ifishoulddie.co.uk/terminal-life-threatening-illness-c40.html
- A website for family carers which offers help and advice for anyone caring for someone with a long-term or terminal illness: *http://www.carers.org/*

GLOSSARY

by Madeline Bass, RGN, BSC (Hons)

Abdominal exploration: a surgical investigation through an incision, or through key-hole surgery using cameras.

Abdominal sounds: the normal sounds produced by movement of the bowel and gut.

Acetylcholine: a neuro-transmitter. This is a substance which the body produces at the end of each nerve cell which then stimulates the next nerve cell to continue the message.

Acidosis: increased acid levels in the blood which is caused by partial or complete renal failure.

Acute intestinal obstruction: This is when the gut suddenly blocks either internally, such as from a tumour or the gut twisting, or externally such as from a tumour pressing on to the gut.

Adrenaline: a substance produced by the body in times of threat or stress. One of its actions is to speed up the heart rate. If the heart stops unexpectedly, adrenaline is one of the drugs used to try and stimulate it to begin working again.

Advance Directive: now called Advance Decision: These are now legally recognised documents, with specific wording, which refuses treatment in specific circumstances, witnessed. They have to be written whilst the person still has mental capacity and can only come into effect when the person loses that capacity. They must be signed and witnessed to become legal. If overruled by a healthcare professional they could face charges of neglect or assault.

Amyotrophic Lateral Sclerosis (AMS): a form of Motor Neurone Disease (MND): MND affects the nerves which control functions of the body, and is always fatal.

Analgesic: a medication or drug which reduces the feeling of pain.

Aneurysm: a blood-filled swelling of the wall of an artery.

Angina pectoris: lack of oxygen to the heart muscles, which causes pain in the chest and breathlessness.

Anodyne: an analgesic which works by lessening the sensitivity of the nerves or brain.

Anorexia: not to be confused with anorexia nervosa, this refers to lack of appetite.

Anti-coagulants: a wide-ranging group of drugs to dissolve and prevent blood clots forming inside the blood vessels.

Anti-emetics: drugs which suppress nausea and vomiting.

Aperients: oral drugs used to stimulate the bowels.

Arteries: blood vessels which carry oxygenated blood.

Arterioles: the smallest arteries in the body.

Ascites: build-up of fluid in the abdominal cavity.

Asphyxia: suffocation, dying through lack of oxygen.

Aspirating needle: a needle used to remove fluid from a part of the body.

Aspiration: being wrongly taken into the lungs, e.g. food entering the lungs. Aspiration will lead to pneumonia if not prevented and treated.

Atheroma of the arterial circulation: swelling of the walls of the arteries, caused by debris such as fats, cholesterol, calcium and connective tissue.

Atrial response: action of the atria, the two smaller chambers of the heart. The right atrium pushes blood into the right ventricle, where blood is then pushed to the lungs to collect oxygen. From there it returns to the left atrium which pumps it into the left ventricle. From there it is pushed via the aorta around the body.

Auscultations: examination by listening.

Bedsores: also called pressures sores: these occur when the body does not move around enough, e.g. due to accident, illness, disability or injury. This causes the person to be less mobile. If pressure is applied to an area of the body for too long the circulation is compromised and the skin starts to break down, causing a sore.

Bladder irrigation: certain conditions can cause a blockage of the urethra, e.g. in prostatectomy, bleeding is prevented from blocking the urethra by passing a large catheter, which has two drainage lines, into the bladder: one allows sterile saline to be flushed into the bladder, and the other allows the saline and bladder contents to drain out.

Blood count: a general term referring to the counts of different elements of the blood, such as red blood cells, urea or potassium.

BMA: British Medical Association.

Brompton cocktail: a concoction of many different types of drugs often given to terminally ill patients to alleviate pain.

Bronchitis: inflammation of the bronchi, the smallest breathing passages in the lungs.

Cannula: a very thin tube, thinner than a catheter, which can be inserted into the body, e.g. into a vein.

Carcinogenic: something which causes cancer, e.g. tar in cigarettes is a known carcinogenic.

Cardiac stimulants: drugs which stimulate the heart to work correctly.

Cardiologist: a medical specialist in conditions and problems with the heart.

Cardio-pulmonary: pertaining to the heart and lungs.

Cardiovascular: pertaining to the heart and circulation system.

Carotid beat: the pulse felt from the carotid artery, in the neck.

Catheterise: to place a catheter, which is a small tube, into the body, e.g. a bladder catheter to help drain urine, a kidney catheter to help drain urine directly from the kidneys.

Central line: a small tube inserted into the one of the large veins leading to the heart. Drugs can be administered into this, and blood samples taken from it.

Cerebral arteries: the arteries in the brain.

Chemotherapy: strong poisons used to destroy fast-dividing cells. Since cancer cells normally grow much more quickly than normal cells, chemotherapy may effectively kill them. However some chemotherapy cannot discern between the cancer's fast-dividing cells and normal fast-dividing cells, e.g. gut cells, hair cells. This is why some chemotherapy causes nausea, mouth ulcers, diarrhoea and hair loss. These drugs are dose-limiting: i.e. a person can only have so much of a certain drug at a time.

Cholera: gastroenteritis caused by bacteria. It results in severe diarrhoea. The disease can progress very quickly resulting in shock within twelve hours from severe dehydration. It is extremely contagious.

Clot-buster: a drug to dissolve any clots which have formed in the blood vessels.

Colitis: inflammation of the colon, the large bowel.

Colostomy: when the bowel is surgically attached to the skin so that faeces are excreted into a bag which can then be emptied.

Congestive heart failure: heart failure is when the heart, which is a large muscle, begins to enlarge and get weaker through age or disease. This means it has to work harder to maintain normal heart function. The disease can be controlled at times by certain drugs.

Coronary arteries: the arteries of the heart. There are four arteries which supply the heart muscle with oxygen.

Coronary failure: another term for heart failure.

CPR: short for cardio-pulmonary resuscitation: the full term for resuscitation.

Craniotomy: removal of part of the skull bone during a surgical procedure to the brain.

Cross-matching: this is a process which is carried out to make sure the person is given the right type of blood during a blood transfusion.

Cyanosis: lack of oxygen in the body's tissues leading to a blue colour in extremities.

Defensive medicine: medicine and treatment carried out to prevent complaints and safeguard against malpractice.

Defibrillator: a machine which delivers electric shocks to the heart, to try and reverse fibrillation of the heart muscle.

Dementia: a disease which causes the brain to begin to degenerate. There are over two hundred different types of dementia, the most common being Alzheimer's. The disease is not curable.

Dialyse: pertaining to kidney dialysis, a process where the blood is mechanically filtered because the kidneys are unable to perform this function.

Diuretics: drugs which increase the drainage of urine out of the kidneys, often used to reduce blood volume, e.g. in high blood pressure and heart failure.

Draining filaments: a drain where the end is frayed out into filaments: used to drain wounds or wound cavities.

Duodenal ulcer: an area of the duodenum, which becomes very sore and excoriated. This can cause pain, indigestion and nausea.

Duodenum: first part of the small bowel leading away from the stomach.

Electrolyte balance: electrolytes are substances produced by the body which maintain healthy functioning. Certain electrolytes include potassium and sodium. If the levels become abnormal such as in kidney dysfunction many of the body's otherwise normal functions may go wrong.

Embolism / embolus / emboli: an object migrating from one part of the body to another which occludes a blood vessel, e.g. blood clot.

Encapsulated: a growth confined to a specific, localised area.

Endogenous clinical depression: depression that people are born with. It is thought it may be genetic.

Endomorphs: endorphins, the body's natural morphine-like substances which give the 'feel good' factor.

Endotracheal tube: a tube placed into the lungs via the mouth and throat. It may be used during surgery to help a person breathe. It is usually temporary.

Epiglottis: a cartilaginous flap of skin which lies between the trachea and the gullet. When swallowing food, saliva or fluid, the epiglottis closes over the trachea to prevent food going in to the lungs.

Erythrocyte sedimentation rates: the rate at which red blood cells precipitate within an hour. ESR is a general test indicating the presence of inflammation within the body.

Excoriated: when skin becomes raw, sore, and the top layers are removed.

Exudate: a fluid that filters from the circulatory system into lesions or areas of inflammation.

Feed-pegs: or peg tubes: tubes inserted directly into the stomach through the skin which can allow liquid feed to be given to the patient. Useful when patients lose the ability to swallow such as after a stroke.

Fehlings solution: used to detect sugar in the urine.

Fibrillating: when the heart muscle is rapidly twitching in an uncoordinated way.

Flavine gauze: gauze soaked in flavine, an antiseptic.

Gastrectomy or gastric resection: this is when part or the whole of the stomach is removed.

Gastric intubation and suction: A tube inserted through the person's nose into their stomach (called a naso-gastric tube) which can then be used to drain the fluids away more comfortably and cleanly. A syringe can be attached to the tube and used to remove the stomach's contents by 'suction'.

Gastro-enterologist: a specialist in the gastro-intestinal tract, digestion and its disorders.

Glucose and saline infusion: (see 'infusion' as well) an infusion into the vein of a mix of weak saline (salt) and glucose (sugar) solution.

Glyceryl trinitrate: a drug used to treat angina.

Glycosuria: the excretion of glucose into the urine.

Haemoglobin levels: haemoglobin is a protein in red blood cells which carries oxygen.

Hallucinogenic: substances causing hallucinations.

Hardened arteries: arteries are normally elastic to cope with the pressure of blood being pushed around the body: this elasticity allows the arteries to maintain the blood pressure.

Hemiplegic: one-sided weakness of the body.

Hiatus hernia: caused by the upper part of the stomach pushing through the hole in the diaphragm.

Hippocratic Oath: historically, an oath taken by doctors to practise ethically in medicine. It has been taken over by another oath in the USA. In the UK it has been taken over by a different code of conduct.

Huntingdon's chorea: a degenerative disease of the brain, whereby the person suffers physical, cognitive and functional effects. It is hereditary and always fatal.

Hydraulic air bed: a specialised bed used to prevent pressure and bedsores in someone with reduced mobility.

Hypoglycaemia: low blood sugar levels. Can occur in diabetics when they do not take in enough glucose from their diet. **Hyper-glycaemia** is high blood sugar levels, again caused by diabetes. Symptoms build up over several days but if not treated it can affect vision, nerves and circulation.

Hypothalamus: a very small part of the brain, which controls temperature, hunger, thirst and circadian rhythms (the twenty-four-hour body clock).

Iliac crest: part of the pelvic bone.

Iliac vein: main veins of the pelvis.

Infarction: the process of tissue death caused by lack of circulation to the area.

Involuntary reflexes: these are the body's responses to certain things and which cannot be controlled by the mind.

Irritable bowel: a disease in which the bowel becomes irritated by something, either an allergy, disease or drugs, which causes profuse diarrhoea or constipation.

Ischaemic heart disease: death of heart tissue caused by blockage of blood vessels.

IV's: short for intravenous, a term used for anything given via a vein.

Jugular: the largest vein in the body, situated in the neck.

Ketones: a by-product of the breakdown of fatty tissue in the body, usually occurring in diabetics.

Lapatoromy: This is the name of the surgical incision to the abdomen.

Laying out: often called 'Last Offices'. This is the process of preparing the body of someone who has just died for burial.

Leukaemia: Cancer of the bone marrow.

Lasting Power of Attorney (LPA) – Health and Welfare: the only legally recognised way a person can make a medical decision on behalf of another. This power only comes into effect when the person loses capacity, i.e. the ability to make a decision. It must be registered (proven by a hologram sticker on the document, and an official rubber stamp) and must be seen by the medics and people treating that person at the time. The person acting as the attorney can only make decisions within the remit of what they think the person they are representing would have wanted in that situation.

Lumbar puncture: an investigative procedure in which cerebrospinal fluid is removed for analysis.

Mastectomy: removal of all or part of the breast.

Mersalyl: an early diuretic which contained mercury.

Metastasis: a single site where the cancer has spread, a single secondary. Metastases is the plural and means multiple secondaries.

MRSA: Methicillin-Resistant Staphylococcus Aureus: a highly contagious and resistant bacterial infection requiring strong skin cleansers, and antibiotics.

Multiple sclerosis: when the myelin sheath (insulation) around certain nerves is affected which slows down the passage of nerve messages. There are several types of MS, some more progressive and damaging than others.

Nasojejunostomy tube: tube that is inserted through the nasal passage, into the gullet, through the stomach and into the small bowel, the jejunum.

Necrotic: dead and decaying: e.g. necrotic skin is blackened skin caused by lack of circulation.

Neurodegenerative disease: disease which causes deterioration of the nervous systems.

Neurologist: a specialist of the nerves, the nervous system and related disorders.

Oedema: swelling of the tissues of the body caused by poor circulation.

Oestrogen / Progesterone: these are female steroids, better known as female sex hormones.

Oncologist: a doctor specialising in treating cancer.

Oncotic pressures: when blood is more concentrated and attracts water into the circulatory system.

Open heart resuscitation (direct manual compression): heart compressions applied directly to the heart through an incision made through the skin, sternum and membranes.

Palliative care: care of patients with incurable disease and their families. In chronic disease it will begin when the disease can no longer be assisted by drug therapy.

Paraldehyde: a substance originally used to control convulsions, and as a sedative and hypnotic.

Paralytic ileus: when the small bowel paralyses itself.

Paramedics: specially trained professionals who attend emergencies in the community.

Parenteral: given via external route instead of via the gastro-intestinal route.

Path lab analysis (short for pathology laboratory analysis): analysis of certain body tissues or fluids.

Pathologist: a specialist of pathology.

Pelvic colon: the colon is the large bowel.

Peripheral: on the edges of the body.

Peritoneal cavity: the abdominal cavity, which is surrounded by the peritoneal membrane.

Peritonitis: inflammation of the peritoneum, the membrane lining the abdominal cavity. It can be caused by infection, disease or injury. It needs to be treated with strong antibiotics or an operation, and can be fatal.

Placebo: a substance with no active element or drug, often used in trials against a real drug to see whether the latter is more effective.

Plaques: in Alzheimer's dementia, small clumps of proteins that grow around brain cells and prevent normal functioning.

Pleural aspiration: drainage of fluid, which has built up between the pleural membranes surrounding the lungs.

Pneumococcal organisms: the bacterial cause of pneumonia. There is now a vaccination to protect people from this.

Polyuria: excessive production and excretion of urine.

Positive pressure: when the pressure within a system is higher than that of the environment it is in.

Potassium citrate: a substance used to dilute acidic urine.

Primary progressive aphasia: when words are muddled and mixed up, and speech is then lost altogether.

Prostatectomy: surgical removal of the prostate gland.

Psycho-geriatric ward: now called Elderly Mentally Ill (EMI) wards. This is a ward specially designed to care for elderly people who have mental health problems.

Psychosomatic paralysis: paralysis caused by the unconscious mind.

Pulmonary oedema: fluid congestion in the lungs which may be caused by heart conditions.

Radiotherapy: treatment of cancer using radium.

Remedial therapy: treatment to aid recovery: it tends to be non-pharmacological in nature.

Respiratory drive: this is controlled by a part of the brain which measures how much carbon dioxide is present in the blood and controls how the person breathes.

Retractor: a surgical instrument which is used to hold back skin, muscle or bone to allow better access and vision during surgery.

Rheumatism: a condition of the joints and connective tissue.

Rigor mortis: after a certain period following death, the muscles of the body begin to stiffen.

Sarcoma: a cancer of connective tissue, i.e. bone, cartilage or muscle.
Sclera: the white part of the eyeball, which is made up of elastic fibrous tissue.
Septicaemia: infection in the blood.
Serum: the watery part of blood, which carries the red and white blood cells, and platelets.
Shock: bodily collapse or near collapse caused by inadequate delivery of oxygen to the cells from decreased heart functioning, e.g. from excessive loss of blood.
Sigmoid colon: this links the anus and rectum to the large bowel.
Sloughing: when part of the body becomes detached, usually linked with wounds and skin in humans.
Staphylococcal infection: a particular type of bacterial infection caused by the *Staphylococcus* bacterium.
Statins: a group of drugs used to reduce the blood cholesterol level.
Sternum: the bone that connects both sides of the rib cage at the front.
Stertorous: heavy mouth breathing, characterised by loud snoring or gasping noises.
Suppuration: the formation and production of pus.
Supra-pubic catheter: a tube placed directly into the bladder through the skin, just above the pubic bone.
Surgical shock: similar to normal shock, but caused by surgery.

Thrombosis: a blood clot occurring in a blood vessel.
Tibia and fibula: the two bones of the lower leg, between knee and ankle.
Titrated / titration: when a drug or treatment is given according to how much is needed by the patient before too many side effects, or intolerance, develops.
Total parenteral nutrition: complete nutritional diet given

intravenously. It is mixed in sterile conditions according to the individual's daily blood tests and contains all the calories, nutrients, vitamins and minerals a person needs.

Tracheostomy: a hole made in the throat wall into which a tube is placed into the bronchus, the main breathing tube into the lungs. A **tracheostomy tube** is placed in this man-made hole to keep it patent, e.g. a Durham's tube.

Transient ischaemic attack (TIA): a small stroke with little or no long-term effects on the person. But a doctor should be seen urgently if one occurs because without treatment a major stroke could follow.

Trephining / trephine: when a burr hole is made through the skull, using a drill, as part of a surgical procedure.

Trocar and cannula: a cannula is a thin 'needle' structure often made of plastic which can be inserted into the body. The trocar is the introducer, a thin piece of stable metal, which assists its placement. The trocar is then removed.

Uraemia: high levels of urea on the blood.

Urethra: the tube that transports urine from the bladder during excretion.

Urinalysis: a simple test of the urine to look for any problems.

Urine drainage bag: used to collect urine drainage via a catheter.

Vascular dementia: dementia caused by lack of circulation of blood to various parts of the brain causing the death of those affected parts and therefore affecting mental functions.

Ventricle: the larger chambers of the heart.

Ventricular fibrillation: fibrillation of the ventricles, the two largest chambers of the heart.

Voluntary euthanasia: when someone's life is actively ended with their agreement, and with the help of someone else using specific drugs.

Volvulus: a blockage of the bowel caused by it twisting in on itself.

Warfarin: a blood clot–dissolving drug which tends to be used prophylactically to prevent further blood clots forming.

White cell counts: white cells exist in the blood and fight infection. If a person is not producing enough white blood cells they will be immunocompromised.

ACKNOWLEDGEMENTS

My appreciation and gratitude to all the people who have helped me in writing this book.

My husband, Philip, whose love and loyalty, wisdom and humour have kept me sane throughout
Dr David Hackett, Dr Richard Lamerton, Dr Michael Boyes
Dr Robin Moffat, President of the Medico-Legal Society
Susan McGann, Paul Vaughan and Susan Watt of the Royal College of Nursing
Louise Massen and Madeline Bass
Patricia Schooling, for her several readings and invaluable suggestions
All those who have supported me in prayer, especially Sister Christine and the Community of St John the Divine, Birmingham; Sister Elizabeth and the Convent of Our Lady, Kettering; the Sisters of the Love of God, Oxford
The Chaplains of the Methodist Homes for the Aged, and St Francis Hospice for the Dying
Colin Rivett, Eve Griffin, Jeremy Buckman, Counsellors
Anna Powiecki, Eugenie Furniss and Claudia Webb at William Morris, Endeavour Entertainment, John Saunders, Kirsty Dunseath, Sophie Buchan and the team at Weidenfeld & Nicolson
Carole Lewis, Sue Theobald, Christoper Howe
David Hart, poet, priest and dreamer
Patricia Birch, Joanna Bruce, MBE; Sue, Jayne and Jane, my sister and nieces who are nurses and care assistants
Lydia Hart, Eleanor Hart
Shelagh and her family in Israel, and Steve and Sandy, Wendy and Philip.
— and the many people who have told me their stories but do not wish to be named.

Excerpt from *Nurse on Call* by Edith Cotterill, published by Ebury. Reproduced with permission of The Random House Group Ltd.

Excerpt from *How We Die* by Sherwin B Nuland, published by Chatto & Windus. Reproduced with permission of Random House Group Ltd.

Excerpt from 'Do not go gentle into that good night' by Dylan Thomas from *Poems*, published by JM Dent, a division of the Orion Publishing Group. Reproduced with permission from David Higham Associates.

Excerpt from *Four Quartets* by T.S. Eliot reproduced with permission of Faber.

Excerpt from *Malone Dies by* Samuel Beckett reproduced with permission of Faber.

Poems by David Hart reproduced with permission of the author and Five Seasons Press.

All efforts have been made to obtain permission for the use of the excerpt from *Truman of St Helens* by Shirley Rosen. Anyone with rights to this book is invited to contact the author.

INDEX